THE HISTORY OF AMERICAN NURSING

Edited by
Susan Reverby, Wellesley College

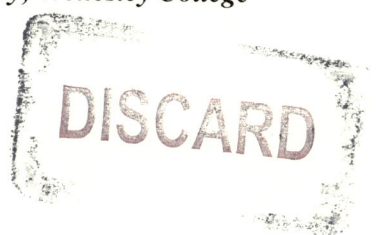

A Garland Series

HOSPITAL MANAGEMENT

Edited by Charlotte A. Aikens

GARLAND PUBLISHING, INC.
NEW YORK • LONDON
1985

362.11
H 794m
1985   dd

For a complete list of the titles in this series see the final pages of this volume.

This facsimile was made from a copy in the Library of Congress.

Copyright © 1911 by W.B. Saunders Co., renewed 1939 by Charlotte A. Aikens

Reprinted by permission of the W.B. Saunders Co.

Library of Congress Cataloging-in Publication Data
Main entry under title:

Hospital management.

(The History of American nursing)
Reprint. Originally published: Philadelphia : Saunders, 1911.
Includes index.
1. Hospitals—Administration—Addresses, essays, lectures.   2. Hospitals—United States—Administration—Addresses, essays, lectures.   I. Aikens, Charlotte A. (Charlotte Albina), 1868–   II. Series.
[DNLM: WX A291h 1911a]
RA971.H59377   1985   362.1'1'068   83–49196
ISBN 0-8240-6500-X (alk. paper)

The volumes in this series are printed on acid-free, 250-year-life paper.

Printed in the United States of America

119531

BOOKS

BY

CHARLOTTE A. AIKENS

Primary Studies for Nurses

12mo of 435 pages, illustrated. Cloth, $1.75 net.

Clinical Studies for Nurses

12mo of 510 pages, illustrated. Cloth, $2.00 net.

Hospital Training-school Methods and the Head Nurse

12mo of 275 pages. Cloth, 1.50 net.

Hospital Management

12mo of 488 pages, illustrated.

HOSPITAL MANAGEMENT

A HANDBOOK FOR HOSPITAL TRUSTEES, SUPER-
INTENDENTS, TRAINING-SCHOOL PRINCIPALS,
PHYSICIANS, AND ALL WHO ARE ACTIVELY
ENGAGED IN PROMOTING HOSPITAL WORK

EDITED BY

CHARLOTTE A. AIKENS

Formerly Superintendent of Columbia Hospital, Pittsburg, and of the
Iowa Methodist Hospital, Des Moines; late Director of Sibley Memorial
Hospital, Washington, D. C.; Member of the American Hospital Associa-
tion; Author of "Hospital Training-school Methods and the Head Nurse;"
"Primary Studies for Nurses;" "Clinical Studies for Nurses," etc.

ILLUSTRATED

PHILADELPHIA AND LONDON

W. B. SAUNDERS COMPANY

1911

Copyright, 1911, by W. B. Saunders Company

PRINTED IN AMERICA

PRESS OF
W. B. SAUNDERS COMPANY
PHILADELPHIA

TO THE

MEMBERS OF THE AMERICAN HOSPITAL ASSOCIATION,

who labor continuously to promote the comfort
and to render more efficient the care
of the sick,

THIS VOLUME IS DEDICATED,

a tribute of appreciation for their unwavering devotion to
hospital ideals and their great service in upbuilding and strengthening American hospitals.

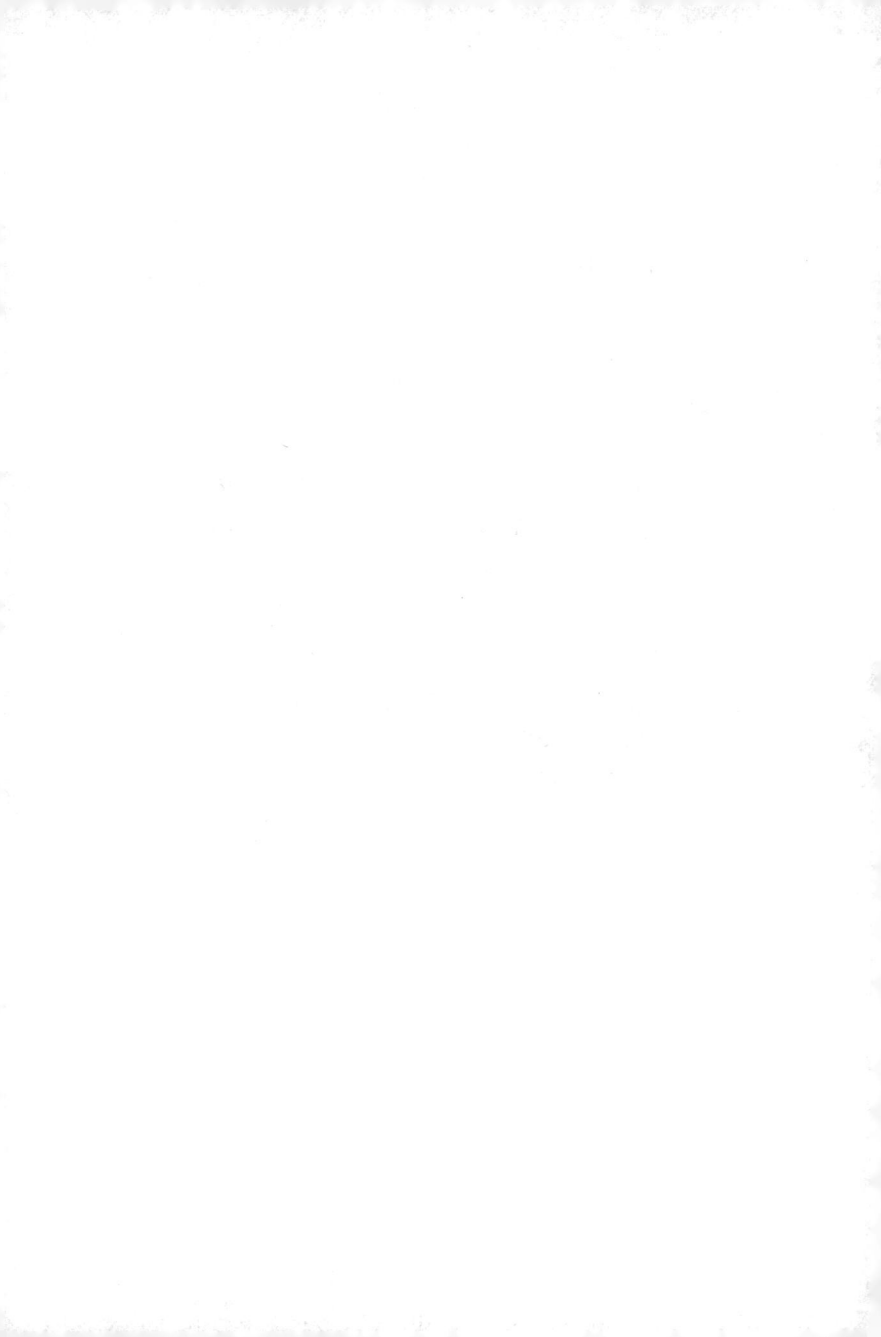

CONTRIBUTORS

Charles Phillips Emerson, M. D.
    Superintendent, Clifton Springs Sanitarium, N. Y.; Author of "Essentials of Medicine."

E. S. Gilmore
    Superintendent, Wesley Hospital, Chicago, Ill.

Henry Mills Hurd, M. D.
    Superintendent, Johns Hopkins Hospital, Baltimore, Md.

George P. Ludlam
    Superintendent Emeritus, New York Hospital, N. Y.

John N. Elliott Brown, M. B.
    Superintendent, Toronto General Hospital, Toronto; Secretary of American Hospital Association.

Edward Fletcher Stevens, A. A. I. A.
    Hospital Architect, Boston, Mass.

Emma A. Anderson
    Superintendent, New England Baptist Hospital, Boston, Mass.

Louise M. Coleman
    Superintendent, Hospital of the Good Samaritan, Boston, Mass.

Charles A. Gill
    Superintendent, Germantown Dispensary and Hospital, Germantown, Philadelphia, Pa.

Warren L. Babcock, M. D.
    Superintendent, Grace Hospital, Detroit, Michigan; President, American Hospital Association.

J. LYMAN BELKNAP, M. D.
> Assistant Resident Physician, Massachusetts General Hospital, Boston, Mass.

RENWICK R. ROSS, M. D.
> Superintendent, Buffalo General Hospital, Buffalo, N. Y.

ELIZABETH HINCHMAN
> Dietitian, McLean Hospital, Waverly, Mass.

CLARENCE W. WILLIAMS
> Engineer; Specialist in Hospital Heating, Ventilating, Etc.; Chairman, Hospital Board N. E. Deaconess Hospital, Boston, Mass.

JOSEPH B. HOWLAND, M. D.
> First Assistant Resident Physician, Massachusetts General Hospital, Boston, Mass.

CARLETON R. METCALF, M. D.
> Assistant Resident Physician, Massachusetts General Hospital, Boston, Mass.

JOHN E. GROFF, PH. G.
> Apothecary, Rhode Island Hospital, Providence, R. I.; Author of "Materia Medica for Nurses."

LOUIS H. BURLINGHAM, M. D.
> Assistant Resident Physician, Massachusetts General Hospital, Boston, Mass.

FRANK T. FULTON, M. D.
> Consulting Pathologist and Visiting Physician to Rhode Island Hospital, Providence.

THOMAS HOWELL, M. D.
> Superintendent, New York Hospital, N. Y.

CHARLOTTE A. AIKENS
> Detroit, Michigan.

PREFACE

As the title page indicates, this volume is designed especially for the use of hospital superintendents, trustees, training-school principals, physicians who are interested in or connected with hospitals; for students of hospital economics, for practical workers who labor in the capacity of professionals or administrators in any part of the hospital field.

Its purpose is to promote system, economy, and a better understanding of the principles that underlie successful, efficient hospital administration. Of necessity, in a handbook and with a wide field to cover, the treatment of the various subjects must be comparatively brief. It makes no pretention to being a complete treatise on institutional administration.

No pains have been spared by those concerned in its make-up to make it thoroughly practical in every respect, and to present the matter in each chapter so clearly that the most inexperienced student of hospital economics or the non-professional executive need have no difficulty in getting an intelligent grasp of the subjects discussed. Throughout its preparation the novice in hospital administration has been kept in view. If it proves of practical value to hospital workers who have strength, sympathy, and ambition to render effective service in the care of the sick, yet lack the well-rounded experience and the ability to take the broad view of their position so desirable, it will have fulfilled its mission.

Besides the writers named who have contributed chapters or sections, numerous others have lent their aid in a practical way to the completion of the undertaking. The editor has aimed to give credit to hospitals rather than to persons.for contributions of photographs, blanks, and forms, and wherever the origin of such material was known, it has been duly acknowledged in connection with its use.

Special thanks are due the Albert Pick Co. for loaning cuts of kitchen utensils.

The volume owes its inspiration to the American Hospital Association. To all the members of that association who have assisted, and to others who have contributed of their professional knowledge and experience, the editor offers sincere thanks. They have been many and exceeding kind.

C. A. A.

DETROIT, MICH., *February*, 1911.

CONTENTS

CHAPTER I
THE AMERICAN HOSPITAL FIELD.................. 17
BY CHARLES P. EMERSON, M. D.

CHAPTER II
THE BOARD OF MANAGERS AND THEIR RESPONSI-
BILITIES.................................... 72
BY E. S. GILMORE

CHAPTER III
THE SUPERINTENDENT............................ 79
BY GEORGE P. LUDLAM

CHAPTER IV
THE MEDICAL SERVICE OF A HOSPITAL............ 97
BY HENRY M. HURD, M. D.

CHAPTER V
A GENERAL HOSPITAL FOR ONE HUNDRED PATIENTS 108
BY JOHN N. ELLIOTT BROWN, M. B.,
and EDWARD FLETCHER STEVENS, A. A. I. A., Architect

CHAPTER VI
THE FURNISHINGS OF A 100-BED HOSPITAL........ 148
BY EMMA A. ANDERSON and LOUISE M. COLEMAN

CHAPTER VII
THE HOSPITAL INCOME AND MANAGEMENT OF TRUST
FUNDS 190
BY CHARLES A. GILL

CONTENTS

CHAPTER VIII
HOSPITAL BOOKKEEPING 207
BY W. L. BABCOCK, M.D.

CHAPTER IX
THE HOSPITAL STORE............................ 236
BY J. LYMAN BELKNAP, M.D.

CHAPTER X
THE KITCHEN 246
BY RENWICK R. ROSS, M.D:

CHAPTER XI
THE DIETITIAN'S PROVINCE AND ITS MANAGEMENT.. 256
BY ELIZABETH HINCHMAN

CHAPTER XII
THE ENGINEERING DEPARTMENT.................... 273
BY CLARENCE W. WILLIAMS

CHAPTER XIII
THE LAUNDRY................................... 283
BY JOSEPH B. HOWLAND, M.D.

CHAPTER XIV
THE PURCHASE AND ECONOMIC USE OF SURGICAL SUPPLIES................................... 294
BY CARLETON R. METCALF, M.D.

CHAPTER XV
THE HOSPITAL DRUG ROOM....................... 317
BY JOHN E. GROFF

CHAPTER XVI
THE TRAINING-SCHOOL AND ITS MANAGEMENT...... 330
BY CHARLOTTE A. AIKENS

CHAPTER XVII
THE OUT-PATIENT DEPARTMENT 378
BY LOUIS H. BURLINGHAM, M.D.

CHAPTER XVIII
THE HOSPITAL LABORATORY 390
By Frank T. Fulton, M.D.

CHAPTER XIX
THE ANNUAL REPORT............................ 398
By Thomas Howell, M.D.

APPENDIX I
TRAINING-SCHOOL REGULATIONS AND SUGGESTIONS... 427

APPENDIX II
HOSPITAL DIETARIES............................ 450

APPENDIX III
MISCELLANEOUS................................. 469

INDEX.. 481

HOSPITAL MANAGEMENT

CHAPTER I

THE AMERICAN HOSPITAL FIELD

By Charles P. Emerson, M.D.

It can, perhaps, be easily understood and pardoned that the author of the present chapter should envy the other contributors to this book that they have but a single subject to discuss. To write on The American Hospital Field is of itself a difficult task, but to write on this subject a chapter which can serve as a suitable foreword to chapters which follow, each dealing more at length with but one division of this general topic, and all written by men who have far greater authority in this field than has the present writer, is a task much harder still. Should the ideas expressed in this introduction prove at variance with those of the other writers, its author begs the reader to accept their opinions in preference to his own.

In this chapter we shall attempt to survey briefly the hospital field as it now appears, and to draw certain conclusions concerning its future development which its history in the past and its present condition may possibly justify. By "hospital field," we mean that sphere in human interest which medical institutions designed for the treatment of the sick do, and probably will, occupy.

The hospital field in America—what to-day are its characteristics? It is the broadest, the most promising, the richest, and yet, perhaps, the least developed and most poorly organized of all the hospital fields of those countries whose institutions we have had opportunity to visit.

One reason why our field may be described as the broadest and the most promising is that American hospitals are not hindered in their present development by their historic evolution. In Europe hospitals were originally erected for the very poor. One cannot fail to see this in Paris, where practically all the great hospitals were, and some still are, also almshouses. With but one important exception, they are all under the control of L'Assistance Publique, a department which controls also practically all institutions, of all kinds, for the poor. In Paris the invalid and the pauper are usually admitted to the same institutions through the same doors and by the same persons. One reads the same official heading on hospital records and almshouse requisition blanks. It is quite impossible there to separate the ideas of "sick in a hospital" and "poor." The famous hospitals of Germany and Austria are, for the most part, municipal institutions, intended primarily for the sick among the poor. It is true that now the number of private wards in general hospitals, and of private institutions for the well-to-do, is increasing, but the prejudice against hospitals as refuges for the poor will probably act in these countries as an obstacle to their rapid development. But in America there is not, and never has been, nearly so strong an association in the popular mind between poverty and hospitals. It has, of necessity, existed in the case of certain hospitals and of certain wards in other hospitals, but this association is not true of hospitals in general, and, where it does exist, it may be traced in some measure to our immigrants from Europe. In this country hospitals are recognized as institutions for the treatment of disease, and they are supposed to provide suitable accommodations for millionaire and pauper. There is a growing belief that a hospital is, or should be, a better place for a sick man than his own

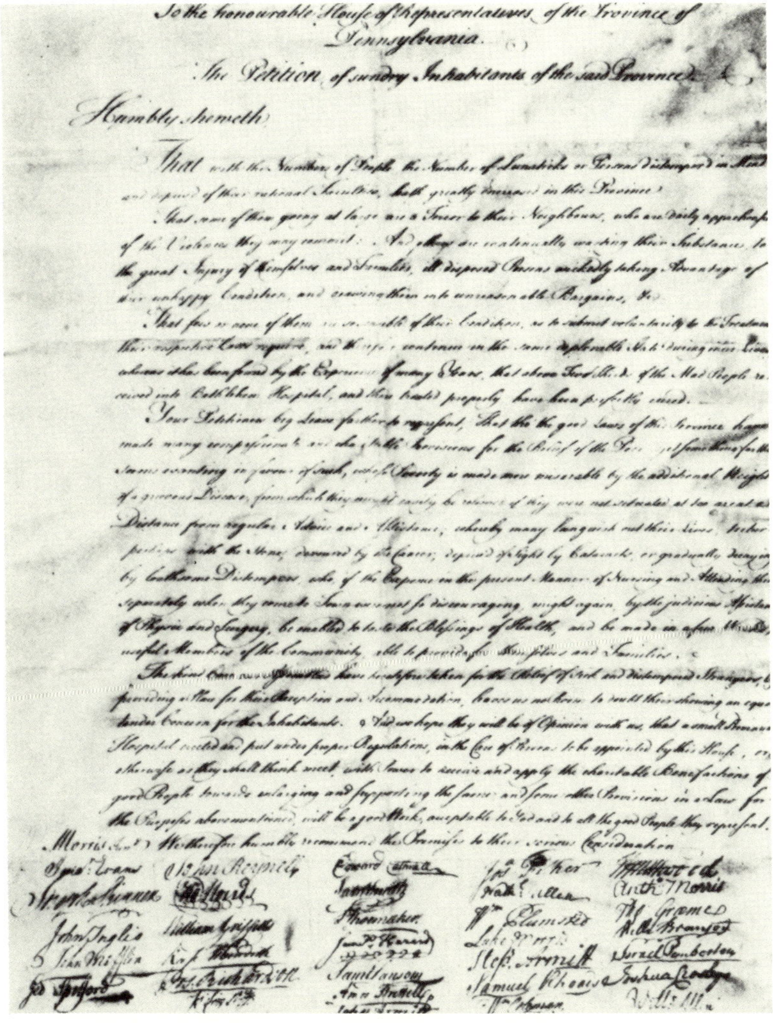

To the honourable House of Representatives of the Province of Pennsylvania.

The Petition of sundry Inhabitants of the said Province,

Humbly Sheweth

That with the Number of People, the Number of Lunaticks or Persons distemper'd in Mind and deprived of their rational Faculties, hath greatly increased in this Province.

That some of them going at large are a Terror to their Neighbours, who are daily apprehensive of the Violences they may commit; And others are continually wasting their Substance, to the great Injury of themselves and Families, ill disposed Persons wickedly taking Advantage of their unhappy Condition, and drawing them into unreasonable Bargains, &c.

That few or none of them are so sensible of their Condition, as to submit voluntarily to the Treatment their respective Cases require, and therefore continue in the same deplorable State during their Lives; whereas it has been found by the Experience of many Years, that above Two Thirds of the Mad People received into Bethlehem Hospital, and there treated properly, have been perfectly cured.

Your Petitioners beg Leave farther to represent, That tho' the good Laws of this Province have made many compassionate and charitable Provisions for the Relief of the Poor, yet something farther seems wanting in Favour of such, whose Poverty is made more miserable by the additional Weight of a grievous Disease, from which they might easily be relieved, if they were not situated at too great a Distance from regular Advice and Assistance; whereby many languish out their Lives, tortur'd perhaps with the Stone, devour'd by the Cancer, deprived of Sight by Cataracts, or gradually decaying by loathsome Distempers; who, if the Expence in the present Manner of Nursing and Attending them separately when they come to Town, were not so discouraging, might again, by the judicious Assistance of Physic and Surgery, be enabled to taste the Blessings of Health, and be made in a few Weeks, useful Members of the Community, able to provide for themselves and Families.

The kind Care our Assemblies have heretofore taken for the Relief of sick and distempered Strangers, by providing a Place for their Reception and Accommodation, leaves us no Room to doubt their shewing an equal tender Concern for the Inhabitants. And we hope they will be of Opinion with us, that a small Provincial Hospital erected and put under proper Regulations, in the Care of Persons to be appointed by this House, or otherwise as they shall think meet, with Power to receive and apply the charitable Benefactions of good People towards enlarging and supporting the same, and some other Provisions in a Law for the Purposes abovementioned, will be a good Work, acceptable to God and to all the good People they represent.

We therefore humbly recommend the Premises to their serious Consideration.

John Inglis

Wm. Plumsted

Luke Morris

Samuel Rhoads

Anth. Morris

Thos. Graeme

Israel Pemberton

Joshua Crosby

Fig. 1.—Original petition for the establishment of the **Pennsylvania Hospital, Philadelphia, Pa.** Benjamin Franklin's handwriting.

home, however rich that home, and consequently private hospitals and endowed hospitals are preparing to accommodate an ever-increasing and ever more varied demand. The institutions which formerly had, in addition to their public wards, a few single private rooms, are now building pavilions with luxurious apartments. There is also a constantly increasing number of physicians and surgeons who insist that their patients become patients in the hospitals with which they are connected, for the double reason that the patient will be better cared for there and that there the doctor can more easily visit him. We may confidently expect that more and more will sickness of all sorts and in all classes of society be treated in hospitals rather than in homes. Of course, the municipal hospitals can of necessity take but little part in this extension of the hospital field, but they, nevertheless, profit by it, as the poor man has little understanding of the difference between an endowed hospital and one supported by public funds, and he goes more willingly to the one if he knows that his rich neighbor goes to the other.

The hospital field in America is very rich and promises to become much richer, because here the erection and the endowment of hospitals are considered rather the duty of private citizens and organizations than the duty of a paternal government or a church. The endowing of hospitals is a philanthropy which appeals to many benevolent and wealthy persons, and will probably appeal to such in the future to a still greater degree; and we see in this country relatively far fewer exclusively municipal or church medical institutions than abroad. In some cities, indeed, the municipal hospitals are relatively unimportant, and seem able to get only those patients that the other hospitals in these cities do not want. Were it considered the duty of the government to build hospitals, as is the case in Continental Europe, our hospital field would of necessity lose the interest of public-spirited men who desire to be identified with this as a charity; and it certainly would be much less varied in its development, and so be capable of a less rich evolution. Under private control also there is the possibility of reaching a much higher grade of excellence, since in no country do municipal hospitals rank, as regards the quality of their work, with the privately endowed institutions, especially those connected with universities.

The American hospital field is very little developed, because this is a very young country, with, on the whole, a scattered population. In any new community hospitals are "after-thoughts."

The history of the development of the hospital field in our several States resembles that in older countries. The first institutions were "homes" or asylums for the helpless—for orphan children, the insane, and the old. In these medical treatment was given by "wholesale" methods. The modern hospital, erected and equipped for the especial purpose of giving the individual sick man the best of individual treatment, is a much more recent institution. At one stage of this development the attempt was made to treat not the individual patients, but the individual disease; that is, hospitals were erected for the care of certain groups of diseases—skin diseases; eye diseases; nose, throat, and ear diseases; cancers; surgical diseases; fevers; pulmonary diseases; diseases of the digestive tract, etc.

But, fortunately, that stage is now nearly passed. A patient can be dissected in the above manner only in the imagination, for one organ almost never suffers alone, but, to some degree at least, involves other organs also. One cannot separate the diseases of the eye from those of the nervous system; diseases of the skin from those of the kidneys and digestive tract; diseases of the lungs from those of the throat, etc. For this reason, a patient is in danger of receiving perilously narrow treatment in any institution which makes a specialty of but one group of diseases. The individual man, whatever his illness, gets that treatment which is best for his individual need in an institution which takes the whole field of medicine to be its province.

5th Mon. 1. 1751

In Pursuance of the foregoing Act of Assembly, the following Persons, Contributors to the Hospital, viz.

John Reynell	Charles Stedman	Alexr. Stedman
Jonathan Mifflin	Richard Peters	Israel Pemberton
Rees Meredith	Samuel Hazard	Caspar Wistar
Saml. Rhodes	Joseph Wharton	John Wistar
Anth. Benezet	John Armitt	Thos. Say
Stephen Anthony	Saml. Preston Moore	Thos. Crosby
Joseph Morris	Thomas Bond	Saml. Sansom
Saml. Powell	Joseph Fox	Cha. Jones
Wm. Griffitts	Charles Norris	Thomas Gretch
Abel James	Benj. Franklin	Jacob Lewis
Anth. Morris	I. Pemberton Jr.	Adam Harker
Wm. Moode	Joshua Crosby	Anthy. Morris

Met at the Statehouse in Philadelphia, and proceeded to the Choice of Twelve Managers and a Treasurer, and the following Persons were chosen by Ballot to continue till the first 2d Day of the Week in the Month called May next, viz.

Managers

Joshua Crosby   Saml. Rhodes
Benj. Franklin   Hugh Roberts
Thos. Bond   Joseph Morris
Saml. Hazard   John Smith
Richd. Peters   Evan Morgan
Iy. Pemberton Jr. Cha. Norris

Treasr.
John Reynell

Fig. 2.—Photographic reproduction of the minutes showing the election of the first Board of Managers of the Pennsylvania Hospital, Philadelphia, Pa. Franklin's handwriting.

THE AMERICAN HOSPITAL FIELD

That the American hospital field is still little developed, extensively as well as intensively, is seen by a study of the rate of increase of medical institutions of all kinds in the United States during the last sixty years. Of 5034 medical institutions in all the states, the date of whose establishment is given in Polk's "Medical Register and Directory" (eleventh ed., 1910), we find the following distribution, so far as their ages are concerned:

```
Established prior to        1851 ......  193, or   3.9 per cent.
Established between 1851–1860 ......  173, or   3.4   "
Established    "    1861–1870 ......  270, or   5.4   "
Established    "    1871–1880 ......  371, or   7.3   "
Established    "    1881–1890 ......  726, or  14.4   "
Established    "    1891–1900 ......1254, or  24.9   "
Established    "    1901–1910 ......2047, or  40.7   "
                                     5034, or 100.0 per cent.
```

From this table it will be seen that, in the rate of increase of medical institutions of all kinds, our country, considered as a whole, shows two points of acceleration—one about 1850 and the second at 1881. During the last thirty years the total number has almost doubled with each decade. But this statement conveys a false impression, for the increase has been by no means uniform in the several states. If we contrast the increase in five of the older northern states (Massachusetts, Connecticut, New York, Pennsylvania, and Ohio) with that of five of the older southern states (Virginia, Georgia, South Carolina, Alabama, and Louisiana), and with five of the newer states (Kansas, Minnesota, Nebraska, New Mexico, and Arizona), we find the following:

		Northern. Per cent.	Southern. Per cent.	New. Per cent.
Established before	1851	7.2	5.5	0.0
Established between	1851–1860	5.2	4.8	0.3
Established "	1861–1870	8.2	4.4	2.3
Established "	1871–1880	10.0	5.9	4.6
Established "	1881–1890	15.6	12.8	15.3
Established "	1891–1900	25.9	20.3	25.8
Established "	1901–1910	27.9	46.3	51.7
		100.0	100.0	100.0

From this table one can see that the rate of intensive increase in certain northern states was accelerated between 1881 and 1890, and that now there is no marked increase. One cannot but see, too, the effect which an influence that depresses the material development of a state (as war) has on the rapidity of hospital construction. The present rapid increase, the country considered as a whole, is due to the growth of population in formerly undeveloped country.

That the institutions on this American hospital field show as yet very little coöperation is not surprising, for the great majority of them are entirely independent as regards origin and control, and are subject to no supervision other than that of the state boards of health, which merely enforce nominal obligations.

It is an advantage, we believe, to have in one city several similar small hospitals, rather than a few large ones, providing they are all well enough endowed or supported to insure good work. Unfortunately, many are not, and, what is still more unfortunate, some of the hospitals in our large cities show among themselves an unfortunate rivalry, and duplicate work in an extravagant manner. If many hospitals in each city could pool their interests, the result would be greater efficiency and greater economy— and yet nothing is more unlikely than that independent, privately controlled hospitals will pool interests. The harder such institutions are pressed for funds, especially if they represent some individual denomination, or some one private benefaction, and still more if they are intended as monuments to certain men or families, the harder will they fight for independent existence; and, in their attempted economy, it is the quality of their medical work which will suffer first. (We refer now only to the hospitals in our large cities.) There may be good reason for the states helping to perpetuate the existence of some of the now inadequately financed institutions, especially those of growing communities, if there is ground for believing that they give promise of growing in the future to strong, efficient hospitals. To combine, were it possible, several

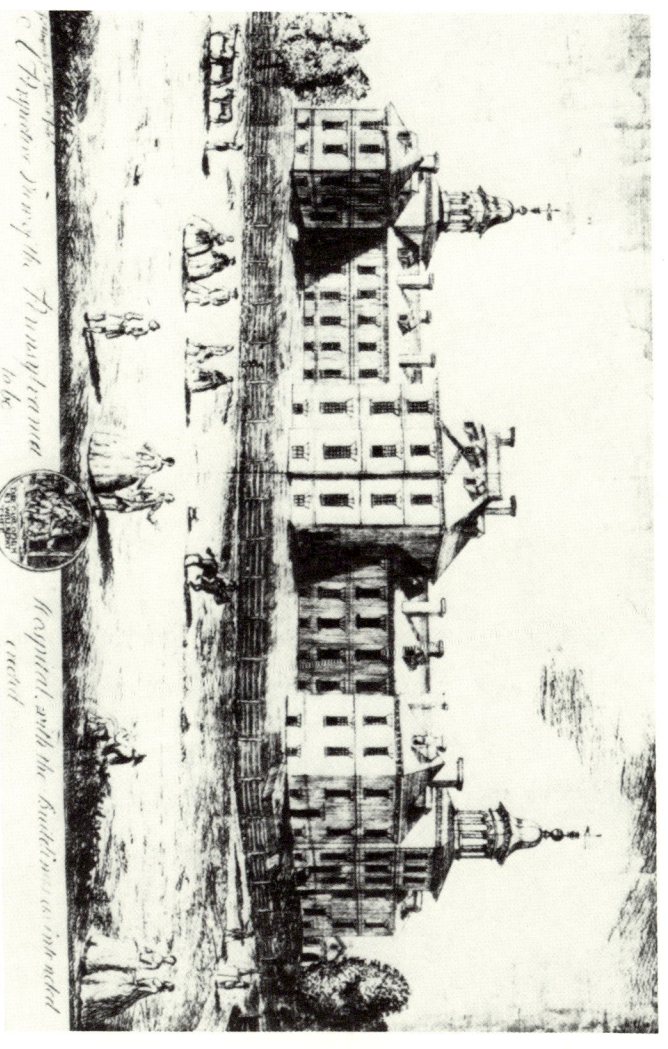

Fig. 3.—Original plan of the Pennsylvania Hospital, Philadelphia, Pa., made in 1754, and used with slight alterations.

weak institutions in a few strong ones in such a manner that they would lose their identity, and no longer represent the beneficence which founded them, would not be desirable, as they would no longer encourage charitable persons, interested in that which they represent, to give to them. I am not sure but that we should desire these privately endowed institutions to decrease in number and variety, and the municipal hospitals to increase; and yet there is little value in an institution so poorly equipped that it cannot do good work.

While all these hospitals and other medical charities differ so much in their origin and in the sources of their endowment, they differ little, generally speaking, in their function. In one city there may be a Methodist, an Episcopalian, a German, a Roman Catholic, and a city hospital. These differ much in the sources of the funds which support them, but not in their clientele. The doors of all are open to all patients, irrespective of creed (though not of color), and usually their internes themselves are appointed to the staffs of all, without regard to their religious convictions (which is unfortunate in some cases), each trying to get the services of those young men best trained in medicine and surgery. If one can find any characteristic difference in the clientele of these several hospitals, it will probably be in the case of those occupying endowed rooms or enjoying special rates. In general, the patients choose among them not according to their name or denomination, but according to a notion of the medical advantages which each has to offer; and it is often for an amusing reason that the sick man prefers one above all the others.

We shall now superficially survey the American hospital field as it appears at the present time. Our authorities are Polk's "Medical Register and Directory for 1910" and the "American Medical Directory," 1909. We cannot claim exact accuracy for these figures, but we believe that they are relatively accurate. Only those institutions are considered whose size is stated in one of these two directories.

In 1909 there were in the United States at least 2547 hospitals for acute medical and surgical cases, and these, it was stated, contained 153,501 beds. It is impossible to distinguish between public and private hospitals, as most of our best hospitals open to the public are truly private institutions, and the doctor who has a private hospital opens its doors as widely as he can to those willing to pay his prices. The American hospital field is not especially related to the poor—it is for all, rich and poor, and our attempt now is to study the total hospital accommodations offered to all classes. Also, it is quite impossible to draw any line between free, part-pay, and full-pay beds, for the bed free to the man from Baltimore, for instance, is a part-pay bed if he happens to come from Virginia; and in some of our best endowed hospitals, the full-pay patients are not charged that which their care actually costs the institution. No attempt is made to distinguish among conditions in large cities, in small cities, and in country districts, since, with modern rapid transit, a patient can, and often does, try in succession, clinics in widely distant cities or even states. There are scarcely any hospitals with a strictly local clientele, and the better its reputation, the wider will be the area from which a hospital will attract patients. For these reasons a grouping by states is the only one we dare attempt.

These 153,501 beds are distributed among the states as follows: From 49 to 100 beds per 100,000 inhabitants, 10 states (Alabama, Florida, Georgia, Kentucky, Mississippi, North Carolina, Oklahoma, South Carolina, Tennessee, and Virginia). From 101 to 200 beds per 100,000 inhabitants, 16 states (Arkansas, Indiana, Iowa, Kansas, Louisiana, Maine, Michigan, Missouri, Nebraska, New Hampshire, Rhode Island, South Dakota, Texas, Vermont, West Virginia, and Wisconsin).

From 201 to 300 beds per 100,000 inhabitants, 15 states (Connecticut, Delaware, Illinois, Maryland, Massachusetts,

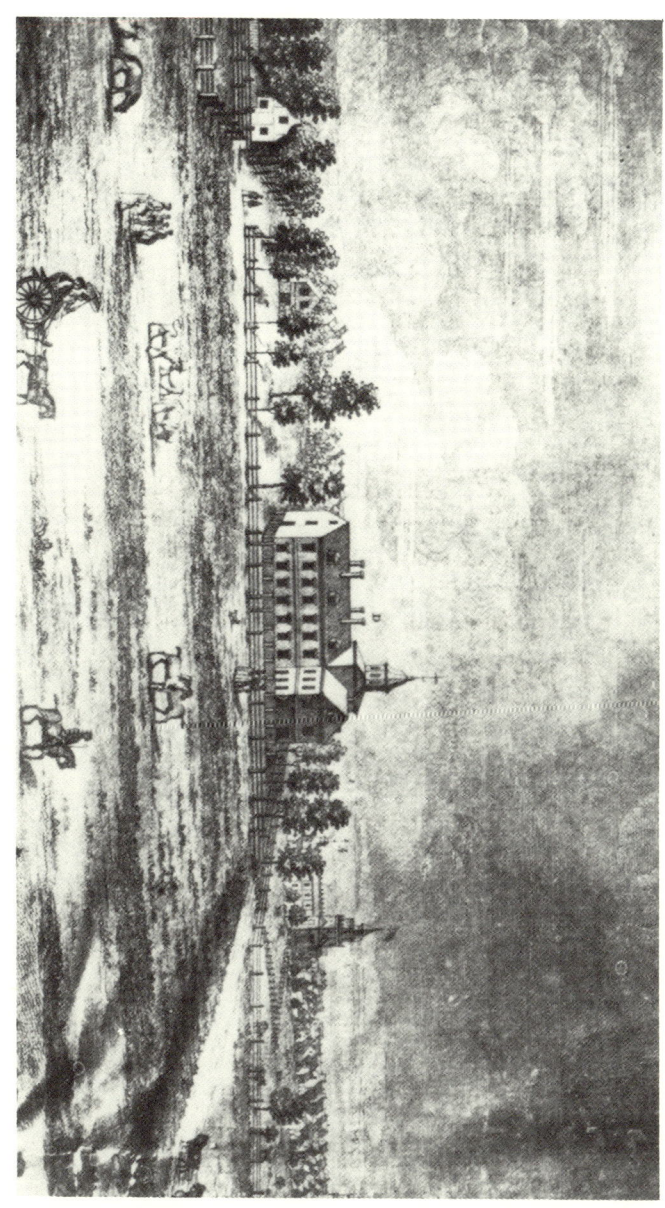

Fig. 4.—East wing, Pennsylvania Hospital, Philadelphia, Pa., completed 1756.

Minnesota, New Jersey, New Mexico, New York, North Dakota, Ohio, Oregon, Pennsylvania, Utah, and Wyoming). From 301 to 400 beds per 100,000 inhabitants, 1 state (Washington). From 401 to 500 beds per 100,000 inhabitants, 4 states (Arizona, Colorado, Idaho, and District of Columbia. For the sake of brevity we shall speak of District of Columbia as a state). Above 500 beds, 3 states (California, Montana, and Nevada).

The Province of Ontario has 204 beds per 100,000 inhabitants, distributed among 53 hospitals (average 81 beds); and the Province of Quebec, 420 beds per 100,000 of inhabitants. In the latter province large institutions are the rule (22 hospitals, average 307 beds).

From the study of these groups of states we can draw some interesting conclusions. The first group is the most homogeneous of all, for its members are all southern states. One can easily understand that, the warmer climate, the slower the appreciation of hospitals by the poor, and especially in states a large proportion of whose population is colored. It is a well-known fact that the wards for colored patients are almost empty in summer, and fill up with the first cold week. But it is important to note, this list includes many of those states in which the number of new medical institutions is at present rapidly increasing. In these states the number of new hospitals built during the decade 1901 to 1910 bears the following relation to the total number of such institutions: Alabama, 55.1 per cent.; Florida, 65.6 per cent.; Georgia, 51.7 per cent.; Kentucky, 30.7 per cent.; Mississippi, 67.9 per cent.; North Carolina, 54.9 per cent.; Oklahoma, 89 per cent.; South Carolina, 40.6 per cent.; Tennessee, 39 per cent.; and Virginia, 42 per cent. That is, of the 571 medical institutions of all kinds in these states, 291, or 50.9 per cent. were built during the last decade. It is evident, therefore, that in these states there is a feeling that they are not adequately provided with medical institutions. They are not all young states, and we mean by this that they are not young if judged by the dates when they began to build medical institutions. In the following pages "young" and "old," when applied to states, will have this meaning. The "age" of a state as given here is the average of the dates of establishment of its three oldest medical institutions now existant. (District of Columbia is counted as a state.) In point of age Virginia is the second, that is, the oldest but one; North Carolina the fourth; Kentucky the ninth; South Carolina the tenth; Alabama the fifteenth; Tennessee the twenty-first; Georgia the twenty-third; Mississippi the twenty-eighth; Florida the thirty-third; Oklahoma, the youngest, the forty-ninth. We believe that the depression following the Civil War largely explains the small number of medical institutions in the Southern states, and, that, judging by the activity of these states during the past decade, we may confidently predict that statistics taken ten years hence will show a different state of affairs from that shown by the statistics just given.

The next group also contains several new states, and, interestingly enough, some of the states with the largest, some with the smallest, territory. The present rate of increase in these states may be inferred from that during the last decade. During the decade 1901 to 1910 the number of new medical institutions bore to the total number the following proportion: Arkansas, 48.8 per cent.; Indiana, 32.1 per cent.; Iowa, 50.7 per cent.; Kansas, 47.7 per cent.; Louisiana, 34 per cent.; Maine, 38.1 per cent.; Michigan, 42.3 per cent.; Missouri, 37.9 per cent.; Nebraska, 50.6 per cent.; New Hampshire, 38 per cent.; Rhode Island, 35.7 per cent.; South Dakota, 48.6 per cent.; Texas, 59.8 per cent.; Vermont, 41.9 per cent.; West Virginia, 64 per cent.; Wisconsin, 34.3 per cent. That is, of the 1471 medical institutions in these 16 states, 647, or 43.9 per cent., were built during the past decade. This group is very interesting. It contains some of the states relatively old, according to the above-mentioned standard (Louisiana was the seventh, Vermont the twelfth, Rhode Island the thirteenth, Maine the fourteenth, and New

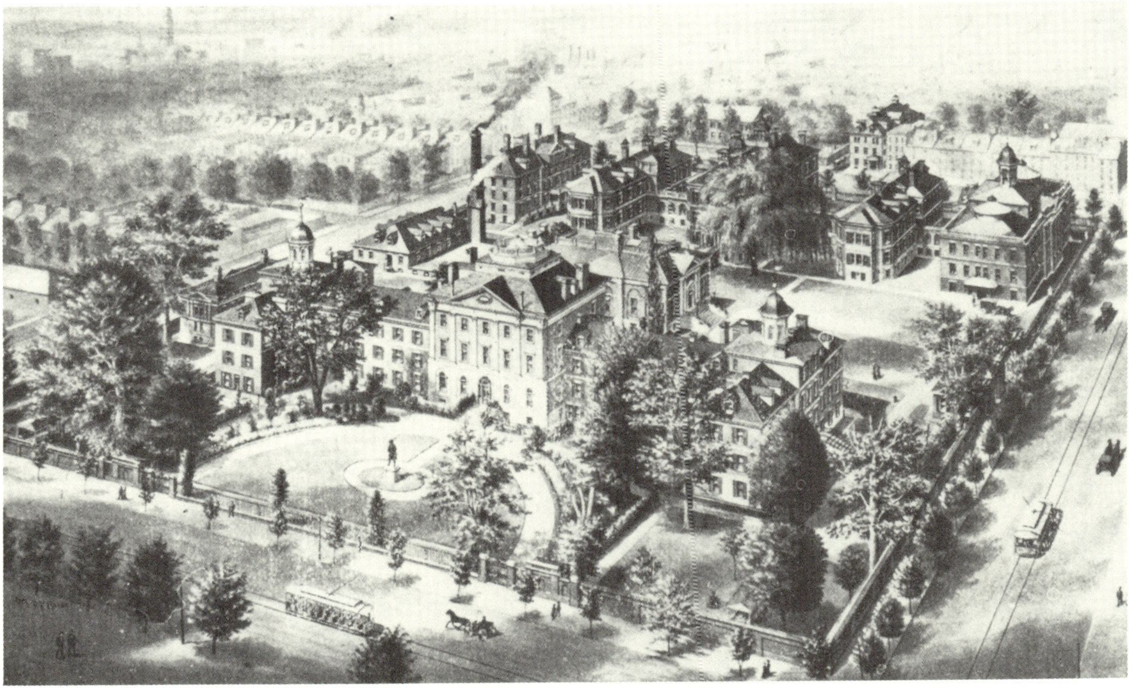

Fig. 5.—Bird's-eye view of Pennsylvania Hospital, Philadelphia, Pa., 1900.

Hampshire the eighteenth); so that it is not merely a matter of ages. Some are, as regards territory, the smallest states, and their inhabitants can easily reach hospitals of neighboring states. Some of them are small states as regards population (yet there are in the Union nine states with lower population than is the lowest of this list), and some are youngest as regards hospital construction (Kansas was the thirty-seventh, Nebraska the forty-second, Arkansas the forty-third, and South Dakota the forty-fourth). We must consider this group as quite heterogeneous, including some states which are young, some just recovering from past decades of depression, and some, owing perhaps to their size, depending on neighboring states for hospital accommodations.

The third group is by far the most interesting of all, for it contains those states with the most highly developed hospital fields. In it are five of the oldest states. In the point of hospital construction Pennsylvania was the first, New York the third, Massachusetts the fifth, Maryland the sixth, and Connecticut the eighth; while Minnesota the thirty-fourth, Utah the thirty-fifth, Oregon the thirty-sixth, New Mexico the forty-fifth, Wyoming the forty-sixth, North Dakota the forty-seventh, are among our youngest states. New York, Pennsylvania, Illinois, Ohio, and Massachusetts are five of the seven largest states in the Union in point of population. During the last decade (1901 to 1910) the number of new medical institutions built in these states bore the following relation to their total number: Connecticut, 29.9 per cent.; Delaware, 30.8 per cent.; Illinois, 37.9 per cent.; Maryland, 25.6 per cent.; Massachusetts, 32.7 per cent.; New Jersey, 25.3 per cent.; New York, 22 per cent.; Pennsylvania, 27.8 per cent.; Ohio, 33.7 per cent.; Minnesota, 49.4 per cent.; New Mexico, 67.6 per cent.; North Dakota, 71.1 per cent.; Oregon, 59.3 per cent.; Utah, 62.5 per cent.; and Wyoming, 61.6 per cent. Nine of these states, Connecticut, Delaware, Illinois, Maryland, Massachusetts, New Jersey, New York, Pennsylvania, and Ohio form a group which, we believe, may be considered as a sort of norm. These states are among the oldest, they have the largest variety of medical institutions, and the increase in the number of their institutions has been the steadiest. It is of interest that their percentages of increase during the past decade are among the lowest of all the states (nine of the lowest sixteen). We may perhaps accept this as that rate of increase most normal under present conditions. If so, then the normal number of beds per 100,000 inhabitants

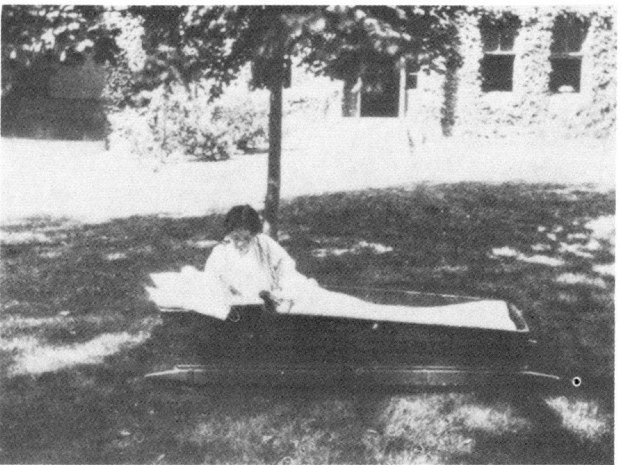

Fig. 6.—Patient's box used in open-air treatment, Massachusetts General Hospital.

would be about 228. It is nothing short of remarkable that in the case of these states the number of beds in hospitals for acute cases per 100,000 inhabitants lies between so very close limits (New York, 209; Maryland, 215; Connecticut, 219; Pennsylvania, 225; Ohio, 226; Delaware, 229; Illinois, 236; New Jersey, 237; and Massachusetts, 263).

The next three groups of eight states contain five which are young in point of hospital construction: Washington

THE AMERICAN HOSPITAL FIELD 29

was the thirty-second, Nevada the thirty-ninth, Montana the forty-first, Arizona the forty-fifth, and Idaho the forty-eighth. The rate of increase in the number of new medical institutions in these states may be judged by the percentage which the number of those built during the last decade is of the total number (Washington, 52.7 per cent.; Arizona, 61.5 per cent.; Colorado, 52.4 per cent.; District of Columbia, 15 per cent.; Idaho, 65.4 per cent.; California, 54.6 per cent.; Montana, 51 per cent.; and Nevada, 62.5

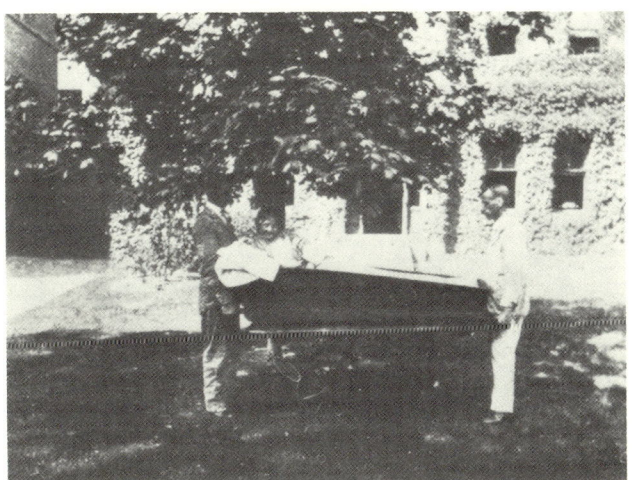

Fig. 7.—Out-door scene, Massachusetts General Hospital.

per cent. Of the total number, 624, of medical institutions in these eight states, 326, or 52.2 per cent., were built during this past decade). We should not expect the same historic evolution of the medical institutions in these states as in the older, since they have the experience of the others to guide them. It certainly is interesting that these young states have now relatively the largest number of beds. So many of their institutions were built during the past decade that one must wait still another ten years before he can tell with any accuracy what this may mean. Is it a temporary condition—the result of a recent overproduction? Or do the guiding minds of this movement, most of them men from older states, unhampered by precedent, at once build more nearly the correct number, and establish a new norm to which the older states should try to conform? It is more than possible that the hospitals built not by the local communities, but by mining com-

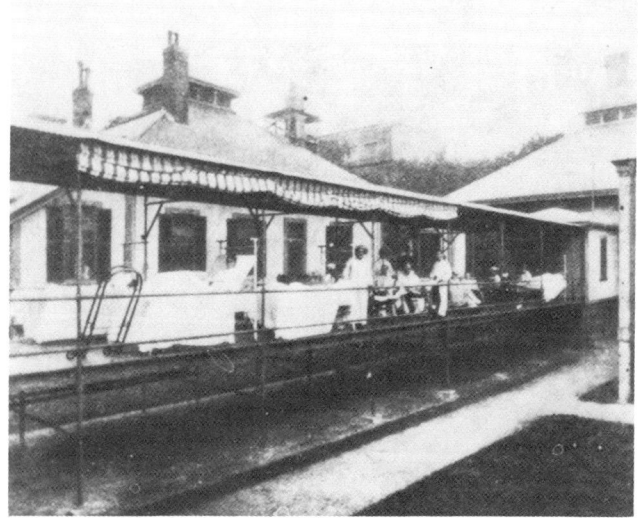

Fig. 8.—Veranda scene, Massachusetts General Hospital.

panies and railroads, may, in part, explain these high figures. These are huge states, territorily, and for the most part sparsely settled. Nevada is the first, Idaho the fourth, Arizona the fifth, Montana the seventh, District of Columbia the ninth, Colorado the seventeenth, and Washington the nineteenth, in a list of states arranged according to population, Nevada having the fewest inhabitants. It will be interesting to watch the growth of the institutions of these states during the next decade.

Of course, it is true that in these newer states there are fewer varieties of institutions, and so the general hospitals must admit many patients who in other states would be cared for in special hospitals; but the study of our tables shows this to be a minor point.

Size is a poor standard by which to judge a hospital. The only correct standard would be that of efficiency in giving each patient the individual care which his case requires. But this standard would be a rather variable one, since it must depend on the local needs which the hospital must meet and on the medical standards of the profession in the locality. Yet some lessons may be drawn from size alone. Of the 2547 hospitals for general medical and surgical cases of acute character, 869, or 34.1 per cent., are credited with 20 or fewer beds; 871, or 34.2 per cent., have from 21 to 50 beds; 474, or 18.6 per cent., have from 51 to 100 beds; 223, or 8.4 per cent., have from 101 to 200 beds; 67, or 2.7 per cent., from 201 to 300 beds; 26, or 1 per cent., from 301 to 400 beds; 12, or 0.5 per cent., from 401 to 500 beds; and 13, or 0.5 per cent., over 500 beds. It is a very interesting fact that each of 68.3 per cent. of our hospitals for acute cases have fewer than 51 beds.

No conclusion concerning the efficiency of a hospital can be drawn from this other than, possibly, one concerning the demand there is for beds in the locality of these hospitals. Excellent individual work may be done in a hospital for five beds, provided the patient is able to pay for excellent professional attention, or, as is far oftener the case, providing excellent professional men and women are willing to give their attention to these five patients. In some of the thinly populated states the reason for many of these small hospitals may be that there is little demand for, or too little money to run, a larger hospital. And yet the question of population would explain but a few of their total number. Of the 869 hospitals with 20 or fewer beds, 483, or 55 per cent., are in the following 12 states: California, 50; Illinois, 26; Indiana, 38; Iowa, 38; Kansas, 36; Massachusetts, 51; Michigan, 47; Minnesota, 48;

New York, 33; Ohio, 50; Pennsylvania, 26; and Wisconsin, 38. It will be seen at once that they are most numerous in some of the oldest and most densely populated states.

The largest hospitals also are in the most populous states. Of the 26 with more than 400 beds, Pennsylvania has 4, New York 9, Illinois 3, and California 2. The rest are scattered.

To discuss the sanatoria of our country is difficult indeed, since under this term are included several different kinds of institutions. (The "American Medical Directory," second edition, 1909, is our authority for their classification.) A sharp distinction can easily be made between sanatoria for mental, nervous, drug, and alcoholic cases, and those for patients with general medical and surgical conditions. The latter sanatoria may take a few of the patients first mentioned, but they do not admit as many as do the hospitals considered in the preceding pages. Surely no law could be more efficient in excluding them from general sanatoria than are the dictates of good business judgment, for practically all sanatoria are private, self-supporting institutions, and are well aware that other patients cautiously shun those institutions admitting mental or drug patients in numbers great enough to attract the general attention of the guests, who are not, as a rule, bed patients and are much interested in their neighbors. For this reason a pretty sharp line can be drawn between those sanatoria which specialize in these cases and those which do not. It is for this reason that some institutions refusing mental and drug cases dislike the name "sanatorium," preferring "health resort," etc., although in some states the word "sanatorium" seems synonymous with "private hospital."

With each decade the sanatoria for general cases are becoming more truly hospitals. Some, indeed, have most active surgical clinics, others just as active medical clinics. Others are hospitals for chronic conditions, especially cardiovascular, renal diseases, joint affections, nervous fatigue, diseases of metabolism—in fact, for all patients not ill enough to require continuous bed treatment. Sanatoria are also convalescent homes. While formerly no small part of their clientele were those presenting no medical or surgical problem, in recent years the summer hotels have diverted most of these patrons, and for this reason sanatoria are becoming, more and more, real hospitals. Formerly many were established as mere water cures, etc., but now practically all are equipped for general medical and surgical work. In two important particulars they differ from the hospitals for the acutely ill—they have not the same local character, but attract patrons from all parts of the country; and their location is in great measure determined not by population, but by natural attractions, as mountains or lakes, or by natural advantages, as springs.

There are registered in our country 643 sanatoria, with a total of 23,071 beds. Each state has at least one, but most of the sanatoria are in a few states. California has 57, Colorado 19, Illinois 28, Indiana 24, Massachusetts 33, Missouri 23, New York 62, Pennsylvania 21, Texas 40, and Wisconsin 22—that is, 51 per cent. of them all are situated in only ten states.

The sanatoria for "nervous," mental, drug, and alcoholic patients are, as a rule, very strictly limited in respect to their clientele, and in this doubtless the mental patients greatly predominate. We could find record of 115 such sanatoria, and these offer 5801 beds. They are most numerous in certain states. California has 5, Connecticut 6, Massachusetts 7, Michigan 5, New York, 12, Ohio 10, Pennsylvania 6, and Wisconsin 5.

The number of special institutions for tuberculosis cases is rapidly increasing. Perhaps there is no better proof of the efficiency of those organizations interested in preventive medicine than is the multiplication of these institutions. We found record of 211 such institutions, with a total of 16,501 beds. Of these, Arizona has 4, California 12, Colorado 21, Georgia 5, Illinois 7, Maryland 7, Massachusetts 17, Minnesota 5, New Mexico 10, New York 24, North

Carolina 11, Ohio 7, Pennsylvania 22, Rhode Island 5, Texas 8, and Virginia 5. The rest are scattered. It will be seen at a glance of how much importance locality has been considered, far too great, in fact, for the out-patient departments in some of our large cities have shown that with good organization of tuberculosis classes and with the aid of visiting nurses, as high a percentage of arrested cases can be obtained in the slums of a city as in the mountain sanatoria. These sanatoria themselves will never be able directly to check tuberculosis, but they have an incalculable value because they show how such cases should be treated, and they teach the patient during the few weeks which he can spend in one of them how he should live during the future months and years. There are also 19 camps for tuberculosis patients, with space for 758 patients. Nearly one-half of these camps are in Massachusetts.

Hospitals for contagious diseases are certainly increasing in number. Although the need of such institutions has long been recognized, there has been comparatively little increase in their number until recently. We can find record of 76 such hospitals, with 6463 beds. Of these, 5 are in Illinois, 4 in Iowa, 9 in Massachusetts, 7 in New Jersey, 8 in New York, and 4 in Wisconsin. The rest are scattered. That we ought to see, and shall see, a great increase in their number is almost without question, for common sense, as well as medical science, teaches that patients with contagious diseases are treated with greatest safety to the public, and with best results for themselves, in special hospitals.

Asylums for the insane are not numerous. There are only 228, but they have a total of 187,930 (!) beds. Of real hospitals for these patients, however, where they receive satisfactory individual study and treatment, there are very, very few. It is, indeed, interesting that there are recorded in the two directories of institutions which we have used 34,429 more beds for the insane than for all patients with acute medical and surgical conditions—yes, nearly 5000 more beds than all the general hospitals, all the sanatoria, and all the institutions for the tuberculous

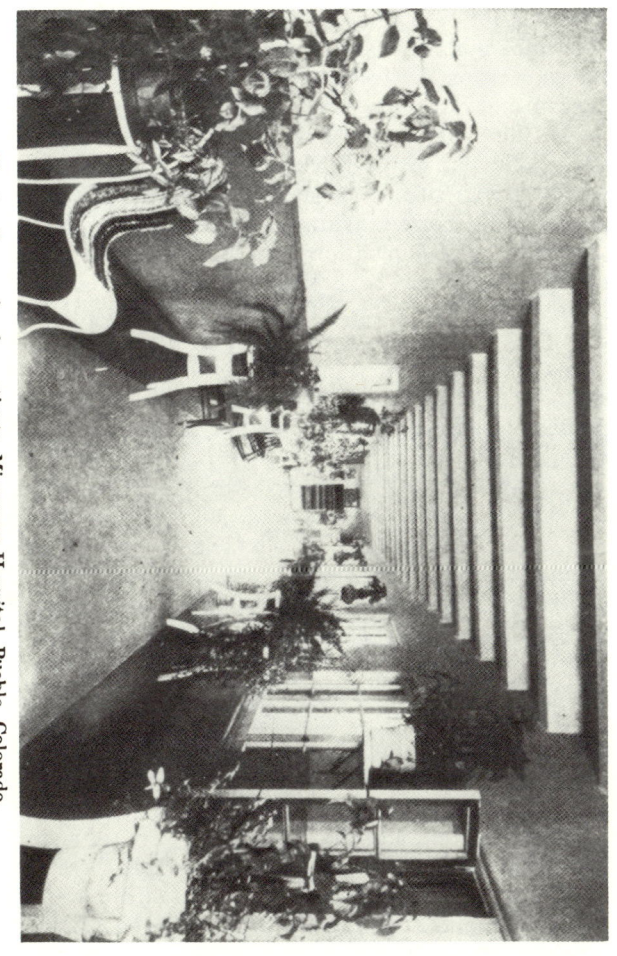

Fig. 9.—Sun-parlor for patients, Minnequa Hospital, Pueblo, Colorado.

patients together have to offer. We know that there are very few insane compared with those needing hospital or sanatorium treatment. If, therefore, hospitals should be more generally used by all classes when ill, how great would have to be the increase in their number and size: Of course, the number of beds in asylums for the insane is little indication of the number of patients needing such care, so many are the districts which "farm out" their insane; but a very much higher percentage of them is in institutions than of the ill but sane. To give some idea of the distribution of these asylums we present the following approximately correct figures:

Per 100,000 of population there are 100 beds, or fewer, in three states (Arizona, Arkansas, and New Mexico).

There are from 100 to 200 beds in 23 states (Alabama, Colorado, Florida, Georgia, Indiana, Iowa, Kentucky, Louisiana, Maine, Maryland, Mississippi, Missouri, Nebraska, North Carolina, North Dakota, Oklahoma, South Carolina, Tennessee, Texas, Utah, Vermont, Virginia, and Wyoming).

There are from 200 to 300 beds in 14 states (Delaware, Idaho, Illinois, Kansas, Minnesota, Montana, New Hampshire, Ohio, Pennsylvania, Rhode Island, South Dakota, Washington, West Virginia, and Wisconsin).

There are 300 to 400 in 5 states (California, Connecticut, Michigan, New Jersey, and Oregon).

There are over 400 in 4 states (District of Columbia, Massachusetts, Nevada, and New York).

It is curious to see what a close general resemblance these groups bear to those of the hospitals for acute cases.

Institutions for incurables are not in as much favor now as formerly, because special institutions for patients with advanced consumption, and the surgical wards of men who dare operate boldly for cancers, have deprived these hospitals of most of their patients. We found record of but 32, 9 of which are in New York, 8 in Pennsylvania, and 3 in Massachusetts. The rest are scattered. All are credited with 2320 beds.

Hospitals for women and children are also in less favor than formerly, as children need special hospitals—buildings which would be unsuitable for women, and the women are better cared for in special hospitals and in the medical maternity and surgical wards of general hospitals. We could find record of but 42 such hospitals, with 3126 beds. Three of them are in Colorado, 4 in Massachusetts, 3 in Michigan, 8 in New York, 6 in Ohio, and 4 in Pennsylvania, while the rest are scattered.

Special maternity hospitals are probably one of the greatest blessings to the women of the poor and will doubtless increase in number. There are now at least 81 such institutions with 2773 beds. Three of them are in California, 6 in Illinois, 4 in Maryland, 3 in Massachusetts, 3 in Minnesota, 7 in Missouri, 10 in New York, 4 in Ohio, 14 in Pennsylvania, and 3 in Texas, while the rest are scattered. Of course, this list includes some institutions for women of which the maternity ward is an important adjunct.

Special hospitals for children are now in great favor. There are at least 61 of them, with 5380 beds, and of these, 5 are in Maryland, 5 in Massachusetts, 5 in Missouri, 3 in New Jersey, 15 in New York, and 7 in Pennsylvania. The rest are scattered.

All these children's hospitals doubtless admit babies, and yet some authorities (especially in Germany) prefer special institutions for patients under two years of age. In this country there are at least 18 hospitals for babies, with 2712 beds, if we count the ward rooms of some of the larger foundling asylums. Four are in Massachusetts, and 7 in New York. The rest are scattered.

The value of special hospitals for eye, ear, nose, and throat cases is a disputed point, for patients with disease of these organs usually need general treatment. While perhaps it would be better to treat such patients in special wards of a general hospital, yet very few general hospitals will admit them, and so these special hospitals fill a very important place. There are 45 such hospitals, with 1610 beds. Some are for eye diseases alone, some for eye and ear, etc., and some for all four groups. Of these, Illinois has 3, Iowa 3, Maryland 3, New York 11, Ohio 4, and Pennsylvania 3, while the rest are scattered. We are struck with the small number of hospitals for diseases of the skin. They are so few that it was not worth while to tabulate them. In the out-patient departments of our large city hospitals the skin clinics are very small compared with those of Europe, which is one of the best of compliments to our poorer classes.

There are very few special institutions for convalescent patients—only 21, with a total of 728 beds. This does not include the convalescent homes in connection with a few of our large hospitals. The majority of these are distributed as follows: Illinois 2, Massachusetts 4, New York 5, Ohio 3, and Pennsylvania 2. The convalescents' hospital is one of the institutions of the future, and we may perhaps measure a state's progress in medical institutions by the rapidity with which such hospitals increase, either as separate institutions or as adjuncts of general hospitals, for they are very necessary and yet do not appeal strongly to the public mind.

In concluding this list of institutions we should like to mention 12 exclusively for epileptics, with space for 5555 patients; more than 147 orphan asylums for over 22,267 children; and at least 515 homes of all varieties, with space for more than 94,115 inmates. Unfortunately in this country the marvelously rich clinical material of these homes and asylums has not been well studied or treated. The medical care of these inmates is "contracted for," or given by busy practitioners whose one interest is to get through. And yet in some of these homes and asylums are larger and more interesting groups of patients than are found in some hospitals where valuable work is being done. These children and infants need and are awaiting adequate hospital care; at present they are treated according to the methods of a generation ago.

This brief review of the field finished, we shall now study its possibilities. Is the field too complicated? New York State has over 40 different kinds of hospitals alone, not counting the several other kinds of hospital institutions. What is the shortest list of the types of hospitals which we shall agree are necessary? In other words, of what necessary members is the medical institutional body composed, and what forms of these types should we consider perfect?

Of first importance are the general hospitals for acute cases, each with the largest number of different departments that it can adequately support. It should certainly have a medical clinic; a surgical clinic (including, or in addition, a gynecologic); an obstetric clinic; a pediatric clinic; a contagious department; a department for skin and genito-urinary diseases; a department for diseases of the eye, ear, nose, and throat; and a psychiatric department. In connection with this hospital there should be a home for the convalescent poor patients.

The ideal institution for these acute cases is a large university hospital, with its many clinics, with accommodations for all classes of patients—the poor and the rich—and with equipment for the treatment of all kinds of diseases. This has the great advantage of its own, or an affiliated, medical school and of a nurses' training-school; it is under one administration; it has well-organized staffs of doctors in residence and chiefs of services who work in harmony. This picture is certainly ideal, for, as a rule, the various clinics of these university hospitals are run almost as independent institutions.

The advantage of the multiple clinics is that a patient seldom belongs to but one service. Nearly all surgical patients need some medical treatment; the medical patients have serious surgical complications, besides skin, eye, ear, and throat conditions, which need the care of specialists; and the medical and psychopathic wards need to be in much closer harmony than they now are. The university hospital is usually a well-endowed private institution whose watchword is quality of work rather than quantity, which limits the number of beds according to its income, and spends more per capita on the public ward patients than do the other hospitals. Theoretically, the university hospital exists not for the sake of the patient, but for the sake of medical advance, for the sake of the medical students and of the pupil nurses. And yet, actually, it is here that the patients fare best, for where the medical students are taught best how to treat, the patients are treated best; where the nurses are taught best how to nurse, the patients will in the long run be nursed best; where the staff consists of doctors who are working on the advancing border of medicine, the patients will in the long run be given advantage of the best in medicine. Only here can truly individual treatment and individual nursing be obtained, for where there are no pupils, but all are experts, there a deadly routine will in great measure prevail. It is for this reason that the free patient in the open ward often enjoys the benefit of better medical skill than is brought to bear on the rich patient in his expensive room. The great difficulty of medicine is not in treating a patient, but in first finding out what the matter with him is, and then in quickly recognizing the complications needing prompt treatment. The stimulus of a group of keen-eyed, open-minded students, who do not know enough medicine to bias them, but who do ask the "why" of everything, helps the doctor to make his most brilliant diagnoses and to suggest his best treatments. Try as hard as he will, he cannot do as well for the private patient with an uncertain condition, who is paying the highest price for the best attention. Of course, the private patient is far more comfortable and less often disturbed than is the poor man, but that is not what he goes to the hospital for.

The city hospital for acute cases is, theoretically, a quite different institution. Since it is maintained at public expense, it will usually be run as cheaply as possible. Theoretically, it cannot limit its number, but must admit all the poor who apply. Theoretically, it should not desire full wards, but should prefer that patients go to the privately controlled institutions and thus reduce its expenses. And, because it is a municipal institution, it must expect to share the political history of the other municipal institutions of the city to which it belongs. This explains why for years there was only one municipal hospital, the Boston City Hospital, whose standards of work were as high (or even higher) as those of the privately endowed institutions.

The question of the strictly private hospitals is a most important one, because on them depends in large measure the further advance in hospital care of the acutely ill medical and surgical patients among the well-to-do. It is generally admitted that better medical and surgical care can be given in a building especially built and equipped for this purpose than in a private home, unless the owner is willing practically to rebuild his house. This is generally understood in the case of surgical patients, but it is just as true of the medical, for the most successful medical care requires the closest study of details. Some doctors have seen the advantage of having private hospitals of their own, so that they can completely govern the treatment of the patient. Others use for this purpose private hospitals which admit the patients of several doctors. These institutions are often semiphilanthropic, as the excellent Deaconesses' Homes. While some private hospitals may be carried on for the convenience of the doctor, and possibly are content merely to pay expenses, yet these private institutions, on the whole, are business enterprises and are not averse to making considerable profit. One need not expect them to make any sacrifice of gain for the sake of scientific excellence, unless they see that it will "pay" to do so. It is remarkable what good hotel accommodations and yet what miserable medical and nursing attention these hospitals provide. The patients, of course, have the care of the doctor who sends them there, but who charge for each visit, and they have private nurses whom they pay well, and whose services are not included in the bill for their room and care. They surely receive very little for the seventy dollars a week which they pay for a fine room and nominal nursing. They receive better care in the private wards of an endowed public hospital, although their quarters may not be nearly so luxurious. But there is a growing need for these private hospitals. Doctors certainly seem to find them profitable, and they must be reckoned with in greater and greater measure.

So different are the apparent reasons for the existence of all these different kinds of hospitals that it is remarkable that those who attend the meetings of our American Hospital Association can find so much in common to discuss. But these differences are more apparent than real. All medical institutions have practically one aim—the good of the patient. Our hospital walls enclose a real democracy. The food and clothes of the rich man may cost much more than do those of the poor man, and yet the latter may be just as well nourished and just as warmly clad. But it is not so with medical care. It is just as expensive to treat typhoid fever well in the case of a poor man as in the case of a millionaire. The medicines cost exactly the same for both. We should not tolerate any cheapening of an operation on a poor man. So far as good treatment goes, there can be no difference in value. All agree that we should give the pauper the very best medical and surgical aid within our power, and for the rich man we can do no more.

Children's hospitals of greater capacity and especially planned for these patients are needed in greater numbers. These little patients are so numerous that it may never be possible to subordinate their wards as one department of general hospitals. Rather we may expect large general hospitals for children, with medical, surgical, orthopedic, and other clinics, with a babies' department, and with large departments for the contagious diseases. Fine examples of such complete hospitals can be seen in Berlin, Vienna, and Paris.

While we may doubt the need of special hospitals for babies, yet most doctors think that these little patients should, at least, have special wards. To many French and German children's hospitals infants are admitted, but are not mingled with the older children; they occupy separate pavilions or at least separate wards. But not all doctors do agree on this point. One large hospital for children in London has a rule against admitting any child under two years of age, and yet its superintendent confesses that one-quarter of its patients are, always have been, and probably always will be, under that age. In some excellent English hospitals the authorities mingle these patients on the ground that, since they are mingled in their own homes, it is more natural to them. Several reasons for separating the babies from the older children are given later, in the paragraph on Hospital Architecture.

That there is a need of separate institutions for orthopedic cases is a disputed point. These patients form a large proportion of the surgical cases in all children's hospitals, but it is agreed that they should be under the care of a specialist, not of a general surgeon. Orthopedic hospitals must be prepared to keep their patients a long time, even over a year, or to have active out-patient departments, with visiting nurses who can closely follow discharged patients in their homes. Such patients need much outdoor life—so many of them are tuberculous—and the best medical care. Many of the separate orthopedic hospitals in America can scarcely apologize for their existence.

Every community, even every town, needs a hospital for contagious diseases and should enforce its use. Only in this way can these diseases be controlled, and only in such a hospital can the victims of these diseases receive the best of care. It is a great economic loss that a whole family should be quarantined, and several children kept from school, because, for example, one child has diphtheria. Nor is it sensible to allow a dozen small foci of infection rather than only one.

There is a great need in this country of convalescent homes, where patients may stay during that long and important period between their acute illness and the return of sufficient strength for them to resume work. Such a home would more likely be connected with a municipal hospital than with one privately endowed, for the convalescent patient does not appeal to the sympathy of the philanthropist nearly as much as does the acutely ill man. A good social service department or a close connection with the city charities will do much to supply this need.

Hospitals for the care of patients with chronic conditions are also sadly lacking. Such patients need hospital attention just as much as do the acutely ill. Many of them must go to almshouses and be treated in the usually inadequate wards of those institutions. I know of no almshouse in this country which corresponds to Bicêtre or Salpêtrière of Paris, in that its patients receive the attention of the foremost medical men. Too often they are at the mercy of very inefficient internes. For those who can afford them, sanatoria are the hospitals for patients with chronic heart, kidney, joint, and organic nervous conditions, but the poor have no share in these institutions. We may devoutly hope that hospitals, not "homes," will be erected for patients with chronic conditions who now crowd the out-patient clinics, and who are welcome in no place where they might get help.

There should be excellent sanatoria for cases with incipient tuberculosis. These are the teachers of the general public and of the patients. There should also be near the great cities large hospitals for advanced cases of this disease. These are the safeguards of the community.

We have in many of the states adequate asylum space. "Insane" is now a legal word, and is applicable only to the patient so abnormal mentally that there is no injustice in depriving him, in some degree at least, of his liberty. But the larger group of the "border-line" cases, patients whose condition is in its early stages or is still indefinite, whom we cannot legally commit, but who are always a potential danger to the community—these need hospital care in special institutions where they can be studied, where perhaps the progress of the condition can be stayed, and they spared the disgrace of commitment. At present general hospitals and the sanatoria for general cases refuse them absolutely, and it is unfair to allow these patients even to commit themselves to a closed institution, for the environment there is not adapted to checking an abnormal mental condition which in other environment might progress no further. Perhaps no group of patients is so neglected as this. Virtually, we encourage or even force these patients to become unmistakably insane in order that they may be cared for.

And we need more sanatoria which will conform to all the best standards of hospitals, and in which the chronic invalid, the convalescent, and the nervously fatigued can find helpful environment and the best of care. There must be also sanatoria for drug cases—small institutions where one man can use all his personal influence on the five or six or perhaps ten patients who need this far more than they need any treatment, medicinal or physical, important though these may be. Sanatoria for nervous (?) and mental cases, which are in fact small insane asylums, have their place, and it is an important one, for the care of those able to pay, but these will more and more form a group apart from other sanatoria. We now speak especially of those open for general medical and surgical work.

The sanatoria have awakened to their opportunities and responsibilities, and find that they have now a responsibility much greater than ever before, and one which only they can well meet. It is not impossible that in them the next great advances in medicine should be made. The general hospitals have studied the serious and late stages of disease, and have come to a temporary stopping point, if we may judge by the interest suddenly awakened in pathologic physiology, the aim of which is really to study the beginnings of disease. But the sanatoria hold the key to this situation, for they have the patients in the early stages of disease, as the hospitals do not, and probably will not, have them. Patients in early stages of disease often are not ill enough to go to a hospital; usually they do not feel ill at all; they have no characteristic symptoms. They are run down, tire easily, and have a vague idea that something is wrong. Sanatoria are literally filled with these patients, and hospitals envy them their opportunities. Sanatoria should not be, as the majority are, chiefly therapeutic institutions, but should be institutions especially equipped for the diagnosis and study of the early stages of disease. May they seize their present opportunity and by their research work prove their right to a very important place in the American hospital field!

Doubtless there was, and surely there is now, a need of the many special hospitals for women—maternity hospitals, etc., and of hospitals for special groups of cases, as eye, ear, skin, etc. Theoretically, it would be better if these special hospitals could be directly connected with, or serve as special departments of, a general hospital, thus freeing for the use of patients much of the endowment, which would otherwise be spent on a separate administration. Although affiliated with a larger institution, they could still preserve their individuality as distinct institutions on special endowments. And yet this is really begging the question. Most of our general hospitals are still far too weak to support such departments. To put it in another way, a far greater percentage of patients with these special conditions will seek hospital care than of patients with more general conditions. It is not yet commonly believed that a patient with pneumonia or typhoid fever can receive better care in a hospital than in his home; but the advantages of these special hospitals is readily granted by the man with, for example, an eye trouble. Our American general hospitals will have to grow into much stronger institutions before they can elbow these special hospitals off the field.

Of course, also, the rare man sometimes does, and more often should, compel the existence of a special hospital. The genius in any specialty will often need, and will usually get, a separate hospital for his particular line of cases. This is well illustrated in the case of Schlossman, of Dresden. As long as this man is active, his hospital may have great value, but the continuance of its existence after his influence ceases is somewhat doubtful.

As stated above, there are advantages in having several hospitals of the same type in one city, rather than a few large institutions representing the sum of them all. But there should be a real need for the total number of beds which all these smaller hospitals represent, each should contain a sufficient number of beds to make economic maintenance possible, each should be well enough endowed or supported to permit it to do efficient work, and, finally, all these should work together in sufficient harmony to prevent unnecessary duplication of work.

The first provision is not difficult to fulfil, for few cities, if any, have numerically too many hospital beds, although many cities have beds which, for good reasons, are usually empty.

The second provision has never received nearly enough attention. In the case of each type of hospital there is a definite optimum number of beds which it can maintain at a certain standard of excellence at a minimum cost per bed. A hospital can be a valuable institution if its capacity is but ten or if it is a thousand patients. But the smaller hospital, granted that it tries to do excellent work, is always at an economic disadvantage. It cannot support a good training-school for nurses or a resident staff of skilful physicians. The reason that very many small hospitals do serve their communities so well is that so many of those officially connected with them are willing practically to give their services. In general, however, our smaller hospitals make a mistake in trying to be miniature copies of large hospitals. It were better that they should try to be good small hospitals.

And the same is true of the other extreme. After a certain number of beds is exceeded, as sometimes, although rarely in America, occurs in municipal and church institutions, either the hospital cannot give the special care that each patient needs, or the whole institution becomes so ponderous that it is difficult and expensive to manage.

The problem we are considering is similar to that which manufacturers have faced and have worked out with some accuracy—that is, the estimation of the optimum number of operatives who, working under certain conditions in a mill, can do the best work at the least cost. Volunteer unremunerated work will hopelessly muddle any mathematical problem in hospital economics, but it is well to have as a standard some number into which this enters little. In the case of a complete general hospital built in the pavilion style, with multiple departments all designed for acute cases, able to pay a capable superintendent, able to pay fair salaries to a resident staff in addition to the interne staff (who get much more out of such an institution than their services are worth), able to make fair compensation to a visiting staff, able to support an excellent training school, what would be an approximation to the optimum number of beds which such an institution could so support that the work would be "worth while" to all concerned, and that every patient would receive that individual care which all such hospitals should guarantee their patients, yet at the smallest per capita expense? We were much interested in studying this problem in Europe, as well as in our own country, and decided that this number would be between 400 and 600. Doubtless good management would permit considerable increase in this number. A hospital for 200 or even 100 patients requires practically the same installation as does one for 400. And yet only 25, or 1 per cent., of our American general hospitals have 400 or more beds. The superintendents of some, at least of the smaller hospitals, will admit that to raise all their pavilions one story and to double their ward space would not mean nearly as great an increase in total administrative expense as it would a reduction in per capita expense. Of course, it might mean a division of services. The chiefs of the services prefer a small clinic which will not take much of their time, and yet they desire to be the only "chiefs" in their subject. But it is now the hospital's point of view, not his, which we are emphasizing. The chief usually has too much privilege and too little responsibility. Of course, a hospital is to be judged by its efficiency in giving each and every patient the best of individual care, not by its per capita daily expense; but the point we make is that for each grade of care there is a minimum expense, and the fact that we have not determined what this is, is proof of our tardy application of business methods to the management of philanthropic institutions. Our conclusion is that the great majority of general hospitals for acute cases in large cities are too small, which probably means too poor, and that the hospitals in smaller cities and in towns would better not try to appear quite so "complete."

In the cases of hospitals for chronic diseases and for insanity each institution now cares for several hundred or even several thousand patients, at a low per capita expense. But there is no claim that individual attention is given these patients, and surely it would be much better if it were. At present they receive wholesale treatment, unless they are fortunate enough to develop some interesting condition.

The third requisite has already been emphasized, but the fourth, that of mutual coöperation among similar but unrelated institutions, requires careful study. In several cities, as Baltimore, the charity organization society in some measure serves this purpose. If the social service departments fulfil their present promises, they will perform this function splendidly. We need in this country a comprehensive but loose system of coördinating the work of medical institutions. This surely might be accomplished even though the medical creeds and founders' purposes of these institutions do not at all agree, provided that those who work in these institutions see advantages in a little voluntary coöperation.

In connection with general hospitals there is one innovation which deserves special mention. We refer to the social service department. This promises to be a powerful lever to upset, and a potent lever to transform, our modern hospital system, especially as regards its relations to the out-patients. There is no doubt that our present system has led to very disappointing results. The chances are that the physical examination of most patients will reveal but few of the troubles which cause their symptoms, that the excellent treatment of their physical ills will cure but few of their complaints, and that medicine is the least important of their needs. The conditions under which a patient lives and works, his family problems, are all quite as important (even far more important in many cases) as are the physical troubles which we find and treat. The hospital doctor assumes that his duty is to the patient's body alone, and that the social aspect of the case is none of his business. But the patient does not understand it so; he assumes that the hospital which receives him is able and willing to treat that trouble of which he comes complaining. That the hospital may keep its part of this tacit agreement which it makes on receiving the patient, it must be willing and able to enter into his home and working life. Only the social service department can do this in a methodic way. Its workers aid wonderfully in diagnosis by discovering many important facts concerning the patient's home environment of which he is unconscious, and they help greatly in treatment by making it possible for the patient to profit by the advice given him, much of which could not otherwise be followed.

The social service department is the "heart" of the institution. To this department a man is not merely an interesting case of cirrhosis of the liver, or a pair of painful flat feet, but is a human being who needs the social worker's advice and encouragement, one whom she can aid by guiding him to the right doctors, whom she can so educate that he is able to make good use of the advantages which the hospital has to offer. The social-service worker can free the patient's mind of much anxiety during his illness by arranging with various charitable organizations for the maintenance of his family, and can plan for his care after he leaves the hospital in case there is no convalescent home available. In fact, in surveying the American hospital field, I see no influence that promises more for the future than the social service department.

As good proof as any which might be cited of the lack of even a loose unity of the hospital organizations in America is the miserable uniformity of their antiquated ward plans. We boast that our medicine and surgery are advancing rapidly. It surely is strange that this advance should not in some degree modify our hospital architecture, for new knowledge usually imposes new duties. Yet with the notable exception of the operating pavilions, our American hospital buildings remain unmodified in their essential features. In Europe it is quite different. There one can trace, especially in Germany and Austria, a definite progression in the plans, for each new hospital is an improvement on its predecessors. Before a building is erected a study is made of other hospitals, and all that has proved good is retained, while an attempt is made to improve on all that has failed. Every important advance in medicine should certainly be mirrored in at least one, perhaps small, detail of hospital construction.

In Germany and Austria hospital buildings are planned by architects who are experts in this line of work—who, in fact, do little else. In America, on the contrary, the plans of a new hospital are left to a board of trustees who are new at hospital work, and to the architect, who, however skilful he may be in planning other edifices, is usually a novice in hospital construction. The chances are that the great majority of our hospitals were their architects' first efforts in this kind of work. For this reason there is little evidence of evolution in our hospitals, and traditional, unsatisfactory types are repeated over and over again. American architects and engineers may justly be proud of their skill in planning and erecting fine residences and business blocks, and they are famous for their daring in attempting new and difficult problems, as, for example, the city sky-scrapers. This skill is strikingly manifested in the construction of parts of our hospitals, but not of its most important parts. The administration building is perfect; the corridors are impressive; the kitchen, the laundry, the hygienic installation, the heating plant, and the ventilation systems are the best in the world. But these are secondary parts of any hospital. The most important part, the wards, the rooms for the sake of which all of the other parts of the hospital exist, these are old-fashioned, conventional, uninteresting, and unsatisfactory. That American hospitals show no new medical ideas in their construction is not surprising. Those who planned them did not get nearly so far as the medical problems; perhaps were not even aware that such problems exist. The architect will "point with pride" to the administration building, but ask him for what group of patients a certain ward is intended, and he will look bewildered. It has never occurred to him that the wards are really the most important part of the institution, or that any one group of patients might need a ward planned differently from the wards for other groups. The result is a row of ward buildings of uniform design, all containing the same number of beds. After these wards are completed, the various services draw lots for "space." There will not be much advance in the hospital care of patients until those who have hospital construction in charge really learn what problems are involved in the treatment of the various groups of diseases, and then try to plan the ward buildings according to the requirement of the different services. What we greatly need in America, since official architects are out of the question, is a library in which plans of various hospitals are collected, where trustees and architects may learn what has been tried in hospital construction. Show American architects what the medical problems really are and the American genius will prove itself by the best of wards as well as of administration buildings.

While, of course, there are few hospitals which can provide special wards for special groups of cases, yet in almost every hospital there are possible a certain differentiation of the patients and a certain adaptation of the buildings to meet their needs. It is not fair to treat in adjacent beds patients with typhoid fever, pneumonia, nephritis, delirium tremens, heart disease, insomnia, and neurasthenia. One patient needs quiet, another fresh air, and a third frequent tub-baths. We may cite the rapid changes in the personnel of each ward as explaining our inability to adjust architecture to the needs of the patients, but we all know that our patients would receive better care if we did group them better, and that we could differentiate them a great deal more than we do if we only tried. There is a remarkable similarity in the work of each hospital from year to year. The hospital for acute medical cases has its "crops" of typhoid cases, its "crops" of malaria and of pneumonia cases; its yearly average of the number of patients with Bright's disease, cardiac disease, joint disease, etc., is fairly constant. Surely a hospital which has been in operation for several years before it decides to rebuild could, did it so desire, adapt with considerable accuracy its buildings to its work.

A much greater elasticity of internal construction of ward buildings is made possible by the use of the steel skeleton. It is now possible to erect a building with some of the inner partitions independent of the general frame of the building, and therefore movable. These, built of cement and expanded metal, can be easily knocked down and quickly rebuilt in a slightly different position at little expense. Granting that only a few even of the inner walls were temporary, this would allow an elasticity of floor plan which would be most heartily appreciated by those using the building. A room originally large could during the winter easily be divided into two or three smaller rooms, and then these partitions knocked down again when summer comes. These temporary walls can be so built that they are as satisfactory in every way from the sanitary point of view as are permanent walls.

Cleanliness not only from the domestic, but also from the sanitary point of view, is now one of the chief aims in a hospital. The tiled floors and plain tiled or cement walls are evidence of this. Some English hospitals deserve careful study. In their wards one sees no cupboards, no closets, no shelves, no ledges. There are movable chests and cabinets for linen, etc. In five minutes every piece of furniture can be moved away from the walls and these be left perfectly bare. There is not a nook or crack where a mouse or water-bug might hide. Mice and cockroaches are numerous enough in some of the finest American hospitals, but not in these English hospitals.

One of the best examples of the attempt to adapt hospital buildings to the character of the work for which they are intended is seen in the construction of pavilions for contagious diseases, which, as a rule, are quite different in style from the other buildings of the hospital group. Different hospitals have met this problem in different ways. In some hospitals are separate pavilions, one for each contagious disease, and a few separate buildings containing but one or two beds for patients ill with as yet uncertain diseases. In one of these tiny buildings the patient remains until the correctness of the diagnosis is assured, after which he is moved to a larger pavilion containing only patients with the same disease he has. The best illustration of this plan is the Wilhimena Hospital in Vienna, but there the architects have carried the idea to an extreme; for there is no advantage in scattering patients all with the same disease, as diphtheria, *e. g.*, among five separate buildings, ratther than caring for them all in one large building. In several of the Paris hospitals the pavilions for infectious diseases are really only open barracks with even incomplete outer walls allowing of free ventilation. Some of them could with ease be moved bodily across the hospital inclosure.

The other extreme is one large building with separate suites of rooms for the different diseases, each suite with a separate external entrance and no inner communicating doors. A good example of this is the children's pavilion of the Virchow clinic in Berlin.

The "box system" is a further development of the idea of special construction. The various forms of this can best be studied at Les Enfants Malades in Paris. But the conclusion of many experiments is that tight boxes are not nearly so good protections as are careful nurses; that, provided the nurse will only imagine that there is a partition between each two beds and will act as if there were, just as good results can be obtained as if this partition actually existed. That is, the carriers of infection are not the air and dust, but various ward utensils and the sleeves and aprons of the nurses.

The highest type of careful internal construction combined with highly trained nursing is seen in the new Pasteur Hospital in Paris, a hospital which admits in adjoining rooms patients with very different contagious diseases. Each room is almost a perfect ward. The authorities of this hospital have yet to see a ward infection.

In all the buildings mentioned above the greatest precautions have been taken to insure perfect asepsis. Practically no wood is used, the ventilation is as free as possible, and the floors and walls allow of perfect cleansing.

Another attempt to adapt construction and plan of the building to the problem in hand is seen in the buildings intended for children. It is due chiefly to the manner of construction, I believe, that in Germany they have only about one-tenth the number of ward epidemics that we have in America or England. In most of the German hospitals terrazzo or tiles are used for flooring, and in a whole hospital one can find scarcely a piece of wood, even in the furniture.

Those children's hospitals, planned by specialists in that subject, differ in all countries radically from those for adults in simplicity of the ward unit. Most superintendents of children's hospitals agree that each child should be under the eye of some nurse or attendant all of the time; that even the sickest child cannot be left even for a few minutes to his own devices. The children's hospitals built on a complex plan, with ward room, sun-parlor, playroom, and perhaps schoolrooms, have been obliged either to provide an attendant for each of these rooms or to keep many of these rooms locked except during stated hours. Other hospitals have tried to make the whole floor one room in so far as possible. We owe it to the English to devise a simple plan. In some of the newer English hospitals the pavilions are so built that even the balconies and toilet rooms are almost a part of the ward-room; even the kitchen overlooks the ward by large windows in the

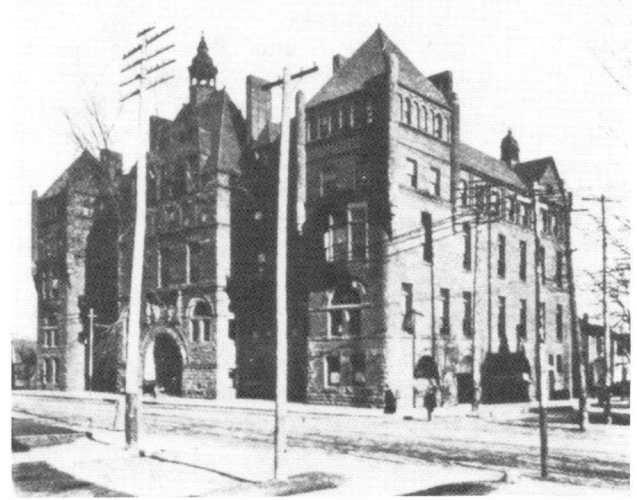

Fig. 10.—Hospital for Sick Children, Toronto.

partitions. The wall decorations, the low window-sills, the mirrors so arranged that the children whose beds face the walls may see outdoors, the few and very simple toilet rooms, the water-taps opening only by keys—all are witnesses to a special plan of construction.

The hospitals for infants are now built on a somewhat different plan from those for children. The wards are so arranged that the infants and nurses can be divided into small groups which need never come into contact with each other. Certain rooms are kept at constant high tem-

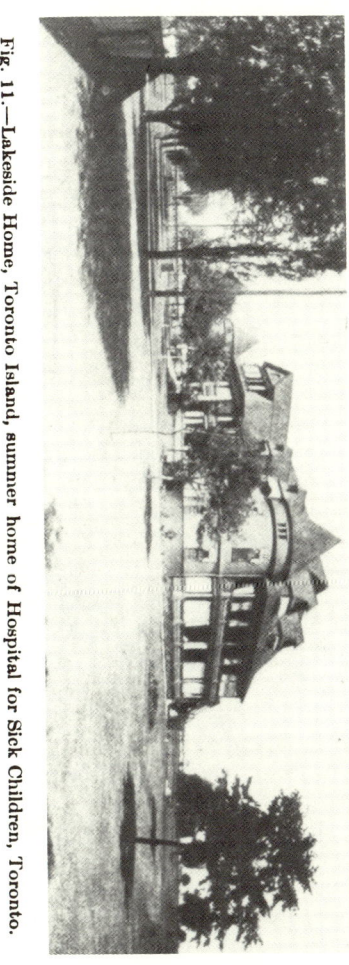

Fig. 11.—Lakeside Home, Toronto Island, summer home of Hospital for Sick Children, Toronto.

perature and at constant humidity. The diet kitchen, in which milk is modified and the other foods prepared, is very large, with fine refrigerators. There are special rooms for the cleansing of the feeding utensils. The service rooms and changing rooms are built with almost the same care as is the modern operating-room.

The buildings for acutely ill medical patients deserve very careful study. The size of the ward-rooms is a subject of considerable discussion. Some, especially the patients and their friends, as well as those doctors who like to group patients according to their condition, prefer the small wards (that is, rooms containing not over six patients), while the nurses and the hospital administration prefer larger wards, because in them it is easier for a small staff of nurses to care for the patients. While there may be differences of opinion concerning detail, yet most will agree that the pneumonia patients should be nursed in outdoor wards or in rooms opening onto a porch; that the room for typhoid cases should be especially equipped for hydrotherapy; that each neurasthenic, of whom there are many even among the poor, should be in a box with opaque walls (in Professor Déjérine's clinic in Paris and Professor Bruce's clinic in Edinburgh canvas screens are used); that the patients with dysentery need special accommodations; that the anorexia patients need a special diet kitchen service; that the insomnia patients should not be mingled with noisy patients; and that the malaria patients should be in well-screened rooms, etc. We are quite sure that there is an optimum temperature for the treatment for each group of diseases, and, this is even more important, that accurate control of the humidity of the air in the room is desirable for the best results of the treatment of some diseases. It certainly is true that patients with pneumonia, typhoid fever, pulmonary emphysema, cardiac dilatation, and acute bronchitis would all do better if separated in rooms in which different temperatures and humidities prevail.

There is no medical authority for the practice of maintaining one constant temperature in all the wards of a general hospital.

Experience has shown that in hospitals with a training school for nurses the ward unit in wards intended for the acutely ill should be about thirty. There should be at least two small rooms for those very ill. Again, in a building for acute cases the ward kitchen and the ward service room should be at the center of the pavilion, for it is from these two points that the most of the trips of the nurses to the patients radiate. In such a pavilion there is practically no need of a special dining-room, for a large lavatory for the patients, or a sun-parlor. There should, however, be a large porch onto which practically all the beds may be wheeled.

The ward for chronic medical cases and for convalescents may suitably contain at least sixty beds. At the center of this pavilion should be a lounging room. Since the majority of these patients will probably go to a ward dining-room for their meals, a rather small diet kitchen can easily serve all the bedridden patients. The service room in this pavilion may be smaller than those of the buildings for acute cases, but the lavatory should be much larger.

The pavilion for women might differ from those for men, as women appreciate a privacy which men do not need or especially desire. The box system offers certain advantages for the women's wards.

Finally, there are certain rooms in the ward pavilion which are usually put in dark corners available for nothing else, which deserve even more of the attention of the architect than do the corridors, the reception room, and the offices. Of these, the service rooms, the rooms in which the bed-pans and urinals are emptied, sterilized, and kept, and where the soiled linen is disposed of, are by far the most important. It is in these rooms that many epidemics among patients are spread, and here that nurses contract typhoid fever, etc. These rooms should be models of sanitary construction. Other rooms deserving most careful attention are, the ward kitchen, the refrigerators, and the store-rooms; even the closets for brooms are important medically.

There is a tendency to relegate clinical chemistry and microscopy to some laboratory in a basement or in some distant corner of the hospital inclosure. The result is that, even though the doctor or student is willing to do this work, not nearly enough clinical chemistry and microscopy is done, and not nearly as much is done as would be were each doctor able to work in his own ward during his spare minutes. All that is needed is a table, a sink, and a gas-fixture in one of the small rooms on the same floor with the patients.

The attention of architects has already been called to the surgical wards, and they are now building recovery rooms near the operating-room. These should be so arranged that the nurses may be able to keep sharp watch over all these patients until they are "out" of the ether. Later the patient with a clean wound may be nursed in almost any sunny, well-ventilated, quiet room, for he does not need nearly as careful hygienic attention as, for instance, does the patient convalescing from typhoid fever. But the surgical patient with a discharging abscess needs a pavilion very similar to that for the acute medical cases, but with, in addition, a dressing-room, and this dressing-room should be as carefully built to permit of perfect cleanliness as is the operating-room itself. We do look forward to the day when that great waste of money now spent for marble, glass, and tiles in the fine operating-rooms, those expensive creations of architects and hospital trustees which are not appreciated by the surgeons, will cease and this money will be used for the ward kitchens and service rooms. These are the proper rooms for expensive tiles and marbles, even though they are never shown to visitors.

The newer hospitals still follow the pavilion plan; that is, they are groups of small buildings connected, as a rule, by corridors. The most cogent of the reasons which originally led to this method of construction was to make difficult the spread of hospital epidemics, which formerly were so terrible, but which we no longer fear. Of course, the multiple pavilion plan has strong arguments in its favor. It is almost necessary in the university hospital, each "service" of which has an almost complete separate "clinic"; small buildings are easily ventilated by a "natural" system; the bed patient can easily be wheeled upon the roof of the corridors connecting the pavilions; and the rooms are not shaded by the balconies of the floor above. But in recent years engineers have learned how to ventilate a high building satisfactorily and safely, and efficient elevators are easily installed. The danger of lessening the amount of sunlight in each room by overhanging balconies is a real objection, but can be met in buildings of few floors by terracing the floors. On the other hand, the multiple pavilion hospital is a very expensive one to heat and a difficult one to keep clean. Medically, there is little to say in its favor.

Roof-gardens, sun-parlors, etc., are evidently quite important in the care of chronic cases, but the tendency now is to omit them in buildings for acute cases, and to make each floor of such a building a unit complete in itself, with ample porch room.

The fresh-air treatment of disease is proving more and more an advantage to the patient. Physicians insist that patients with certain diseases be treated out-of-doors— not only cases of tuberculosis, but cases of pneumonia, whooping-cough, anemia, insomnia, and those convalescing from almost any acute medical or surgical trouble. Hospitals with open-air wards and sleeping porches are now in construction and there is little doubt but that in the future many more will be.

And now we reach that subject which is becoming one of the most important among our hospital problems: the training-school for nurses. It is the duty of the writer to consider them only in so far as they are related to and affect the whole hospital field; but their relation to this field is not a minor but a most important one—in fact, the development of this field depends quite as much on the nurses as it does on the doctors.

For the sake of comparison we would mention some of the highest types of the nursing systems of other countries. There are, doubtless, poorer systems in each country than those we mention, but these we need not consider. We do not intend to catalogue all systems, but to mention certain prominent types. First, there are the Sisters of all Roman Catholic countries and of Roman Catholic institutions in Protestant lands, who work with, but not quite under the authority of, the medical men; second, the nurses of the public hospitals of Paris who (except in the Boucicault, a Roman Catholic institution) are government employees and accept the position for indefinite service; third, the nurses of northern Germany, many of whom receive their training in the hospital where they expect to remain; fourth, the nurses of German Switzerland (*e. g.*, Basel), who are trained in special small hospitals designed for the training of nurses, and who enter the service of the city hospitals as graduates; and, lastly, our American and English hospitals, where the nursing is done by pupil nurses who take a three years' course with the view to receiving a degree which will entitle them to practise private nursing. Doubtless each system has its advantages, but one should remember that they are very different systems, and that we should not expect the results of all to be the same.

At this point allow me, please, to call your attention to the great difference there is between institutional nursing and private nursing. America, but not American hospitals, should be proud of her private nurses, and the hospitals of northern Germany of their institutional nurses, but American hospitals can be proud of neither, for they have neither. They must bear patiently with the faults of pupils who leave their service when just beginning to be useful to them.

In America, nurses' training-schools and medical schools vary much more than they do in Europe. Some are excellent, others are very poor. Doubtless the majority of training-schools had an origin similar to that of the medical schools (which formerly were paying investments for the teachers); that is, the hospital kept a nursing school in order to get cheap nursing. But the demands on the trained nurse are now believed to be so exacting that her education, like that of the medical student, is more expensive to the institution training her than are her services worth to this institution; and the belief is gaining ground that only those hospitals have now a moral right to maintain a school which are willing that the school should be an expense to them rather than an economy. We are led to believe that in time the fate of the majority of our smaller training-schools will resemble that of the smaller proprietary medical schools, and that endowed schools will control the training field.

But we must not, for one minute, believe that, even though these larger and richer schools were to dictate who should dress in white and write "R. N." after their names, all the smaller hospitals would give up their "schools" and employ these graduates. How could they? Not 1 per cent. of our hospitals can afford to do this, and the less able a hospital is to conduct a school which will conform to the standards of the few, the more will it need to get inexpensive nurses, and untrained young women working for a diploma are the cheapest labor the hospital (or any other institution) can get. No; either such schools will continue or such hospitals will cease to preach that it is their duty to sacrifice themselves in order to serve the community by training its nurses for it, and will employ permanent institutional nurses, as do the hospitals of Paris and Germany; women who "wouldn't do" as private nurses, but who can keep in order and nurse the patients in a large public hospital far better than do the timid young ladies of gentle breeding, who, as soon as they get over being scared, shocked, and "torn by pity" and really begin to know how to help their patients, move on to another department of nursing. Upon these smaller hospitals, so much in the majority in all, and all there are in some, states, depends the development of the hospital field. There are not yet nearly enough hospitals to cover this field, and for a long time to come those which now exist and the many soon to be established must struggle on, their existence made possible in great measure by the self-sacrificing service of all those officially connected with them.

But granting the need of a university education for a nurse, where may she expect to receive the best training, and what effect will her training have on the other work of the hospital which trains her? The most of the pupil nurses enter a training-school in order that they may become private nurses. A very few schools can serve as "normal schools," training the teachers and superintendents for other hospitals; these can encourage their students to enter public service as school nurses, orthopedic, tuberculosis nurses, etc., and can boast with reason that those of their graduates who at once take up private work are the exception. But the great majority of pupils have no such aims in view. They want to earn their living as private nurses. Where will these get the best training for this work? Certainly not in the public wards of a general hospital. And yet it is here that the hospital, for economy's sake, needs them the most and uses them the most. But there is a great difference between keeping a room with twenty-five negroes quiet and orderly, and keeping one private patient comfortable; between serving ten trays in a public ward and clearing up all traces of the meal before one o'clock, and serving one tray in so attractive a manner that the patient is tempted to eat all there is on it. To account accurately for every dish, knife, and fork in a large ward and to have all ward requisition blanks filled and handed in before five o'clock is quite different a thing from making one sick-room pleasant. Our general hospitals, of course, have private wards, but here so many graduate nurses are on duty that the pupil nurses get relatively little training in private nursing. We believe that the best training in private nursing is obtained in the schools connected with large private hospitals or sanatoria, which have an active surgical department, and which are affiliated with the schools of general hospitals. In the former institutions they are trained in general nursing, and in the public wards of the affiliated institutions they learn that which cannot be taught in the home school. Women thus trained know at graduation much more of private nursing than do the graduates of those schools whose pupils work for the most part in the public wards.

It certainly is true, although this is not generally understood, that all the work of a hospital with a large training-school is in many ways conditioned by the school, and that such a hospital cannot do all things as well as it can train nurses. This influence has even determined the size of the hospital pavilions. Undoubtedly, this was originally an unconscious influence, but it has nevertheless stereotyped the form of pavilion now most popular. In planning hospital wards one of the first units to decide upon is the nursing unit; that is, the product of the number of patients one untrained pupil nurse can care for and the number of pupil nurses whose work one head nurse can supervise. In our American hospitals practically all the ward nursing is done by inexperienced pupils. The supervisors, or head nurses, do not themselves take care of the patients, although they are directly responsible for the nursing of each. Experience has shown that in the case of the acutely ill patients one head nurse can supervise the care of about thirty patients, and in the case of the "chronics," the care of about sixty. If the ward contains a smaller number of patients, the head nurse finds too little to keep her busy; if more, then there is sometimes need of two head nurses in one ward, and this is by no means an ideal condition. Experience has shown the desirability of having each floor constituting a single unit, and, as a matter of fact, in many American hospitals each floor of each pavilion has space for just about thirty-five patients. Hospitals whose nurses are all institutional nurses with long service in those particular hospitals can handle the patients in much larger units—even double that of our American hospitals. And one working in some European hospitals cannot fail to see the advantages of this larger unit.

In another way the presence of the training-school conditions the work of the hospital, for training-school hospitals are apt to be failures as research hospitals. One would be unwise to attempt in our hospitals the elaborate problems in metabolism, for instance, which are so successfully conducted with the aid of graduate nurses in Germany, and in many hospitals of Paris and Switzerland, where the nurses are experienced and can be depended on in matters of detail. It is quite unreasonable not to expect that of the three, four, or more inexperienced nurses, who have during the day and night something to do for the patient whom they are studying, all new in the ward, and all fearful of committing some worse blunder than mixing the diets or confusing the specimens for the chemical laboratory, some one will not in the course of a week make that little mistake which will ruin a whole week of laboratory work. For this reason much of the too little metabolism work in America is done with private ward patients who can afford special nurses. We need more hospitals where research work can be done. In fact, this is the great need of our universities, and the training-school to them is no blessing. In the development of our hospitals of highest grade it would, therefore, not be wise for all to attempt to train nurses. Indeed, there is always danger that the training-school may exert an influence unduly strong over the scientific work of the institution. Since so much of the work must be done by pupil nurses who "are there to learn how to nurse," the head of the training-school has a dangerous power of vetoing projected plans. Her decision that her department is not equipped for certain work will usually at once preclude it. The case, for instance, of a new treatment proposed for trial sometimes resolves itself into the question of what the nurse in charge thinks of that particular treatment. If it appeals to her, she will take the trouble to see that her staff is equal to that new duty; but if it does not appeal to her, then there are always reasons enough why it should not be tried. I cite these influences of the training-school not at all in a carping spirit, for I believe that our training-schools are one of the finest features of our hospital field, and surely the graduates of these schools as superintendents make possible the many new hospitals our country needs; but that hospital which proposes to give nurses specialized training should specialize in the training of nurses, just as is now done in Switzerland. We need also hospitals which have other objects in view.

Finally, may I be pardoned if I venture a few remarks on that subject most difficult of all to discuss, the hospital superintendent and his relation to the hospital field?

The personnel of our American Hospital Association is an interesting study. At its meetings one comes into contact with doctors, business-men, clergymen, and women, many of whom were formerly superintendents of nurses' schools—persons very differently trained, yet occupying nominally the same position in their respective hospitals. Can their actual duties, we ask ourselves, be the same? Doubtless in a large measure they are, for in every hospital there is much which only the superintendent, whatever his "previous condition of servitude," can do. But the duties of the administrative head of a hospital are so complex that in their discharge one can use almost any preliminary training to good advantage. Do we at our association meetings get the benefit of this difference in the training of our members?

I am confident that in no country is the position of superintendent as difficult as it is in America, since here so much is expected of him. The trouble is that we have so few really efficient hospitals. The majority are like a five-horse-power engine trying to do the work of a twenty-horse-power machine, and the extra strain comes on the superintendent, to whom, in large measure, is due the credit if his hospital "makes good."

In the university hospitals of Germany, in the hospitals of German Switzerland and of Paris, there is but one head of each clinic or division of the clinic, and in all that concerns the professional care of the patients this man rules supreme. The superintendent of these hospitals is usually a business-man. If he is a medical man, we hear little about it. But these chiefs, and, in their absence, the next in rank in the university, make almost daily visits to their clinics and sometimes visit them twice a day. The students accompany the professor on his ward visit on certain days only, and then only for the first half of the visits. These professors have their full clinic well in hand. In some hospitals even no patient can leave before the professor in person has discharged him. But in America our chiefs of clinics visit their public wards about three times a week, and then consume most of the time demonstrating to the students a few interesting cases. The care of the patients who are not interesting for teaching purposes usually falls to the resident men, who are, for the most part, men of limited experience. In some hospitals the superintendent, if he is a doctor, theoretically, has the responsibility of the medical care of all his patients, but practically that is impossible. In hospitals with no rotation of services and with a staff system demanding more than three years of resident service, the superintendent may rely on his senior residents, who in turn supervise the internes, but such hospitals are very rare. But in hospitals with rotation of services, and, as is usually the case in these hospitals, with interne residency of two years or less, the superintendent has the assistance of even partially trained men, and, the less trained these internes are, the more they resent any medical suggestions from the superintendent, appealing to an absent chief in cases of necessary interference. Some of the superintendents of our medical hospitals feel the limitations of their position very keenly, and do what little they can under an almost heart-breaking strain. They doubtlessly often regret their medical training and envy the nurse superintendent, who perhaps feels the same limitations in a less degree, and the clergyman and the business-men, who must feel them still less. Certainly the chiefs of services in our large city hospitals could do much to improve hospital treatment if they only would consider their position more as one of duty and less one of opportunity. Another plan is, we are told, now being tried in Germany. In some hospitals the superintendent, a medical man, has charge of a certain department of the hospital, in which he is also chief of service. This superintendent can thus keep his medical or surgical interest alive, and can, if he will, exert a very potent, if indirect, influence on all staffs by running one ward at least in a model way. We cannot help feeling that in America the future of the hospitals rests more with the superintendents than it does in any other country. They are the teachers of their boards of trustees, and the ones on whom the brunt of the staff burden falls.

But cannot something original be expected from our superintendents? Must all that is individual in each, all that his previous training affords, be crushed out by a deadly weight of hospital routine? Will the subjects discussed at the meetings of the Hospital Association continue to represent the greatest common divisor of the thoughts and opinions of the doctor, the nurse, the clergyman, and the business-man? The duties of the superintendent can doubtless be ably performed by suitable representatives of all of these professions, and each be busy enough, but may we not look forward to contributions which are products of the special training and interests of the representatives of these so widely different professions, and which would be valuable to all superintendents? Surely the nurse superintendents of England have evolved splendid hospital furniture, of which we, who still buy from manufacturers' catalogues, are quite ignorant. There is much in a clergyman's experience and point of view to fit him peculiarly for the position of hospital superintendent. The business-man who is a superintendent should be able to show those of his brother superintendents who have not had his training how to improve the business methods of their hospitals. And the medical man—why does he not write papers on the duties of a medical director which will help those superintendents who have not a medical education? As it now is, these various heads of hospitals discuss vacuum cleaners, windows, elevators, etc., all of which their housekeepers understand better than they. That the responsibilities of American hospital superintendents are especially heavy would indicate that their opportunities are correspondingly great; and surely on them depends in great measure the development of the great American hospital field. May our American superintendents improve their opportunities, so much wider than those of similar coworkers in other countries. May they coöperate in their work, each for the sake of his fellows, developing in himself and in his hospital that for which his talents and his training especially fit him.

If the growth in the number of new medical institutions during the next decade proves as rapid as that of the past ten years, we shall see several hundred new hospitals opened. Of what sort will they be? The present decade is for most states the period of new institutions and will probably be followed by the evolution from these of efficient institutions; for ours is medically a very new country, and there are not nearly enough trained superintendents and trained supervisors of nurses to undertake the direction of all the hospitals which we now have, much less of those already projected. But more hospitals there must be to fill the needs of the communities, and so for years there must be much self-sacrifice, much underpaid work lovingly done, for our patients. Let us strive that the seed sowed be good seed. Let the standards of even the small hospital with slender financial resources be high, and a good hospital will surely be the result. It is not more money that our institutions need above all else, much as they need this, but higher ideals. In this "business age" we must not lose sight of the fact that our hospitals are gaining less morally than they are financially. That institution which studies how it may, with the means at its disposal, give the best (not "good enough") care it can to each patient, that hospital the "human side" of which feels anxious for its patients, as well as for its doctors and nurses, is the hospital which will grow to the position of greatest influence among its fellows.

There is another duty which faces our hospitals. Not only should they do their best for all their patients, but they should also be willing to aid other hospitals in their work. There is probably not one superintendent with a cortex of any depth who does not devise some little improvement in the detail of his institution, who does not think of some way of meeting some one problem better than it has ever been met before. Is it not his duty both to use this idea, trifling though it may seem, in his own hospital, and to help others to use it also? That which would help our hospitals greatly is a closer friendship among their executive heads and a much freer exchange of ideas. May the spirit of jealous rivalry among institutions designed to serve suffering humanity cease, and may the body of medical institutions consisting of varied yet interrelated members grow strong in the spirit of mutual helpfulness.

CHAPTER II

THE BOARD OF MANAGERS AND THEIR RESPONSIBILITIES

By E. S. Gilmore

BOARD of Managers, Board of Trustees, Board of Directors, and Board of Regents, are terms practically synonymous, used to denominate that body which comes into immediate governing relation with any corporation. For the purposes of this chapter the term, " Board of Managers" will be used to represent such governing body.

Boards of managers of hospitals are either appointed or elected. If the hospital is a state hospital, the board is usually appointed by the state executive. Sometimes, however, state institution boards are elected either by the legislative body or the people direct. If a private hospital, the board is usually elected by the hospital association membership. The hospital association is composed of people in sympathy with the hospital, who are enrolled as members, and who meet annually for the election of the board of managers and for the perpetuation of itself. The association is the final authority with full power to inaugurate policies and control and instruct its creature, the board of managers.

The hospital association and the public hold the board of managers responsible for the proper conduct of the hospital. This responsibility the board cannot evade. Public opinion, and the courts as well, have decided otherwise. The board of managers, generally, is too unwieldy a body to permit of frequent meetings and active work, so it in turn elects its officers and appoints its committees and works through them.

BOARD OF MANAGERS AND THEIR RESPONSIBILITIES 73

The officers of the board of managers are the president, vice-president, secretary, treasurer, and auditor. The president of the board is the head of the hospital; upon him devolves the appointment of the committees, and in a large measure the direction of their work. To him the public carries its grievances, and from him expects redress. The superintendent of the hospital reports to him more frequently than to the board, and desires his counsel and assistance. He presides at all meetings, signs all legal documents and directs the policy of the hospital. The

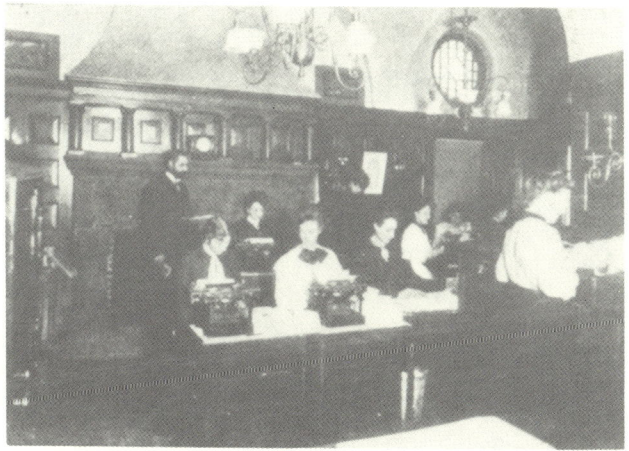

Fig. 12.—Main office, Hospital for Sick Children, Toronto.

success of the hospital depends in the greatest measure upon the president.

The vice-president is charged with the duties of the president during the absence of the latter

The secretary is the record keeper of the board of managers. He attends to its correspondence and compiles the minutes of its meetings. Legal documents usually require the signature of the secretary, together with that of the president.

The treasurer is the custodian of the hospital funds.

It is a convenient custom to have a banker for the treasurer, that all funds may be deposited with him, and that checks drawn for the hospital may pass under his inspection. Some boards of managers require the treasurer's signature to all checks issued by the secretary or superintendent. Most hospitals prefer to have checks drawn upon the treasurer by the superintendent and approved by the secretary, auditor, or accountant.

The auditor has for his duties the inspection of hospital accounts and preparation of financial reports for the board of managers.

The numerous needs of a hospital call into creation committees differing in name and duties. These committees generally consist of the executive, advisory, finance, publicity, medical, and training-school committees. When conditions require it, there are such committees as endowment, nominating, visiting, buildings and grounds, etc. Usually, however, these are appointed by the president as temporary committees, to be discharged upon completion of the work for which they were definitely appointed.

The committee charged with the most important duties is the executive committee. This committee is composed of the most active and influential managers. It should meet regularly and consider all phases of the hospital work. It should direct the superintendent and through him control each department of the hospital. It should report to the board of managers at stated periods, and ascertain the wishes of the board. For most practical purposes the executive committee is the board of managers.

The finance committee is especially charged with the raising of funds for endowment of the institution, and to meet the expenses incurred in the care of free patients. Any matter pertaining to the finances of the institution comes within its province. The publicity committee has for its special duty the advertising of the hospital.

The medical committee provides a medical staff and is especially interested in the medical side of the hospital management. It sits to consider suggestions from the medical staff. In an active hospital, membership on the medical committee is not viewed in the light of a sinecure.

The training-school committee deals with the problems of the training-school for nurses, now so prominent a part of every hospital. The curriculum of the training-school, the selection of the superintendent of nurses, and matters of discipline may properly come within the province of this committee, where need for appeal from the superintendent of the hospital is evident.

The work of all these committees should, so far as possible, pertain to such things only as require the attention of the trustees. All details of hospital management should rest with the superintendent. The best conducted hospital is that in which the superintendent is held directly responsible for its management, and his authority is not questioned except in the gravest of occasions. If a hospital have a superintendent not capable of such responsibility, the wisest thing is to dismiss him, and get one who is. Carrying things over the superintendent's head to the president or executive committee, either by the medical staff or any one else connected with the hospital, is destructive to the morale of the institution. Trustees miss a proper conception of the dignity and importance of their office who deem it their duty to superintend the hospital. The superintendent must, of course, expect criticism; being human, much of it he will merit; but the board of managers is wisest that sends the critics back to the superintendent for settlement of difficulties, except when it is clearly evident that right or policy dictates otherwise.

In the hope that this chapter may come to the notice of one who is contemplating starting a hospital, it may be useful to speak of some things which retard a hospital's growth.

Absence of printed rules and by-laws contribute largely to confusion. It is very desirable that all the by-laws and such rules as are fundamental for the government of the hospital officers and employees should be printed and that all interested in the hospital, including the trustees, become conversant therewith. Ignorance cannot be pleaded as an excuse for wrong-doing. The rules and bylaws should be revised and reprinted as often as there are sufficient changes to warrant such action. The insertion of a few blank pages for the addition of rules as occasion requires will help in keeping this part of the work up to a proper standard.

One of the dangers which beset a hospital board of managers is the turning of all board affairs over to one man. This means that the hospital has the experience, wisdom, judgment, and assistance of only one man, when it is entitled to that of all the board members. Any manager large enough to perform all the work of the entire board is also large enough to desire the help of his fellow-members. If he does not desire it, he should be compelled to accept it.

Another danger is the retention on the board of "dead timber." Any one unwilling to accept or unable to perform his share of the responsibilities of hospital management should not be allowed to take the place of one who is willing and able to do so. The member who seldom or never attends a meeting is a good member to be dropped.

The first duty of any manager is to acquaint himself with the needs and conditions of the hospital. In addition to a careful study of the local conditions, he can receive material aid by visiting other hospitals, reading hospital journals, and attending hospital conventions, notably those of the American Hospital Association. This will broaden and equip him for a better performance of his duties.

Another duty of the board of managers is to see that a proper system of accounting and reporting is installed. This will not only prevent the disaster attendant upon the shortcomings of a dishonest or careless or inefficient superintendent, but will be an incentive to careful and methodic men of wealth to contribute to an institution which shows a systematic effort to provide and to account for all disbursements.

BOARD OF MANAGERS AND THEIR RESPONSIBILITIES 77

A question sometimes arises as to the desirability of the superintendent attending board meetings. To the writer its seems that none but a short-sighted and small-minded board would fail to take advantage of the gain to be had by the superintendent's presence. There will come times when the personality of the superintendent or some contemplated action regarding him is under discussion. At such times he will voluntarily retire or should be asked to do so if necessary. But ordinarily the board can profit by the superintendent's more accurate knowledge of the hospital details, and the superintendent can profit by a more accurate knowledge of the board's desires. Both results work in harmony for the hospital's advancement. Besides that, it can be stated as a general proposition that a superintendent unworthy of his board's confidence and support is unworthy to retain his position.

The hospital receives its charter, its right to exist, from the state. It follows necessarily that the hospital must owe allegiance to the state. It is bound by the same laws that govern other corporations and owes cheerful obedience to such laws. Inasmuch, however, as a hospital is expected to receive and care for citizens and wards of the state who reach its doors in need of immediate medical and surgical care, whether such citizens or wards are able to recompense the hospital for the expense incurred or not, the hospital naturally expects, and is entitled to, some consideration from the state not given to the ordinary corporation. Such consideration usually takes the form of freedom from taxation.

Sociologists compute in dollars the value of a man to the state. The hospital, then, that is saving lives, returning to their families as bread-winners those who, with their families, otherwise would be a care upon the community, is rendering the state a valuable service and may justly claim some recompense at its hands.

Hospitals also give great value to the community through the advance in medical and surgical science, possible only through the care of the sick under hospital conditions. It also is teaching its internes how to meet the emergencies they will be called upon to command when they enter their work of relieving sickness and preventing death. A similar service it is rendering to a larger class, its nurses, who will go into the homes of the state and give their tender ministry of comfort and compassion and helpfulness, healing, soothing, sweetening, giving the child to its mother and the mother to her child, restoring failing strength to him who is the support of the home, creating a debt which neither the state nor the home can ever repay.

CHAPTER III

THE SUPERINTENDENT

By George P. Ludlam

The modern hospital should be recognized as a composite institution or organization, with a definite aim, but with sufficient elasticity to admit of ready adaptation to changing conditions, and an equally ready response to ever-increasing demands. Its definite aim is the care of the patients. This is distinctly its "raison d'être." Whatever else it may do along the line of legitimate work, it should never lose sight of this first duty, nor allow other demands to interfere with or overshadow it. Indeed, except in so far as these other demands relate directly or indirectly to the better or more intelligent care of the patients, it is questionable whether they should be allowed to have any place in the hospital scheme. Yet medical and surgical science has developed so rapidly, this development has resulted so largely from experimentation and research, and the hospital has presented so large and productive a field for such investigation, that it has become exceedingly difficult to draw definite lines which will mark the hospital's limitations. Thus, in addition to its being a place for healing, it has become an educational center. This feature is becoming more and more prominent with the advancing years, and in so far as it has to do with the more intelligent, hence more successful, care of the sick, it finds a legitimate place in the hospital plan. The plan of organization, then, should be sufficiently elastic to permit the absorption or adoption of these educational features as they develop.

The government of a hospital should be located definitely and finally in a board of trustees or managers. This board must be supreme in all matters of management and control. It may have in its membership representatives of the different interests which go to make up its working force, but it should not share its responsibility or authority with any of these interests. Its government should be by legislation, and all delegation of authority which results in its concentration in one man or one woman should be avoided.

The ground covered in hospital management is so large in extent and so diversified in interest, that the work will be divided, and its several parts referred to appropriate committees, which will operate within clearly defined limitations, and report their findings to the board for final approval.

The committee with which this chapter has to do is the executive committee. It should be large enough to permit frequent changes in its personnel without disturbing its autonomy. It should have general charge and management of the hospital, including the buildings and grounds, and of all departments, officers, employees, and inmates, subject always to the rules and regulations of the board of trustees. It should make rules for its own government and that of the hospital. It should meet frequently and statedly, should direct the superintendent as to his duties, and as to matters referred to him, should audit bills for payment, should attend in a general way to the discipline of the house and to needed repairs and alterations, should appoint the house staff, manage the training-school for nurses, and should keep a book of minutes, wherein should be entered in detail the action on all matters which have come up for consideration. Said minutes should be presented to the Board of Trustees at its regular meetings, and, when approved, become finally operative.

The executive committee should refer so much of its duty and responsibility as it may deem wise to the superintendent, who thus becomes the chief executive officer of the hospital, exercising the functions of his official superiors, whom he represents, and to whom alone he is responsible.

He should meet with the executive committee, and report in detail regularly on all matters which have been the subject of his official consideration or action, and should refer to the committee all such matters as were deemed of too large moment for settlement by his authority.

He should have control, subject always to the higher authority of the executive committee, of all departments of the hospital, including the out-patient department, should hire and dismiss all employes, should purchase supplies, admit and discharge patients, arrange the rates for those who are unable to pay the full rates, decide upon the applications for free admission, be responsible for the good order and discipline of the house, and by constant inspection and supervision keep himself well informed of, and in close touch with, the condition of the house, the conduct and behavior of officers and employees, and should qualify himself to act judiciously and intelligently on all matters which come before him for decision.

While his immediate official superiors are the members of the executive committee, yet his duties are so comprehensive as to bring him into direct contact with all branches and details of hospital work. Hence it would be well for him to attend regularly the meetings of the board of trustees, and be ready to give information on matters which come up for consideration. Many matters come up for discussion or settlement in the board of which the superintendent should have full and intimate knowledge, as the duty of executing them will ultimately fall to him, and of which he cannot have as intelligent knowledge as he would have if he were acquainted with the history of each item from its inception. This is a point which is too frequently overlooked, and, as a consequence, the superintendent is often to that extent handicapped in his work.

His relations to the medical board are necessarily

close and intimate. While it should have no direct share in the executive control of the hospital, yet the department which is the sphere of its work is the one main department to which all are subordinate or contributory, namely, the care of the patients. This is without question the most serious and important part of the hospital work, and the responsibility for it falls wholly and directly upon the medical board. Hence, in a large measure, the superintendent is the executive officer of that board also, not in any sense as independent of the executive committee, but rather in conjunction with that committee. Hence it is his duty to see that the requirements of the physicians and surgeons are promptly supplied, that all suggestions from them receive prompt attention, that, in so far as possible, their needs are anticipated, and he should be in constant communication and consultation with them to insure the smooth working of that part of the hospital for which they are directly responsible. In all matters which are purely professional they should be supreme, acting always under the rules and regulations established by the board of trustees or executive committee. All matters coming under their observation as touching their work, calling for the exercise of the executive authority should be referred by them to the superintendent.

The training-school for nurses should be distinctly one of the departments into which the hospital is divided, and the superintendent's authority should extend over it in the same way as over other departments. Neither here, nor in any department, should he interfere in any arbitrary or dictatorial manner, but should exercise his authority in the department through its duly appointed head, with frank recognition of the authority exercised by such head, with a full appreciation of the importance in the maintenance of discipline in the hospital, and of loyally upholding and sustaining the heads of departments. The tendency to divorce the training-school for nurses from the regular hospital plan, and to erect it into a separate body, in a measure independent of the general executive authority, is a mistake to be avoided. It should take its place side by side with the other departments, and should be governed and controlled by the same authority as controls in all other departments.

While the hiring, discharging, and disciplining of employees is distinctly the superintendent's prerogative, he may delegate so much of it to heads of departments in so far as concerns the employees of the several departments as he may deem wise, especially including those filling minor positions. At the same time he will do this conditionally, so that at no time can his right to interfere immediately and directly be questioned.

The superintendent will recognize as a most serious and important part of his duty his attitude toward the public. Upon his careful and discreet conduct in this direction will depend very largely the success of his administration. To a degree which it would be difficult to exaggerate the hospital is dependent for its success upon the good will and favorable regard of the public, and the superintendent is, in large measure, its representative in this direction. A courteous demeanor, a tactful handling of difficult situations (and their name is legion), an ability to refuse impossible and improper requests without giving offense, an enforcement of hospital rules in a manner that will convince the individual that he is not being personally discriminated against, a maintenance of an even temper, even under most trying conditions, a cheerful and cordial response to requests wherever this is possible, a refraining from disabusing the mind of the individual who fancies that he has brought about by his own influence a situation which would have been established in any event by the operation of the regular routine, in short, an ever present appreciation of the fact that the public is an important factor, a sort of unofficial partner in the hospital scheme—these features must conspicuously characterize the superintendent's attitude and conduct in this direction. He should remember that even when he is acting clearly within his authority, when all the facts as such are distinctly in his favor, indeed, when his official position cannot be assailed at any point, it is still possible and quite easy to maintain this position, and assert this authority in a manner, so far as the public is concerned, to offend the sensibilities, and alienate the friendly regard of those whose good will is important, and to this extent to deprive the hospital of one of its most valuable assets. The hospital authorities want results. They do not want explanations of failure to reach results. The superintendent who is the subject of frequent complaints, and who must be continually explaining his attitude and justifying himself, will soon reach the end of his usefulness.

It would be impossible to formulate a code of rules which would be of universal application. Conditions vary so widely that what would be possible and necessary in one hospital would be wholly inapplicable in another. Starting with certain fundamental rules or definitions of the duty and authority of different officials, each hospital must work out the details to suit the exigencies of its own conditions. The following may serve as such startingpoint. The assistant officials are not mentioned, since they always perform such duties as are assigned to them by the principal, or represent that principal and act for him in his absence.

The Superintendent.—He shall be the chief executive officer of the hospital, and shall have charge of the hospital and all the premises.

He shall have authority over all the departments, and shall be responsible for the good order and discipline of the house.

He shall hire and dismiss all employees, relegating so much of this authority to the heads of departments as he shall see fit.

His decision as to the admission and discharge of patients shall be final.

He shall keep books of account covering receipts and expenditures, purchase all supplies, approve all requisitions for the distribution of supplies, examine and approve all bills, and send them statedly to the treasurer for payment.

He shall also keep books of record wherein shall be entered the names of all patients, their age, residence, occupation, date and terms of admission, date of discharge, elopement, or death, with diagnosis of disease or injury, and result of treatment.

He shall make frequent inspection of the hospital and premises in all departments, and shall be responsible for the conditions prevailing therein.

He shall collect all dues from patients, shall take charge of all valuable property brought by them to the hospital, returning the same to them on discharge, shall receive money paid to the hospital, other than that paid directly to the treasurer, and shall remit all such receipts promptly to the treasurer.

He shall conduct all official correspondence, and issue all official certificates, except death certificates or insurance claims, where the signature of the attending physician is required.

No autopsies shall be made except on his express authorization in writing.

He may suspend from duty any house officer or member of the house staff who may violate any of the rules of the house, or otherwise misbehave, and shall report the case in writing to the executive committee at its next meeting for final disposal.

Superintendent of the Training-school for Nurses. —The training-school for nurses shall be a department of hospital work conducted and controlled by the executive committee in like manner with all the other departments.

The superintendent or principal shall be appointed by the Board of Trustees, and shall discharge the functions of her office subject to the general authority of the superintendent of the hospital. With this reservation, the school shall be under her direct supervision and control.

Her authority shall extend over all that pertains to the instruction, duty, and discipline of the pupils.

She shall receive and pass upon applications for admission to the school, shall decide upon the fitness of probationers to become pupils, and shall assign pupils to duty, making such changes from time to time as may be necessary to secure for them a practical experience in all the branches of ward work.

In cases of misconduct or inefficiency, she may suspend the delinquent from duty.

Her action in all these matters shall be subject to the final decision of the executive committee, to which she shall report regularly and in detail.

She shall have supervision over those parts of the hospital as are occupied by patients, and also of the nurses' home, shall be responsible for the good order and cleanliness of those parts, and shall have authority over the housemaids and cleaners who are regularly assigned to work there.

All requisitions for ward supplies, except medicines ordered by the staff, shall be submitted to her, and approved by her before being sent to the superintendent of the hospital for final approval.

She shall reside in the hospital, and take her meals in the dining-room with the pupil nurses.

She shall be the official head of the nursing department, and all who are engaged in that department in any capacity shall be subordinate to her authority, subject to the general restrictions already noted.

Matron or Housekeeper.—She shall be immediately under the direction of the superintendent of the hospital.

She shall have charge and be responsible for the good order and cleanliness of the dining-rooms, kitchens, laundry, linen rooms, sewing room, and all parts of the hospital assigned to her, making daily inspections in the same.

She shall have charge of all domestic arrangements, except such as are assigned to the nursing department, and shall hire and discharge, subject to the authority of the superintendent, all servants employed in her department.

She shall prepare the ménus and order the meals for all the dining-rooms, including the patients', following in regard to the latter the dietary prescribed by the medical board.

She shall make requisitions for all supplies needed in her department, including food supplies, submitting all requisitions to the superintendent for his approval.

She shall have immediate charge of the distribution of food supplies and shall see that these are of good quality and are economically used.

She shall perform such other duties as may be assigned to her by the superintendent.

Steward.—The steward shall receive all supplies delivered to the hospital, including food supplies, shall have charge of them, shall be responsible for their safe keeping and proper and economic distribution.

He shall verify quantities, weights, and measures of goods delivered, and shall enter the same, with costs, in a proper book of record.

He shall issue supplies from the store-room only on the written requisition of duly qualified officials, and shall keep a record of such issues.

He shall perform such other duties as the superintendent may direct.

Engineer.—The engineer shall have charge of the engines, boilers, dynamos, elevators, and machinery of all kinds, and also of plumbing and electric apparatus and fixtures.

He shall make weekly reports to the superintendent of the quantity of fuel consumed, and shall be responsible for its economic use.

He shall make all ordinary repairs in his department.

He shall have control over all assistants, stokers, coal-passers, or other employees in his department, and may hire and discharge them if so empowered by the superintendent.

He shall report frequently to the superintendent on the condition of his department, and shall report promptly on all matters requiring immediate attention.

He shall be under the authority and control of the superintendent, and shall perform such duties as may be imposed by him.

Apothecary.—The apothecary shall be a graduate of a college of pharmacy, and shall have the immediate care and custody of all drugs, medicines, and other articles belonging to his department, and be responsible therefor.

He shall compound and make up all medicines which may be prescribed.

He shall deliver no medicine or other article unless the same be duly entered upon the prescription or order books, or ordered in writing.

He shall put up medicines intended for each ward separately, and shall annex to them labels containing the names of the patients for whom they are respectively prescribed, with written or printed directions for the use of them, and shall deliver them promptly to the nurses of each ward.

He shall keep the pharmacy and everything belonging to it in good order, and the same shall be open from 8 A. M. to 7 P. M. in his charge.

He shall be under the general supervision and control of the superintendent, and shall follow his directions.

He shall also perform such other duties as the executive committee or the medical board may require of him.

He shall not be absent without the permission of the superintendent.

He shall not be required to reside in the hospital.

House-staff.—There shall be a house staff for each of the divisions of the hospital service.

It shall consist of a house physician and house surgeon, with as many assistants for each as the exigencies of the service require.

They shall be appointed by the executive committee on nomination by the medical board.

These nominations shall be based upon competitive examinations, due notice of which, as to time and place, shall be publicly given, and all appointees shall have received the degree of Doctor of Medicine from a recognized medical school.

The service shall be at least eighteen months, and shall be divided as nearly as possible into equal periods, each period representing a grade of service.

The staff shall be advanced from a lower to the next higher grade upon completion of a term in that grade, by the executive committee on recommendation by the medical board.

They shall reside in the hospital, shall not practise outside, and shall give their entire time to their hospital duties.

So far as possible, the duties of each grade shall be clearly defined, and occupants of higher grades shall not substitute those in lower grades for the performance of any duty especially incumbent on themselves except by permission of the hospital authorities.

The house physician and house surgeon shall visit their respective wards at least twice a day, morning and evening, and as much more frequently as the condition of the patients demands.

They shall record all orders and prescriptions for their administration in books kept in the wards for that purpose. They shall also prescribe the diet of patients, under the immediate direction of the attending physician or surgeon.

They shall keep the clinical histories of the patients in such manner and under such conditions as may be fixed by the medical board.

In any medical or surgical case of emergency, whether a recent admission or a development of a case under treatment, they shall immediately notify the attending physician or surgeon.

They shall not admit, discharge, nor transfer patients from one ward to another. That is the exclusive duty of the superintendent.

They shall be present at the usual hours of attendance of the attending physicians, and accompany them on their rounds. The house physician or surgeon shall never be absent at the same time with his first assistant. He shall not be absent more than two evenings in each week, and when so absent shall return to the hospital at a reasonable hour.

The house surgical staff shall not take part in autopsies.

They shall not accept gifts or fees, or compensation of any kind from or in behalf of patients for professional services rendered. They may accept fees for testifying in court, and for making out proofs of claim in life insurance in cases of patients who have been treated in the hospital.

They shall examine applicants for admission to the hospital, and shall report the result to the superintendent.

Orderlies.—Orderlies are attached to the nursing department, and are under the immediate control of that department.

They shall be hired and discharged by the superintendent of the training-school, subject to the approval of the superintendent of the hospital.

The hours of duty for day orderlies are from 6.30 A. M. to 7 P. M.; for night orderlies, from 7 P. M. to 7 A. M.

Each class will remain on duty until the relief arrives. They shall do such work in the wards and render such services to patients as may be directed by the nurse in charge of the ward.

They shall not receive any gift, fee, or compensation of any kind from patients or others in their behalf for services rendered.

Ambulance.—Each ambulance shall be accompanied by a surgeon and a driver in uniform.

In reaching the patient, the surgeon shall determine the nature of the injury or disease, shall administer such temporary relief as may be necessary, and take the patient without delay to the hospital.

If the patient falls within a class not treated at the

hospital, he is to be taken to another hospital, where the proper service is maintained or to his own home.

A record book of the service shall be kept by the surgeon, in which shall be noted the time and place of call, the time of reaching the patient, that of return to the hospital, together with patient's name and diagnosis. If no patient is brought, the fact shall be stated in the record, and the reason assigned.

On arriving at the hospital from a call, the surgeon shall superintend the removal of the patient to the reception ward, and immediately notify the house physician or house surgeon, according as the case may be a medical or surgical one, and then, before attending to any other duty, make proper entries in the record book. The house physician or house surgeon, thus notified, shall, without delay, make a thorough examination and assume charge of the case.

Pathologist. — The pathologic department shall be under the charge of the pathologist, who shall have such assistants as may be necessary to secure prompt and efficient work in the department.

He shall assign work to his assistants in his judgment, but shall not assign to them any work which is especially incumbent on himself.

He shall have charge of the autopsy room and laboratory.

He shall be personally responsible for the work of his assistants, both as to its prompt performance and accuracy.

He shall be responsible for making of autopsies, and the investigation of material derived from them; for the examination and report upon tumors and all other tissues that may require investigation, and for all bacteriologic work.

He or a qualified assistant shall be on duty throughout each day.

He shall not be required, nor shall his assistants, to reside in the hospital.

No autopsy shall be made without the permission of the superintendent, expressed in writing.

Clinical Registrars.—Clinical registrars shall be appointed by the executive committee on the nomination of the medical board.

They shall have the supervision of the clinical histories of the patients, under the direction of the attending physician or surgeon on duty.

They shall examine the histories at least once a week.

They shall give instruction to the house staff as to the method of keeping the histories so as to secure a uniform system throughout the hospital.

On the discharge of a patient, they shall examine the clinical history in the case, and note their approval of it before it is turned over to the custodian for filing or binding in permanent form.

These histories, while the property of the hospital, having been compiled from the confidential statements of the patients, shall not be given to persons outside the hospital without the patient's consent, unless under compulsion of a subpœna or other legal process.

Ward Patients.—The admission and discharge of patients are wholly within the jurisdiction of the superintendent.

The examination of applicants for admission shall be made by a physician especially employed for that purpose, or, in the absence of such an official, by a member of the house staff.

All acts of any member of the staff, attending or resident, in the direction of the admission or discharge of a patient, shall be regarded as a report or recommendation to the superintendent, and shall become operative only when stamped with his approval, except that any member of the board of trustees or of the medical board shall have the constitutional right to order the admission of a patient, subject to the rules of the hospital governing admission.

Patients shall pay the established hospital rates, unless they are modified or rescinded by a member of the board of trustees or of the executive committee, or by the superintendent.

All patients on admission shall be furnished with ward cards. These cards shall be placed in a rack over the bed assigned to the patient, and on the patient's discharge shall be returned to the hospital office, properly filled out as to diagnosis and condition, and signed by the house physician or house surgeon. No patient shall be admitted to a ward without a card.

Patients to be operated on shall not, except in emergency cases, be anesthetized before the arrival at the hospital of the operating surgeon, and no patient shall be taken to the operating theater to await operation until after the operating surgeon shall have notified the nurse in charge of the ward that he is ready to receive such patient.

No patient shall leave the house without the permission of the superintendent, nor engage in any immoral act, nor have immoral literature in his possession, nor bring any liquor into the house.

No patient shall smoke tobacco in any part of the house except such as is specially designated for the purpose, nor use profane or obscene language, nor indulge in any offensive or objectionable behavior.

No male patient shall go into any of the women's wards, nor any female patient into those of the men, without the permission of the superintendent.

No patient shall enter the dead house, engine room, kitchens, laundry, nor any of the nurses' or servants' apartments under any pretense whatever.

No food or drink brought by friends outside the hospital shall be given to a patient without the permission of the house physician or house surgeon.

All articles of value should be turned into the office for safe keeping. If kept in the wards, it is at the owner's risk.

Convalescent patients shall render such help in the general work of their wards as their condition will warrant, in response to the demands of the nurses.

All patients shall receive the regular house diet unless otherwise specially ordered by the attending physician or surgeon.

Liquors and other stimulants shall be given only on the order of the house physician or house surgeon, and entered in a special book provided for that purpose.

Patients may receive visits from a clergyman by making their wishes known to the superintendent through the nurses of their wards.

Visitors to patients will be admitted on such days and at such hours as may be designated by the executive committee. Members of the immediate family circle of patients may be admitted on other than the regular visiting days, in the discretion of the superintendent.

When the patients have been reported as in serious condition or *in extremis*, friends will be admitted as freely as the patient's condition, or the exigencies of the hospital work will permit.

If visitors bring food or drink surreptitiously into the wards, the privilege of visiting will be revoked. All such articles must be left with the doorkeeper.

The ordinary length of a visit is half an hour. This time may be extended by the nurse in special cases in her discretion. All visitors must leave the hospital promptly on the expiration of the visiting hours.

Private Patients.—Patients occupying private rooms must pay weekly in advance the rates established by the executive committee. These rates may not be modified, nor rescinded in any case without a specific order by the executive committee. These rates cover the ordinary care and attention provided by the regular hospital routine. They do not include the services of the attending physicians and surgeons and anesthetizer, nor of special nurses, nor special articles of food, drink, or medicine not found in the hospital dietary, nor kept regularly in the hospital stock. These extras will be furnished by the hospital on order of the attending physician or surgeon at the patient's expense.

The fee to be paid by the patient to the attending physician or surgeon or anesthetizer, is a matter or arrangement between themselves, and should be settled before the professional services begin.

A private patient entering the hospital in regular course, and not sent by any member of the attending staff, shall be assigned to the attending physician on duty at the time of his admission. He may, however, have the privilege of selecting any other member of the attending staff. In either case he becomes the private patient of such attending physician as if originally sent in by him.

If special nurses are required, they shall be furnished by the hospital at established rates at the expense of the patient.

Transient cases, operated on and going away immediately after operation, shall be charged a reasonable fee for the use of the operating theater and attendance.

Private patients returning to the hospital after discharge for additional advice or treatment shall be charged a reasonable fee. They shall secure an order from the office covering each visit.

The hospital will not provide for the washing of personal clothing.

The hospital is not responsible for money or valuables brought by private patients.

When parent and child occupy a room together, the child being the patient, only one rate shall be charged if the child is under four years old, and half the rate additional if the child is between four and twelve.

Visitors to private patients will be admitted between 9 A. M. and 9 P. M. without restriction other than that imposed by the patient's condition, subject always to the orders of the attending physician or surgeon.

The hospital will not furnish meals to visiting friends, but rooms not required by patients may be occupied by relatives or friends. When so occupied, they shall pay the fixed rates of the rooms, and be subject to all the rules of the hospital.

Out-patient Department.—The out-patient department shall have classes or clinics corresponding to the service in the in-patient department, so that patients may be passed from one to the other as conditions demand.

It shall have as many special clinics, in addition, as may be desirable.

It shall be in charge of the assistant superintendent of the hospital, or of a chief of clinic, and shall be conducted as a department of the general hospital work.

Each class or clinic shall be in charge of a principal, who shall have as many assistants or deputies as may be necessary, all to be appointed by the executive committee on nomination by the medical board, and to hold office during the pleasure of the committee.

It shall be open for stated periods in the forenoon or afternoon, or both, of each day, except Sundays and holidays.

A small fee for treatment or surgical dressings shall be charged. All cases of alleged inability to pay shall be passed upon by the officer in charge, and his decisions thereon shall be final, but due diligence shall be exercised to prevent the abuse of the charity by unworthy applicants.

Complete records shall be kept, giving name, age, civil condition, diagnosis, and result of treatment in each case.

The professional staff of the out-patient department shall not, under any circumstances, demand or receive compensation for services rendered, nor shall they divert patients from the department to their own offices, or to those of other physicians for private treatment, nor to other hospitals.

Each member of the attending staff shall register in a book, provided for the purpose, the hour of his arrival and departure on each day of attendance, and if his arrival is delayed, or his departure hastened before the expiration of the hour of service, the reason shall be recorded.

The department shall be conducted for the treatment of such patients as have been discharged from the hospital wards, because no longer requiring treatment therein, yet requiring some professional care before final discharge, and for others whose condition does not require treatment in the wards, and who are unable to pay for proper professional care privately.

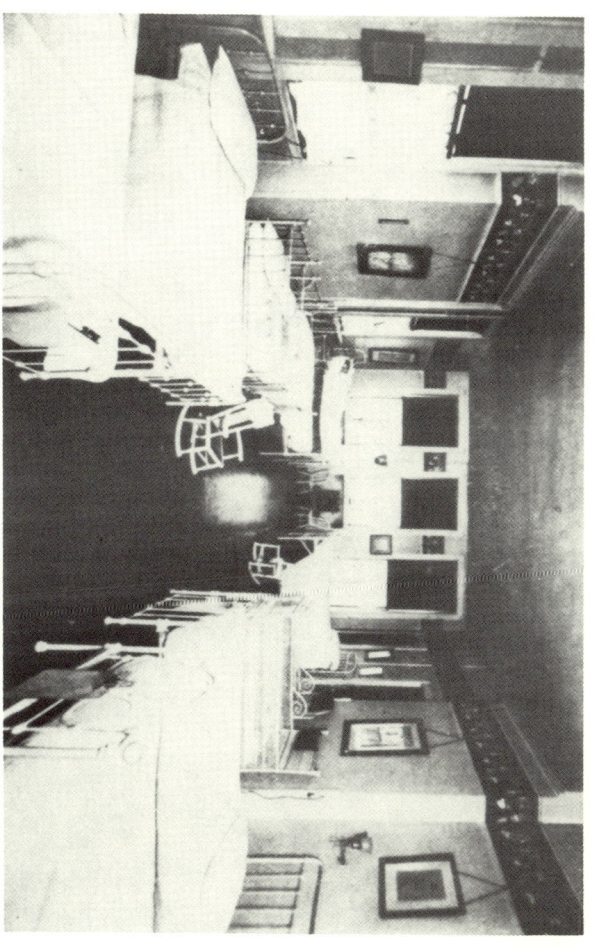

Fig. 13.—Children's ward. Eleven beds. Huron Road Hospital, Cleveland, Ohio

CHAPTER IV

THE MEDICAL SERVICE OF A HOSPITAL

By Henry M. Hurd, M.D.

The organization of a medical service for American hospitals has changed very materially during the past century. At first this organization was provisional and became attached to the larger hospitals to suit special conditions. For example, at the opening of the Pennsylvania Hospital, the first of our hospitals, it was recognized from the start that a hospital position was one which involved labor and self-sacrifice on the part of the staff, and brought no emolument. The physicians, therefore, who assumed the duty of extending medical aid to the patients of this hospital were actuated wholly by philanthropic motives and felt that in this way they could bring relief to a large number of persons who, if left in their own homes, would be destitute of proper care and nursing. They gave their time and services without any prospect of pecuniary returns.

For this reason, and in view of the fact that it seemed unfair to ask one man to do this large amount of gratuitous work, three persons were appointed to relieve each other in such service. Out of this circumstance grew the divided supervision of hospitals in America, and the inauguration of a service which, while at first it was simultaneous and coördinate, was taken in rotation afterward by those who received appointments on the visiting staff. This arrangement has remained in force ever since in almost all American hospitals, and continues to have a great degree of influence in the organization of staffs with a divided service, and a rotation of heads of different departments of service.

As hospitals grew and their service became more complicated and unwieldy, further divisions were made of the medical and surgical service, and in some larger hospitals subdivisions for the various specialties were established. Thus, for example, in one of the large hospitals of the United States to-day there are four different surgical and two medical services, besides an obstetric and a gynecologic service. As matters are arranged at present, the members of the visiting staff of almost all large hospitals serve for a comparatively brief period, and at the end of three or four months relinquish their positions to other persons who come in to take their place. In many instances a period of three months covers the entire service of the individual to the hospital during the whole year.

Such an arrangement of the services has many disadvantages. It involves different and contradictory methods of treatment, and in certain respects a diversity of practice which may work to the detriment of the individual patient. For example: a short time ago I had a letter from a hospital manager complaining that there was a lack of uniformity of action on the part of the medical staff of the hospital with which he was connected, whereby a disease like pneumonia, which was treated by one visiting physician wholly in the open air, was treated by a second visiting physician wholly in the house, the former taking all the patients out-of-doors, and the latter, when his service began, carrying the same patients into the house.

If hospitals are to be used for the instruction of physicians and the training of nurses, it is evident that a comparative uniformity of practice is desirable. It should not be forgotten, however, that the divided service has a certain advantage in that it brings new blood to the visiting staff and prevents the tyranny which a single overmastering mind is apt to exercise upon the whole medical service of any hospital, provided he has full opportunity to enforce his views without any possibility of contradiction or change. In some hospitals these appointments are made for a definite period, and in one hospital at least, the Massachusetts General Hospital, the person retires at the age of sixty-four or after twenty-one years of continuous service. When the chief retires, it is usually customary to promote one of the assistants or associates in the same department to the vacancy, by an appointment lower down on the staff. As a rule, as has been said before, these services are from three to six months, and those who are concerned in them receive no compensation, the emolument which comes directly from the hospital position being considered sufficient.

Another form of organization has lately been making its way gradually into popular favor, that of a continuous head of each department, with a service lasting during the whole year. This enables the physician or surgeon to supervise the work of the hospital, and, in a teaching hospital, to carry it forward in an exemplary and uniform manner. In view of the fact that such a service, continuous during the year, constitutes a serious tax on the time and energies of the chief, it has become customary to pay an adequate salary to such heads of departments, so that it may be possible to claim his services, and thus secure an absolute conscientiousness on his part in attending to his duties.

It may be said in passing that in some instances, under the former system, a hospital position was sought because of the advantages which it gave in the community to the possessor, and not because of the opportunity which was afforded to do good professional work. Under these circumstances, in many cases, the work was done in a perfunctory and slip-shod fashion, and much of it was intrusted to young and inexperienced men. Under a single responsible head for each department of the hospital it is possible to accomplish the work much more effectually and economically. There is, it is needless to say, much greater economy in the matter of surgical dressings and apparatus where the requirements of a single surgeon are to be considered rather than of half a dozen. It is also possible for one head of each department to supervise the matter of medical histories, clinical examinations, and the like, much more thoroughly than can be done by a larger number of people. The great objection to such an arrangement arises from the fact that it is sometimes difficult to secure the services of a single chief, uninterruptedly, during the whole year. The requirements of the climate, and the necessity of a long vacation for the purpose of health, during the summer, may require that an associate be appointed who can replace the chief of the department in his absence, and carry out his ideas and enforce his methods. The former method is more wasteful and not as efficient, but has the advantage of giving scope to a larger number of persons with special gifts in the medical profession.

It seems to me desirable that, where a divided service with rotation of the different heads of departments is absolutely necessary, there should be a very careful investigation on the part of the authorities of the hospital as to the attendance of each person, and a system of fines and penalties should be enforced, in order that the work may go on without disastrous absence or neglect.

Admitting Physician.—One member of the resident staff should be a permanent medical officer, with a term of service for life or during good behavior. I refer to the superintendent and admitting physician. He should have charge of all the physical affairs of the hospital, under the authority of the trustees, and should serve as a means of communication between them and every department of service. In addition, he should be the admitting and discharging physician, and should regulate the movement of the population of the hospital. This is not the place to speak of his other administrative duties, but the importance of placing the whole question of the admission and discharge of patients in his hands cannot be too strongly urged. In no other way, except by placing the whole matter in the hands of a permanent official, continuously in office, whose duty it is to carry out scrupulously, consistently, and uniformly the regulations established for the admission and discharge of patients, can the hospital be protected from the admission of patients who are not true objects of charity. Many of the abuses of medical charity have their origin in the zeal of medical teachers who see an interesting case in every applicant for admission, and do not wisely discriminate as to the need of charitable relief. In the majority of instances the interesting case is not a true object of charity, and ought not to burden the hospital. The admitting physician should receive the fullest information concerning all patients from the members of the medical staff, but the ultimate decision as to admission and discharge should rest with him.

The House Staff.—During the past one hundred years serious difficulties have developed in connection with the resident service of a hospital. In many hospitals the period of service of the house staff has been eighteen months, divided as follows: six months as a junior and possibly non-resident medical officer, six months as assistant medical officer, and six months as a resident with charge of the work of the division, under the supervision of the visiting physician or surgeon. These positions have usually been filled by energetic and well-intending, but inexperienced, young men, who, during their first year of service, have usually learned their duties at the expense of their patients, and at considerable ultimate cost to the hospital. After the apprenticeship of one year, they are in a position to do good work for the hospital, and to give efficient service. As soon, however, as they become familiar with their duties, it becomes necessary that they should retire to give place to others equally inexperienced, who must serve a similar apprenticeship before they are fitted to do hospital work satisfactorily.

Attempts have been made to meet this situation by prolonging the whole period of service from eighteen months to two years or even to two and a half years. It is evident, however, that in many instances this prolongation of the period of service has been a serious disadvantage to the individual who comes to the hospital for service immediately upon receiving the degree of Doctor of Medicine, and who only wishes to fit himself for general practice, but has no intention of specializing in any branch of medicine or surgery. For such an individual it is important that he should have a range of service which takes in both medical and surgical service, and perhaps some practical acquaintance with gynecology and obstetrics, but at the most he cannot afford to spend more than one year or eighteen months in securing this service. It seems to me preferable that the terms of service of all the members of the resident staff be readjusted to provide both for those persons who wish merely a routine acquaintance with practical work in important departments, and equally for those who desire to specialize in some one direction. To accomplish these ends I would, accordingly, advise that one year be spent by the student in a divided service which includes medicine, surgery, gynecology, and obstetrics. If, after this year, any individual desires to specialize in medicine or surgery, or any other branch, he may then receive a hospital appointment for at least one more year. If, further, he shows unusual capacity and fitness for any one branch of medical service, he should receive an appointment as resident physician or surgeon with a moderate salary, so that he may be able to occupy the place, and to increase his special knowledge until such time as he is prepared to go elsewhere to assume unusual care and responsibility.

The medical staff of the hospital, therefore, should be organized under competent and efficient residents, men of character and capacity, and fitness to supervise the medical work of those subordinate to them. These residents should be appointed for a period of at least two years, and should be the assistants of the heads of the different departments during their term of service. Under these heads of departments there should be internes sufficient to do the work of each department, who should invariably be men who have had some previous hospital experience. Subordinate to these there should

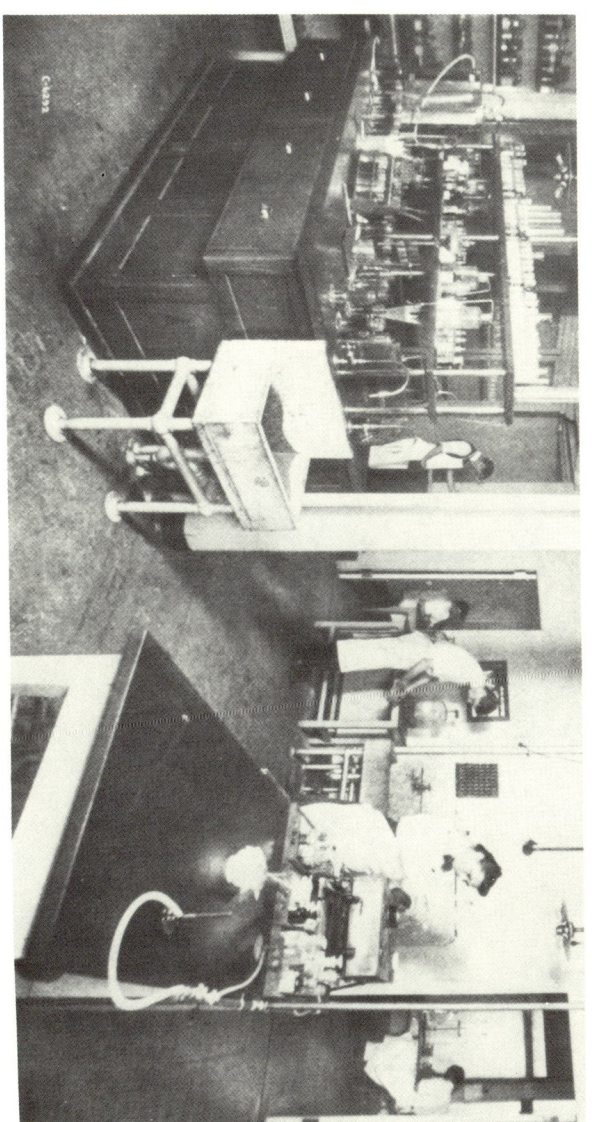

Fig. 14.—A laboratory. Presbyterian Hospital, New York.

be house officers who have just graduated in medicine and who have had no previous experience in hospital work. The latter should engage in making dressings, in the routine treatment of patients, in visiting patients who may apply for admission to the hospital, and in the performance of various other duties under the direction of the resident or some of the internes.

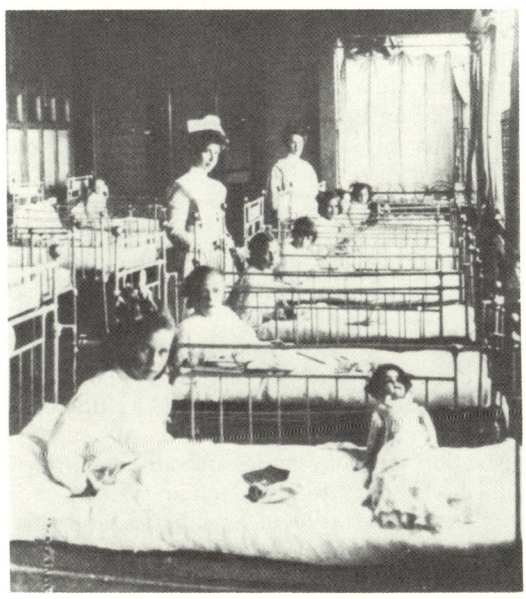

Fig. 15.—Veranda ward at Lakeside Home, Hospital for Sick Children, Toronto.

It is desirable that a hospital should have an active staff in all its separate departments. Thus, for example, a large municipal hospital like Bellevue, New York, should have medical, surgical, gynecologic, psychiatric, and pediatric departments. Each of these departments should be under definite control by a competent visiting staff, and each should be provided with a resident physician, one or more internes, and assistant officers. There should also be appointed to reside in the hospital a bacteriologist to examine body fluids, to be present at surgical operations, to make such examinations as are required in order to throw light upon the operation which may be required for the good of the patient, and a clinical microscopist to make clinical examinations, Widal reactions, etc.

The Anesthetist.—The instruction which has been given to medical students and young physicians in the administration of anesthetics has generally been fragmentary, unsystematic, and fortuitous. Some persons have a natural aptitude for administering anesthetics and are able intuitively to keep in mind the condition of the patient's respiration and heart's action and his behavior toward the anesthetic. They are also quick to observe the thousand and one danger-signals which must always be kept in mind at such a time. The majority of physicians must learn the essentials of a proper administration of anesthetics through careful preliminary instruction, and by the experience which comes from habitual observation of good work. Every hospital, consequently, should have a skilled anesthetist upon the staff, whose duty it should be to conduct and supervise the administration of anesthetics in all operating-rooms. It should be his duty to give regular systematic instruction in the administration of anesthetics, and this teaching should become a routine procedure in every hospital. Many of the untoward effects of ether, chloroform, nitrous oxid, or other anesthetics are to be ascribed to a lack of skill in their administration. Many of the costly drugs are also wasted by unskilled anesthetists, and it is true economy to place this branch of hospital work in the hands of a thoroughly well-trained anesthetist and hold him responsible for the proper conduct of this important adjunct of modern surgery.

X-ray Expert.—A physician skilled in the use of the x-ray should be attached to every hospital, and in daily attendance to give treatment to skin affections, to examine fractures and dislocations, to search for aneurysms, heart lesions, and pulmonary diseases, to locate and disclose the presence of nephritic, hepatic, and vesical calculi, and to give other examinations requiring expert knowledge and technical skill. He ought to be a permanent officer of the hospital with an adequate salary, and his work should form part of the ordinary routine of the hospital. The danger of x-ray burns is great, and can only be avoided by skill and experience. Many malpractice suits have arisen from misinterpreted skiagraphs, and the need of a skilled

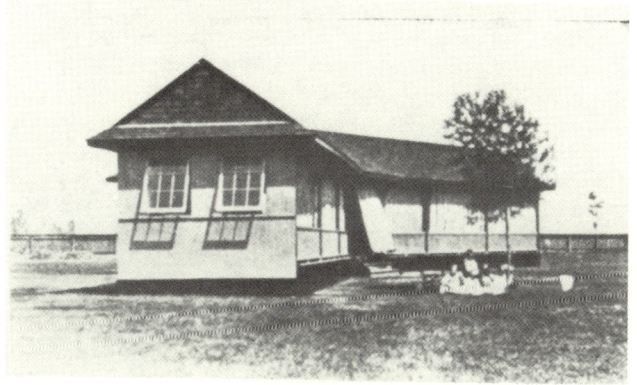

Fig. 16.—Tuberculosis Building at Lakeside Home of Hospital for Sick Children, Toronto. It has accommodations for 14 patients and nurses.

expert in actinography is apparent to all who have had practical experience in the difficulties of x-ray work.

There should be an officer in charge of the medical and surgical histories, to see that they are properly taken, that all details are supplied, and that they are indexed and bound up in such a manner as to be accessible and to contribute to the sum-total of the medical knowledge.

In institutions where there is not a divided service and resident physicians who are more or less permanent, with a comparatively long tenure of office, a chief of staff should be appointed whose business it should be to coördinate and to bring into proper relation the work of the different departments. This chief of staff, as far as possible, should be free from all bias and tendency to favor one service more than another. He should organize the work for the benefit of all, and should see that the work of each department receives a proper recognition on the part of the hospital authorities.

In many hospitals under visiting physicians who take but little interest, the work is haphazard and unsystematic, and does not accomplish the good which can be expected for the community. The privileges of the hospital

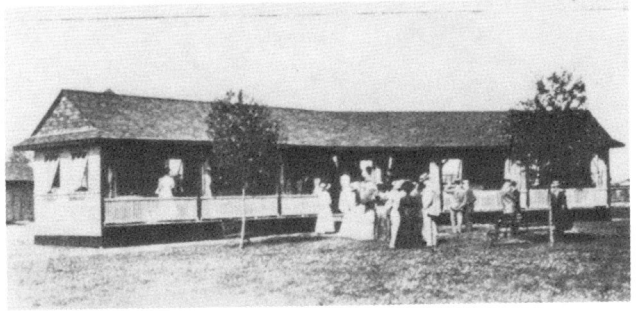

Fig. 17.—Another view of Tuberculosis Building at Lakeside Home, Hospital for Sick Children, Toronto.

cannot well be given to any physician in a large city. It is desirable that they be reserved for those members of the medical staff who, in the judgment of the trustees or managers of the hospital, are personally considered fit to undertake and to assume the professional work of the hospital.

To extend the privileges of the hospital beyond this is to bring expense to the hospital and confusion and disorder among the members of the medical staff, and tends to defeat the true object for which the hospital has been founded.

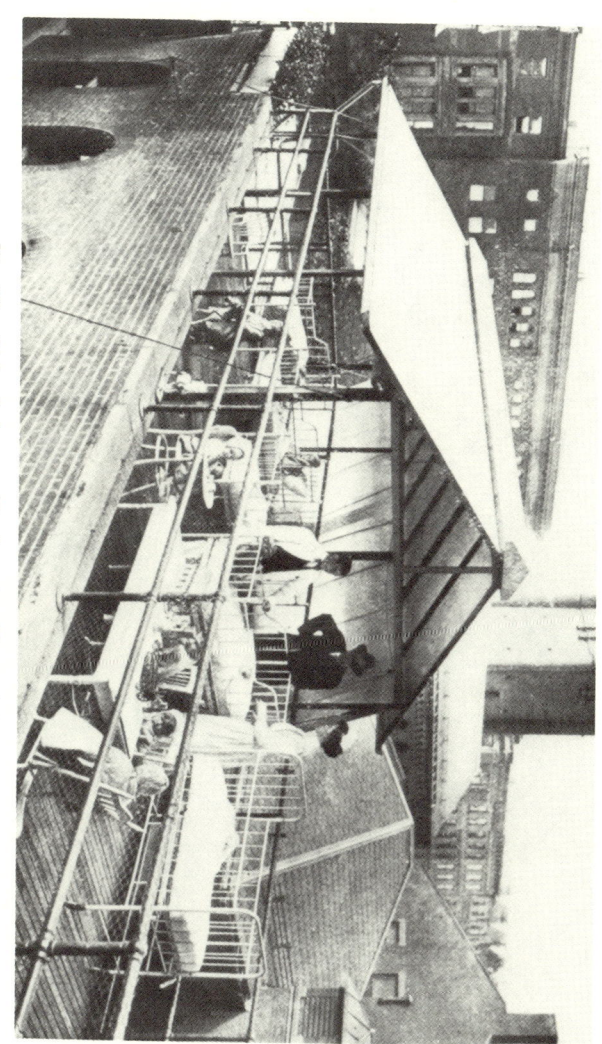

Fig. 18.—Airing balcony. Presbyterian Hospital, New York.

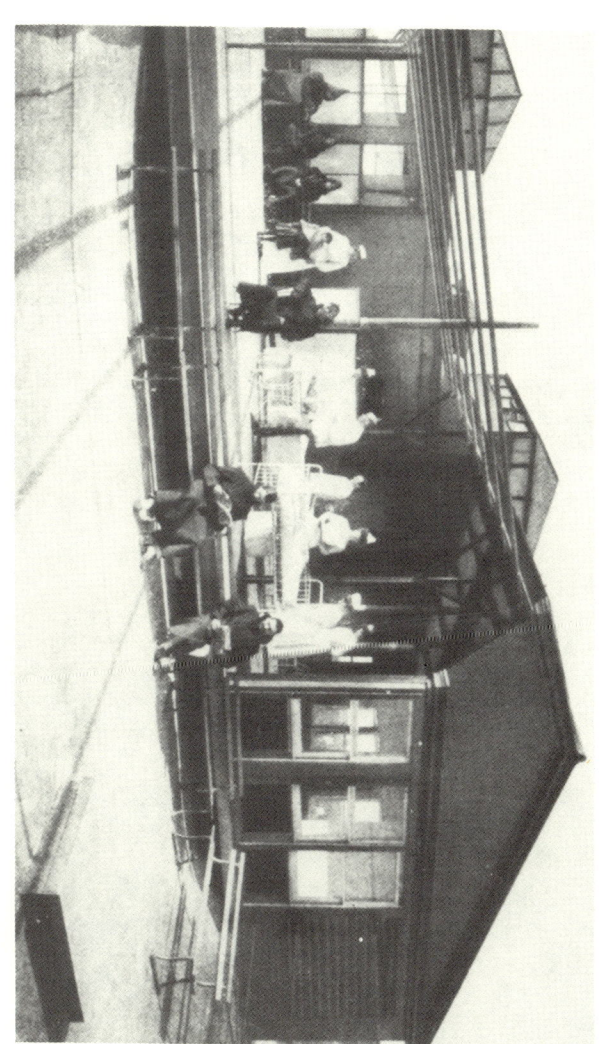

Fig. 19.—Airing balcony. Presbyterian Hospital, New York.

THE MEDICAL SERVICE OF A HOSPITAL 107

In a hospital in the country or in a small town the situation is different. Here it is desirable that the hospital be so arranged that physicians of the community who are of reputable standing and are trusted by their patients and neighbors should have the privilege of sending their patients to the hospital and of looking after them. They also should have the privilege of charging moderate fees for their services in connection with their hospital work.

CHAPTER V

A GENERAL HOSPITAL FOR ONE HUNDRED PATIENTS

By John N. Elliott Brown, M.B. and Edward Fletcher Stevens, A.A.I.A. Architect.

GENERAL CONSIDERATIONS

Site.—Hospitals should be so built that an abundance of pure air and sunlight will be available for all the patients; distant enough from streets and railways to be free from noise of traffic; and, if possible, in such a position as to command a view of pleasant surroundings. If these ideal conditions cannot be fully realized, every effort should be made to see that they are secured as nearly as possible.

It must be admitted that hospital opinion is divided between the central and suburban location. The chief point in favor of the central location is that it is good for business (if we may use the term), convenient for accidents and emergencies. It is generally more convenient also for the medical staff and medical students. (A teaching hospital should preferably adjoin its medical college, a point to be considered in the choice of site.) The superintendent of a large hospital in Chicago confesses that he dislikes the central location of his hospital. Where a hospital, though central, adjoins a park, no strong objection is urged against its position if street noises are not too disturbing. Placing the patients' welfare uppermost, we have no hesitation in saying that a hospital placed beyond the noise of the traffic of the city, and completely removed from the vicinity of its smoke and germ-laden atmosphere, is the ideal spot. Sir Henry Burdett, the great British authority, advocates that all sick people requiring hospital attention should be cared for in such a location, in what he terms the "hospital city."

Let us consider the arguments which lead up to the conclusion that such a site is the best place for sick people.

Nowadays, much less reliance is being placed on drugs than formerly. Fresh air, sunshine, rest, proper diet, together with good nursing, have very largely taken their place. We are already utilizing as much as possible such means are are at hand—balconies, roof-gardens, and grounds.

A prominent hospital superintendent recently published the following in relation to the treatment of a large class of diseases:

"One almost feels forced to the conclusion that the simple, common-sense remedies, such as nutritive diet, fresh air, sunlight, mental and moral suggestion, rest or exercise, as may be indicated, are as efficacious as anything that has been advocated," etc.

The value of light as a therapeutic and germicidal agent is unquestioned. An eminent specialist in light therapy directed one of his patients, a lady suffering from lupus (obliged to go to the mountains for her holidays, beyond the reach of Röntgen and Finsen rays), to expose the ulcer to the direct rays of the sun for a certain portion of each day. She did so, and the ulcer healed.

The perfect site, therefore, should afford air of the utmost purity, a maximum of sunshine, and perfect quietude —three most desirable adjuvants in the cure cf disease.

There is only one word to be said in respect to the size of the site, and that is that it should be as large as possible. The Beverly Hospital, Massachusetts, has ten acres; Evanston Hospital, Illinois, five acres; Worcester, Massachusetts, seven acres; the Municipal Hospital, Philadelphia, forty-eight acres, with a farm nearby; William Backus Hospital, Norwich, Connecticut, twenty acres; Wolfsboro Hospital, New Hampshire, twenty-five acres; Agnew Hospital, California, three hundred and twenty acres. We should like to have a farm near our ideal hospital.

A large site outside of the city limits can be purchased, as every one knows, very much cheaper than an urban site; so where the amount of money available for a new hospital is limited, the amount saved by building in the suburbs can be applied to construction and equipment. The average length of patients' stay in such a hospital is some days less than in a hospital in the city.

Style of Building.—The battle still wages over the style of building, as it does over most questions relating to hospitals; and the last word has not yet been said. Twenty years ago, when our knowledge of bacteriology began to influence hospital construction, the one-storied pavilions, separated from one another by corridors, over high, open basements, were much in vogue, particularly on the continent of Europe. This continental influence did not influence the larger centers of the British Isles, and has not influenced construction very markedly in America. The notable exceptions are to be found in the Johns Hopkins Hospital, Baltimore; the Presbyterian Hospital, Philadelphia; a hospital in Colorado, and another in Mexico.

Dr. Gilman Thompson, in a paper published recently, expresses his high appreciation of the construction of the Policlinico, Rome; the Virchow and the Moabit Hospitals of Berlin; and the Boucicaiaut Hospital, Paris. The Virchow covers 96 acres; it has 53 separate buildings, with a capacity of 1650 beds. The cost was $2250 per bed, which corresponds to $2500 and $3000 in this country. A favorite arrangement in these continental hospitals is a pair of pavilions connected with a double-storied service building—these comprising a unit. Dr. Thompson likes this arrangement of buildings, as it permits of a better classification of patients, is cheaper in construction than the "sky-scraper" variety, and has much to do with a pleasanter and quicker convalescence.

On the other hand, in many of the large cities in Great Britain and America of late years the tendency has been to construct multi-storied hospitals in a central location, recently exemplified in the construction of the New Jefferson Medical College Hospital, Philadelphia. This building, eleven stories in height, was completed in 1908 at a cost of one million dollars. It accommodates 300 patients. Such hospitals, while possessing many virtues—being of first-class construction, compact and concentrated, convenient for business, for administration, and for medical students, yet they lack the virtues we have referred to above. In the continental variety, on the other hand, the enormous extent of ground covered makes the heating, the porterage of food and other supplies expensive, and supervision more difficult.

The chief points, of course, to be kept in mind in considering the style and size of the hospital building or buildings are the extent of the site, the number of patients to be accommodated, the character of the diseases to be treated, whether medical students are to be trained in them or not; and the amount of money at the disposal of the building committee. In all hospitals construction ought to be fire-proof.

One of the most unique hospitals we have seen is the new Royal Victoria Hospital, Belfast. It is but one-storied, contains 300 beds, and was constructed for $1500 per bed. The wards, eighteen in number, lie side and side direct, each with an A-shaped roof, through which sufficient light seems to be admitted. The administration building and the nurses' home are adjacent three-storied buildings. The kitchen is in the basement, the outpatients' department is connected by corridor, and the superintendent's residence, the laundry, and the pathologic department are detached buildings. Heating and ventilating are provided for by the Plenum system, which works very satisfactorily.

For a general hospital to accommodate 100 patients, the writers are neither in favor of the sky-scraper nor of the one or two-storied pavilion, but rather of the opinion that the building of medium height, say three or four stories, is the best. The argument on this point is one relating to maintenance. The very high building is only necessary when building in a congested portion of the city.

Heating.—One of the writers (Dr. Brown), while in Glasgow, was impressed with the Reck system of heating, as exemplified in the Western Infirmary, and takes the liberty of quoting a description of it from Dr. Donald Mackintosh's recent work on Hospital Construction and Management. It is economic and satisfactory.

"In the Reck system a circulator is used which causes a strong and rapid circulation of the water throughout every part of any apparatus to which it may be fitted, so that by its use all the recognized benefits of hot-water heating may be obtained without any of the disadvantages. As generally arranged, a heating apparatus on this system is fitted with flow and return pipes, having connections to the various radiators, in much the same manner as an ordinary gravity system. The water is partially heated by low-pressure steam in a "reheater" similar to a calorifier; to this "reheater" the flow and return pipes are connected. Before the flow-pipe starts on its course through the building to distribute the heat to the radiators it is taken up to a point above the highest radiators and connected to an expansion tank.

The patent circulator is fitted on the flow-pipe several feet below the expansion tank. Through it low-pressure steam is introduced, and this causes the water in the pipe between the circulator and the expansion tank to boil, thereby reducing the specific gravity of the ascending column of water. The connection of the flow-pipe to the expansion tank is made in such a manner that the steam injected by the circulator is separated from the water and discharged into the space above the water-line in the expansion tank. The flow-pipe descending from the expansion tank on its way to supply the radiators contains hot water only, entirely free from steam. A condenser is fitted on the ascending flow-pipe just below the circulator, and the steam discharged above the water-line in the expansion tank is condensed by the partially heated water coming from the "reheater."

It will readily be seen that between the contents of the portion of the ascending flow-pipe which contains water mixed with steam, and those of an equal length of the descending pipe which contains no steam, there will be a considerable difference in weight, and an overbalancing effect is obtained which is sufficient to cause a circulation about four times as fast as that in an ordinary gravity system.

A system to provide heat from hot water is considerably dearer to install than one to provide steam, but the maintenance is not much, if any, more. The heat provided is preferable.

Most of the larger hospitals in America are heated by steam. Steam can be carried from a power-house which it is often economic to combine with the laundry, some distance from the main buildings. The same boilers may be used to generate steam for power, electric light, ventilating fans, also for sterilization and disinfection. Heat, if wanted, can be secured more quickly than by the hot-water plant. It is generally conceded that the heating and ventilating systems should not be dependent one on the other.

Ventilation.—The ventilation of hospitals may be generally divided into several sorts.

First, we have natural ventilation by means of windows and openings through the walls to the outdoor air. These facilities, plus the fireplace, constitute the favorite kind of ventilation in a number of the larger hospitals in London, England, and New York. Dr. Gilman Thompson strongly favors this system of ventilation.

The Western Infirmary in Scotland is heated and ventilated by what is known as the direct-indirect system.

The radiators are placed along the walls, and immediately below there is an opening cut through the external wall to the outside air; this permits of a free passage of air from the outside through the opening and up through the radiator into the ward. This opening is controlled by dampers, so that the volume of air can be regulated. The air is extracted through flues with outlets near the ceiling—all the branch flues connected to one main trunk in which is placed an exhaust fan. This system gives satisfaction there. The only objection heard to it in that country was that if there were any mal-odors near the ward, they would be sucked into it. This is not a strong objection, because the sanitary towers, so common there, are practically cut off from the ward. The objection to its use in colder climates is the danger that the water in the radiator may freeze and burst the pipes, should any of the nurses or employees close the valves.

Then there is the Plenum system. This consists in pumping fresh air through water trickling down moist curtains, and in winter over hot-water radiators, forcing it into the ward about the center of the side walls and out through openings near the floor into flues which connect with a shaft ending in a protected turret at the top of the building. Supplementary hot-water coils are placed contiguous to each ward, as may be found necessary, the heat from which may be utilized or not. This system we have heard condemned strongly in London, England, in New York, Chicago, and other American cities, but it appears to be working satisfactorily in the new hospital in Birmingham, a large new hospital in Paisley, and perfectly in the Royal Victoria Hospital in Belfast. The superintendent of a large new hospital in Chicago, where we saw a much similar system in operation, vigorously denounced it. Some hospitals in the old country where the Plenum system has been tried have abandoned it because nurses and patients developed anemia. In one of the Glasgow hospitals where it is used the superintendent is not enthusiastic over it.

The City of Worcester Hospital has what might be called a Plenum system plus exhaust fans, the foul air being drawn down into chambers in the basement. Four to eight thousand cubic feet per patient per hour are pumped through the wards. The twenty-five motors which run the fans are one-half to two horse-power each. By this system, of course, the hospital is heated and ventilated at one and the same time. The Worcester people say the results are eminently satisfactory.

In the new Toronto General Hospital the heating system and the ventilating system are to be separate and distinct from each other. Each room throughout the building will have sufficient direct radiation to provide the proper temperature during the coldest weather. The system of ventilation for the wards has been designed on the lines of what might be termed natural ventilation, in contradistinction to mechanical or artificial ventilation— the incoming air, if so desired, can be heated to a required temperature; the air then passes on and up through flues of large area into the wards, the inlet into the wards being so arranged as to give the best distribution of air. In the exhaust flues there are aspirating coils which induce the flow of air in that direction. The flues are practically twice the size to that which would be required if mechanical means were adopted. There is also installed in the air-supply flues to the wards a large fan which can be used when occasion demands—for instance in damp, murky days, or to occasionally flush through the wards.

The principle of exhaust or positive ventilation has been applied to all ward kitchens, sink rooms, bathrooms, etc. —a partial vacuum is created and the flow of air is through these rooms and through the exhaust flues and out into the open.

Dr. Christian Holmes, of Cincinnati, who has made wide observations, favors a system of natural ventilation supplemented by the exhaust fans.

Attention might be called to some points in connection with the simpler system of heating and ventilation, such as the direct-indirect radiators set up from the floor on brackets. These radiators should be smooth castings with the sections set far enough apart to permit the passage of the hand between the sections. The cold air is brought to the under side of the radiators from the outer air through a cast or galvanized iron duct in which a controlling damper is placed.

To prevent the cold air from coming directly into the room, a removable shield is fastened to the front of the radiator. In this way all the virtues of a direct-indirect radiator are obtained and still every portion of the radiator can be readily cleaned.

Direct ventilation can be secured by making the stool cap to the window project about 4 inches above the stool and making a coved intersection with the stool, so that when the window is raised a few inches direct draft is prevented.

Ventilators should have no register faces and should have the openings smooth and curved at bottom to prevent the lodgment of dust, etc.

Floors.—Most ward floors are made of hard wood, maple being the favorite; a few have oak; some have pine. A number of hospitals put linoleum over the wood and are partial to it. In several hospitals the maple is laid over the fire-proof concrete. An occasional ward floor is of cement, terrazzo, or tile. Terrazzo is used in the children's ward in the Worcester. The new Jefferson Medical College Hospital has used a preparation called magnesite. It is liked because it is non-absorbent, easily cleaned, resilient, and wears well. For operating-rooms the favorite floor is tile. Next in popularity is terrazzo. A few have marble; and among the list of remaining floors we find florette, monolith, asbestolith, asphalt, asbestos, stone, murall, and carbolite; while many of the old-fashioned hospitals still use hard wood, either bare or covered with linoleum. The junction between the walls and floors should be coved; indeed, there should be no angles nor ledges anywhere.

The use of battleship linoleum cemented directly to the concrete flooring is coming much into favor for ward use. It wears well, keeps its color, is easily cleaned, is easy on the feet, and is almost noiseless. We cannot refrain from commending the ward floors of the New York Hospital, New York—colored tiles in pattern. These tiles have been in place some thirty years, and seem as good as ever.

Windows.—Windows should extend from the ceiling to within twenty inches of the floor, thus allowing no dead air space at the ceiling and permitting the patients to see the outside world. Transoms, when used, should occupy the upper portions. Aprons should be provided to cover the triangular space made at each end of the transom when open, so that there will be no lateral inflow of air, the current from outdoors impinging against the ceiling only. There should be space enough between each two windows for a bed. In some institutions this space is made wide enough for two beds. The older writers recommend windows quite close to the corners of the ward. This permits of the corners of the ward being flushed out with fresh air. Following this idea there should be openings which can be closed by gratings, so that fresh air can be admitted close to the floor line.

Doors.—There is nothing better than the perfectly plain door without panels, with the outer veneer cut from around the rim to form continuous grain. There should be no threshold.

All door-jambs should be set before plastering. The plaster should be brought to the face of the jamb. No casing should be applied. The base also should be set in the same way, coved at the floor, this base to return around the door-jambs.

Where transoms exist, the transom bar should be made the thickness of the doors and transom sash.

Size of Public Ward.—The number of patients in a public ward in hospitals runs from forty down to four. The favorite sized ward is twenty—many superintendents giving that as their idea of the right number. Some superintendents recommend a twelve-bed ward. A few superintendents agree with Ochsner and Sturm that a still smaller ward is more desirable—that no ward should hold more than four to six patients. It would appear to us, in view of the present-day economies demanded, that twelve should be the minimum number of patients in a public ward and the maximum about twenty. This view is supported by a number of nurses whom we have interviewed on the matter. We do not think we can afford in a large hospital to build a ward running north and south, in which the sun will shine morning, noon, and night, to hold less than twelve or fourteen beds. When the ward comes to be smaller than that, we must introduce the corridor, which shuts out half the sunlight.

Reverting to Dr. Brown's paper, read before the American Hospital Association, Sir Henry Burdett, in his annual "Hospitals and Charities" (page 125), in referring to this point, says:

"Dealing with the size of wards, the American view is that a ward of twenty beds is the best. Some superintendents prefer a ward of twelve beds, and a few consider the contention of Ochsner and Sturm in their recent book that a smaller ward, one of four to six beds, is more desirable. Judging by the Seaman's Hospital, Greenwich, we should say that Ochsner and Sturm are wrong in their contention, which is not likely to be adopted by any one who is possessed of an intimate knowledge of hospital administration. We imagine that the ward of twenty beds has come to stay."

Direction of Wards.—Ninety out of one hundred superintendents who replied to our queries recommend that wards should run north and south. This permits the free entrance of sunlight, of which no ward can get too much. In northern United States and Canada, where we have so much dark weather from November to May, we are glad to see as much of the sun as possible, love to see it flood the wards, bathing the patients from head to foot. Rarely do we find them complaining of too much of it, and when we do, it is very easy to place a screen so as to put their eyes in shadow or to pull down blinds or awnings.

Dr. A. D. MacIntyre, former superintendent of the Kingston General Hospital, in a paper on fumigation, read at a meeting of the Canadian Hospital Association (after pointing out the futility of the ordinary method of the gaseous fumigation as usually carried out) said: "We should should use all means of disinfection, such as taking the fixtures out of the room and exposing them to the sunlight and fresh air, then thoroughly wash the walls, floors, and woodwork. Keep everything exposed to the sunlight and fresh air, or in absence of the latter to diffuse daylight. These are the agencies that have thus far tided us over in spite of faulty fumigation, and we would certainly give the credit where it is due."

Arrangement of Ward Dependencies.—A great feature in the arrangement of ward dependencies is to have them convenient, in order to save labor and make the necessary work as easy and pleasant of performance as possible. A London Hospital, and a new one being built in Paisley for sick insane people, have the bath-rooms opposite the center of the ward. This arrangement, though somewhat lessening the amount of sunlight, to my mind, is most convenient for nurses and orderlies. In the old country generally, these conveniences are placed in sanitary towers at the distal end of the ward. Some authorities hold this to be more desirable than having them placed near the diet kitchen, linen closet, and other dependencies of the ward, in which case nurses and orderlies, bearing urinals and bedpans at meal hours meet other helpers bearing the meals of the patients, an objectionable procedure.

The toilets should be capacious. We have a most favorable recollection of observing in the old Pennsylvania Hospital, Philadelphia, that the closet is large enough and its doors wide enough to admit a bed. The beds are on wheels and can easily be moved by the orderlies into the closet when the patient wishes to use the bedpan.

The reason is obvious. For a similar reason, Dr. Mackintosh, of Glasgow, holds that the separate divisions of the closet used by ambulant patients should be completely divided off from one another from floor to ceiling.

Our general public ward would be at least thirteen feet high and twenty-eight feet wide, with a balcony running from it in such a way as to obstruct as little as possible the entrance of sunlight. The length of the ward, of course, should depend on the number of patients to be accommodated. The door or doors leading to it should be wide and conveniently placed. The bottom of the door, of course, should be flush with the floor of the ward and the balcony. The floor of the balcony, if it runs along the wall, as in the new pavilion at Bellevue Hospital, New York, should be of glass or some material which will allow as much light as possible to enter the ward below.

Roof-gardens are desirable, but only for such patients as are able fairly well to look after themselves. All bed patients and other patients requiring observation preferably should be under the convenient supervision of the nurse who is in charge of the ward to which they belong. A recent observer states that enough outdoor accommodation should be provided to accommodate at least one-half of the patients in the hospital. We should say all if such an arrangement be possible.

In arranging for using the roof, provision should be made for pantry and toilet accommodation, also for a convenient room into which the bed may be run while a dressing is being done. Awnings or other overhead shelter should be provided. In this connection one should remember to have doors of rooms and elevators plenty wide enough for the passage of beds.

Operating-Rooms.—The operating-rooms of the hospitals as to size may be divided roughly into three classes. Here are some of the dimensions of the larger: 50 x 50 feet; 50 x 180 feet (total superficial area); 44 x 45 feet; 60 x 60 feet; seats 500, seats 100. Next in size: 25 x 32 feet; 23 x 35 feet; 30 x 16 feet; 32 x 40 feet; 28 x 30 feet;

30 x 40 feet; 40 x 40 feet. The smaller and most common are as follows:

16 x 18 feet.	15 x 12 feet.	22 x 16 feet.	20 x 20 feet.
14 x 17 "	14 x 17 "	20 x 20 "	18 x 24 "
12 x 15 "	20 x 20 "	18 x 20 "	20 x 20 "
30 x 15 "	16 x 18 "	14 x 20 "	19 x 20 "

The favorite operating-room is about 20 by 20 feet in dimension. In private hospitals where students are excluded a smaller operating-room will suffice. Terrazzo or tiled floors and tiled wainscoting are most desirable. As subsidiary rooms there should be provided an anesthetic room, a sterilizing room, an instrument room, a surgeon's wash-up room with conveniences, and a surgical supply room. Some hospitals have a recovery room near the operating-room; others have their recovery room off the main surgical ward. Our preference is to have it in connection with the ward.

Where the operating department is under the charge of a special nurse who has nothing to do with the treatment before and after operation, our preference is to make provision for sending the patient to a quiet room adjoining the surgical ward to which he belongs. In cases where the nurse who has charge of the patient during the operation, as well as before and after, $i. e.$, where the surgical unit system obtains, the recovery room may be near the operating-room and also near the main ward.

Operating-rooms are often ventilated by the same system which is used to ventilate the whole building. Many hospitals have a separate system for the operating-room, in which fans are used, on the Plenum and exhaust principle. There should certainly be a Plenum fan and an exhaust fan.

The favorite lighting for an operating-room is from a north window and a skylight. These are sometimes combined by the use of a window similar to that used by photographers facing the north star.

Duplicate instrument sterilizers are convenient in the

operating-room. The hot and cold water sterilizer may stand in an adjoining room, connected with the operating-room by means of pipes and taps. The dressing sterilizer should be in a separate room from the operating-room.

The tendency to-day is against the old-style operating-room, with its amphitheater arranged to seat a multitude of students. This witnessing the spectacle was not very helpful in teaching students the art of operating, and we predict will soon be a thing of the past.

There is a new operating-room in a hospital in Naples, about sixteen by sixteen. Running around its wall, about six feet from the floor, is a balcony, from the edges of which are glass partitions sloping up toward the center of the ceiling. Students leaning against a railing behind this look almost directly down upon the operation. By this arrangement they may see more of what goes on than is possible in any sort of theater.

In America most hospitals have their operating-rooms massed in one place in the hospital proper or in a separate pavilion. In the British Isles one occasionally sees an operating-room attached to each surgical service—a part of the unit. The writers are of opinion that when the cost of maintenance covering a period of years is considered, an operating-room attached to each unit will be found to work for economy. The initial outlay for instruments, furniture, etc., will be greater, of course, than that for equipping a number of operating-rooms en suite.

If there is to be any plumbing in the operating-rooms, it should be so arranged that all parts of the fixtures are get-at-able—not only the exterior, but the interior of all fixtures and pipes. The trap should be placed so high that the water-line will be within reach of the finger and made perfectly smooth. Then there can be no more danger from plumbing fixtures than from any piece of equipment.

The Hospital Unit.—The hospital unit, adverted to in a former paragraph, is a feature one notices in the old country hospitals more than he does in the United States and Canada. In several of the British hospitals we were interested in noting on one flat a large ward of some twenty patients for men, with sanitary towers at the distal end of the room; and the nurses' room, kitchen, linen closet, etc., at the near end. On the same story, not far away, similar provision is made for females suffering from similar diseases. Between the two is a small unit of three rooms—the house surgeons' quarters. If the cases are surgical, an operating-room is attached. A small clinical laboratory is also convenient. These 40 to 50 patients are looked after by one sister or head nurse; they are in charge of one house surgeon and in the service of one visiting surgeon and assistants. It is easy in such cases to keep track of the supplies which are given out to the officers in charge of such a hospital unit, and comparisons may be made weekly or monthly with other similar units. This arrangement makes for economy in administration.

Kitchens.—Kitchens are found in basements, top floors, and occasionally half-way between basement and attic. In some of the larger institutions they occupy separate buildings. The favorite location, where there are a number of pavilions, is in a separate building, in which one often finds the officers, employees, and sometimes the nurses' dining-rooms. In such case the kitchen is connected with the patient's building by corridors, the food being carried on trucks bearing jacketed hot-water food containers destined for the serving room of the ward. In the multistoried building, where the kitchen is located in the basement, a convenient arrangement is to send the food directly from the kitchen by automatic food elevators to each serving room.

One of the main arguments for the kitchen on the top floor is the avoidance of kitchen odors through the house. Situated here, it is also more easily ventilated and usually better lighted, and hence more sanitary and more easily kept clean. The offset is porterage up and down of that portion of the provisions which constitutes the waste and refuse, and the carrying up and down of the kitchen employees.

The diet-kitchen may be placed alongside the general kitchen with advantage. The proximity of these kitchens should tend to centralization of food supplies and an economy in their use. In the smaller hospitals the dietitian may supervise both.

Laundries.—In American hospitals the laundering is done sometimes in the basement, sometimes on top floors, and sometimes in separate buildings. In the larger hospitals the favorite location is a separate building, placed somewhat centrally to the adjoining buildings. In many cases it is located in the same building as are the boilers and engines, and in some instances is placed in a building which also contains the kitchen.

Provision should be made for a washer in which infected clothing and used gauze may be washed and sterilized under steam pressure.

Care of Private Ward Patients.—In our experience administration is made difficult where private ward patients are housed in the same building in which public ward patients are, particularly where they occupy the same flat and are requisitioned for by one head nurse.

Where all classes of patients are accommodated under one roof, it is better to have all private ward patients ministered to on a separate floor from the public ward patients.

Most superintendents act as hosts to the millionaire as well as to the pauper. The care of patients who pay for more than the cost of maintenance constitutes one of the modern problems of hospital management, both in America and the British Isles. Here we charge our patients about all they can afford. They leave the hospital reading the motto over our door, "I was sick and ye visited me," sometimes, with a smile.

A phase of the opposite situation was presented to one of the writers rather strongly by an executive officer of one of the large hospitals in London, England. Over the door the sign, "Supported by Voluntary Contributions Only," met the eye of the curious cis-Atlantic visitor. This gentleman informed me that a considerable number of the patients treated had sufficient money to pay or in part pay their way, but the hospital, although greatly needing the money, received nothing or very little for the care given them.

This problem of looking after the patients who can afford better accommodation than the public wards has been dealt with in the most satisfactory way by the St. Luke's Hospital, New York, and the St. Luke's Hospital, Chicago, in the erection of hotel pavilions in which all such patients are cared for by themselves. In the Province of Ontario, in Canada, the question has been best solved by the National Sanitarium Association, which has provided both in Muskoka and in Weston (a suburb of Toronto) two separate sanatorium buildings. The one at each place is used for free patients only, and for the support of these two free institutions strong appeal is made to the public for funds. The other two buildings are remote only half a mile from the corresponding free institutions, and take paying patients; the profits from the two latter institutions are applied to the maintenance of the two former.

Cost of Hospitals.—The following schedule gives the names of a number of hospitals, the number of beds, the cost of the building, and the cost per bed:

Name of Hospital.	Beds.	Cost of Building.	Approximate Cost per Patient.
Rochester City	139	$230,000	$1,654.67
State Hospital, Hazelton, Pa.	110	120,000	1,000.00
Germantown Dispensary	150	210,000	1,400.00
Cincinnati Hospital	500	900,000	1,800.00
Bridgeport, Conn.	140	224,000	1,600.00
Homeopathic (Allan)	350	600,000	1,701.42
Manhattan Ear, Eye, and Throat.	150	506,676	3,377.84
Allegheny General	350	600,000	1,742.85
Grace Hospital, Detroit	150	200,000	1,333.33
Worcester, Mass.	280	563,440	2,012.28
National Jewish	132	315,000	1,386.37
Presbyterian, Chicago	275	250,000	909.09
Lincoln, New York	500	350,000	700.00

Name of Hospital.	Beds.	Cost of Building.	Approximate Cost per Patient.
Central, Maine	80	127,937	1,599.21
St. Mark's, Salt Lake City	150	180,000	1,200.00
Newark, New Jersey	340	300,000	882.35
Clifton Springs, New York	400	300,000	750.00
Lowell, Mass	150	145,000	966.66
Wesley, Chicago	175	268,425	1,142.85
Blank Hospital, N. H.	30	30,000	1,000.00
Mount Sinai, New York	480	1,800,000	3,750.00
Grand Hospital, Colorado	85	95,000	1,117.64
St. Joseph's, Glace Bay	75	60,000	800.00
Backus Hospital	65	250,000	3,864.15
New Britton	60	38,000	633.33
Beverly Hospital	45	100,000	2,222.22
City Hospital, St. Louis	600	395,424	659.04
Meth.-Epis. Hospital, Brooklyn	200	800,000	4,000.00
Charlotte Hospital	40	150,000	3,750.00
Lacrosse Hospital	51	391,183	7,670.25

This represents an average cost of about $2000 per bed. With the advance in price of building material and labor, the cost of construction to-day would average, we believe, about $3000 per bed.

Questions In Re Hospital Construction.—In gathering material for this article, one of the writers sent out the following questions, the publication of which may be of interest:

1. Name of hospital.

2. At what date did the erection of your hospital commence?

3. What is the estimated cost of your hospital?
   (a) Site.
   (b) Building.
   (c) Equipment.

4. How many patients does it accommodate?

5. What is the location of your hospital with respect to your city?

6. How do you like it?

7. What is the acreage of your grounds?

8. What is the type of construction of your hospital? Do you like it?
   Can you send me a picture of it?

9. In which direction do your wards run, how is the light admitted, and from which direction does the sunlight enter during the various portions of the day?

10. What is the average number of beds in each of your general wards for the poorer classes?

11. What, in your opinion, should be the number of beds in a general ward?

12. Would you kindly inclose a rough sketch showing a general ward and its dependencies (bath-rooms, sink room, laboratory, etc.), giving dimensions?
    (a) Medical.
    (b) Surgical.

13. Do you have private and semi-private wards?

14. Do you approve of them in a general hospital?

15. Please state briefly your system of ventilation?

16. How do you like it?

17. What other plan, if any, would you prefer, and why?

18. How is your hospital heated and what are the virtues of your system?

19. What artificial light do you use, and why do you prefer it?

20. What sort of floors are in your building?

21. What is your favorite floor, and why?
    (a) Operating-rooms?
    (b) General wards?

22. What is your favorite preparation for walls?
    (a) For operating-rooms?
    (b) For general wards?

23. What is your roof made of?

24. What are its virtues and defects?

25. Where is your kitchen, and what provision in construction is made for sending the food quickly to the wards and obviating kitchen odors in the building?

26. Would you send us a plan of an ideal kitchen, showing its position in relation to the room for receiving food supplies?

27. Where are your dining-rooms located with reference to the kitchen?

28. What is the location of your officers', servants',

nurses', and convalescent patients' dining-room in relation to the kitchen?

29. How many operating-rooms have you, and are they adequate for your purpose?

30. How many accessory rooms have you to your main operating theater, and how are they located with reference to it?

31. How is your operating theater lighted?

32. How is it ventilated?

33. What is its size?

34. What is the relation of your operating-room to—
   (a) Out-patient department?
   (b) The emergency department?

35. What would be your idea of having these three more or less amalgamated if you were building a new hospital?

36. Is your out-patient department in a separate building?

37. Is your preference to have such a department in a separate building or in the main building of the hospital?

38. Would you inclose a rough sketch of what you consider an ideal arrangement for receiving 100 out-patients a day (who suffer from general complaints), showing how you would separate the various rooms?

39. Is your obstetric department in a separate building?

40. Are the gynecologic patients in a separate building? If not, would you prefer it so?

41. What provision is made for patients suffering from diseases of the eye?

42. Do you have separate wards for ear, nose, and throat cases?

43. What arrangement have you made for treating erysipelas, whooping-cough, chicken-pox, and the minor contagious diseases?

   (a) Patients developing the diseases in the hospital?
   (b) Patients brought to the hospital with them?

44. What arrangement, if any, have you made for treating scarlet fever?

GENERAL HOSPITAL FOR ONE HUNDRED PATIENTS

45. What for diphtheria and measles?
46. Have you made any provisions for tuberculosis?
    (a) Cases developing in your wards?
    (b) Cases from outside?
47. What provision have you made for convalescent patients?
48. What provision do you think should be made?
49. What system of calls have you installed and how do you like it?
50. What provision do you think should be made?
51. What special provisions have you made to minimize the amount of noise?
52. Would you give us an idea, by sketch if possible, of an ideal arrangement for administration offices to accommodate a superintendent, a superintendent of the training-school, an admitting officer, and an accountant and their assistants?
53.. What provision in your construction have you made for the collection (and storage until removal) of garbage?
54. Where do you house your domestics?
55. Why do you favor this plan?
56. Where is your laundry, and do you like its location?
57. Where are your pathologic laboratories?
58. Where do you think they should be placed in a teaching school to be most convenient for the use of—
    (a) Internes?
    (b) Students?
59. What provision have you made for the disposal of the dead, pending removal of remains?
60. Please let us know of any faults or defects in the construction of your hospital and also please tell us of any special ideas you have in respect to hospital construction generally.

DESCRIPTION OF PLANS OF 100-BED HOSPITAL

As a site for a building required for 100 patients we would suggest an area of at least three or four acres, sloping slightly toward the south. If there be no natural woods on the north side, trees should be planted so as to form, in future, a protection from the cold winds from that direction. If the site be suburban, it would be well to secure 25 to 50 acres in area adjoining it as a farm, on the rear of which should be a commodious farmhouse with barns and stables nearby. This piece of ground, in charge of a practical man, would be very valuable to the hospital in producing supplies of vegetables, fruit, and grain needed. The poultry, pigs, and other animals required for meat might also be kept, the pigs being fed on the refuse food and slops from the hospital. The cinders and ashes from the boilers of the hospital might be used for the construction of drives, pathways, etc. Near the farmhouse a small convalescent home, with room for six or eight patients, might well be provided. The regular hospital employees, many of whom have no homes other than the hospital, and who perform long hours of duty, might be occasionally transferred to the convalescent home or farmhouse for recuperation.

In the group of buildings for which sketches have been prepared to illustrate a 100-bed hospital, the following points have been kept in mind:

(1) A place where as many natural advantages can be secured as possible.

(2) A set of buildings to treat as many sorts of diseases as possible, including contagious.

(3) Provision for ample out-of-door treatment.

(4) Provision to save steps of nurses and other hospital workers.

(5) A minimum number of utilities consistent with efficiency.

(6) Provision for special treatment of medical cases.

It is assumed that the site is practically level, with street to the north.

The group (Fig. 20) is planned so that the center of administration and the center of domestic service is so placed that the service is rendered with the least outlay of strength on the part of the attendants.

Underground passages connect all buildings, furnishing connections for the carrying of food and supplies and for pipes and conduits.

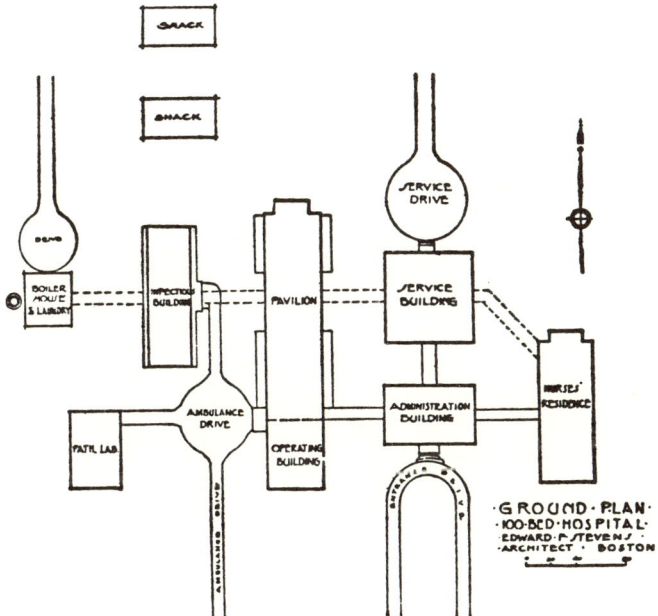

Fig. 20.—Ground plan, 100-bed hospital.

Administration Building.—In the center of the group, facing north, is the administration building. This is three stories high, with basement. On the ground floor (Fig. 21) are located the main business office, the superintendent's office, the waiting room, the medical library, and across the corridor from the superintendent's office is the office for the superintendent of nurses. This office controls the corridor to the nurses' home. A room for the visiting staff and a toilet complete the floor. A main stairway and elevator control the upper stories.

On the basement floor (Fig. 22) are the rooms for male employees, a recreation room, a staff dining-room, and serving room. Basement corridors connect to the kitchen, nurses' home, and pavilion.

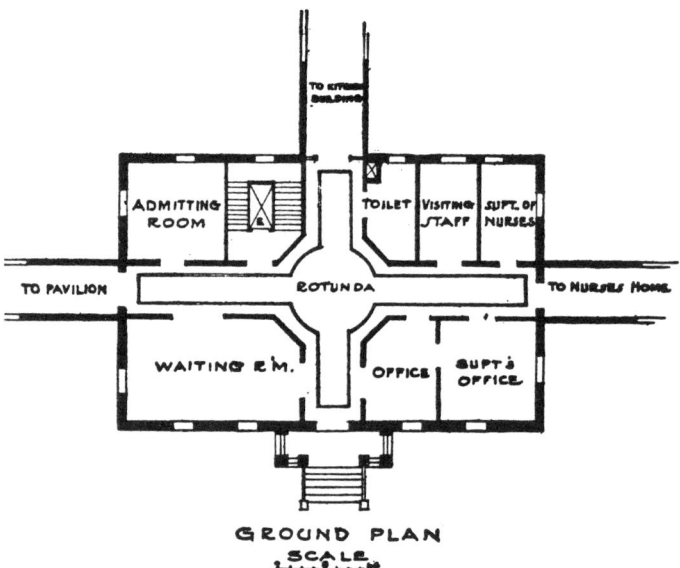

Fig. 21.—Administration building, ground floor.

The first floor is devoted to the maternity department (Fig. 23) with a 6-bed ward on the west side of the building, a private room, sterilizing and toilet rooms, diet-kitchen, a delivery room facing north, a baby room with toilet, blanket warmer, and supply closets. The delivery room and baby room are located on a private corridor and shut off from the other portion of the floor.

The children's department (Fig. 24) is located on the second floor, consisting of a 12-bed ward, with balcony on

GENERAL HOSPITAL FOR ONE HUNDRED PATIENTS

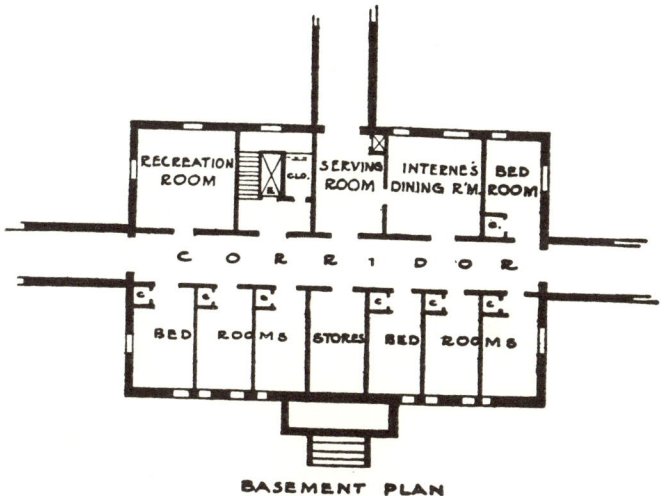

Fig. 22.—Administration building, basement plan.

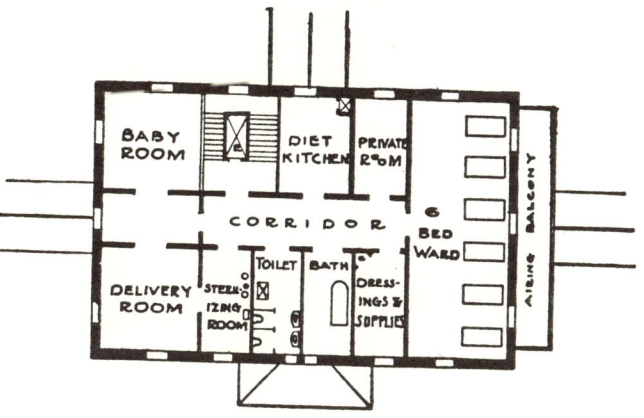

Fig. 23.—Administration building, first-floor plan.

the west, private room, surgical dressing room, a room for nurses and supplies, and a diet-kitchen. On this floor are

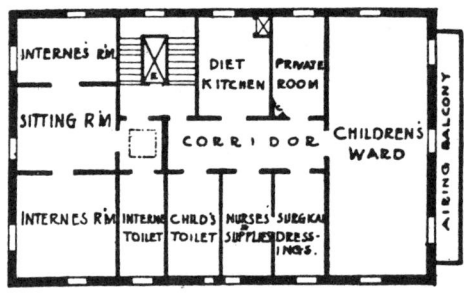

SECOND FLOOR PLAN
SCALE

Fig. 24.—Administration building, second-floor plan.

provided rooms for the internes, consisting of two chambers, a sitting- and bath-room.

Operating Building.—The operating building is located at the north of the pavilion, separated from it by the

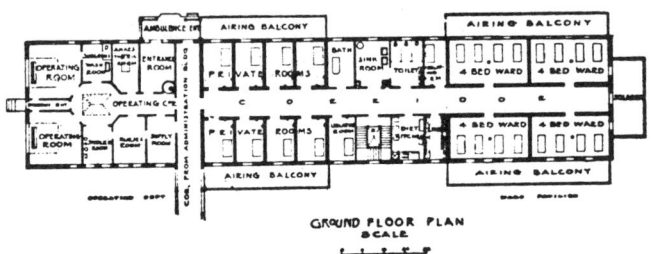

GROUND FLOOR PLAN
SCALE

Fig. 25.—Pavilion, ground-floor plan.

main cross corridor. The ambulance entrance is so arranged that a patient can either be taken to the operating building or to the pavilion through the main corridor.

Two operating-rooms (Fig. 25) are provided, each with north light. Visitors' entrance between the two rooms enables visiting surgeons or students to enter the room without passing through the working corridor. The sterilizing room, nurses' room, instrument and supply room, the surgeons' scrub-up room, and the anesthetizing room are located around an octagonal rotunda.

In the basement of the building (Fig. 26) is the outpatients' department, consisting of waiting-room, eye and ear treatment room, and extra storeroom. A circular stair connects this department with the operating department.

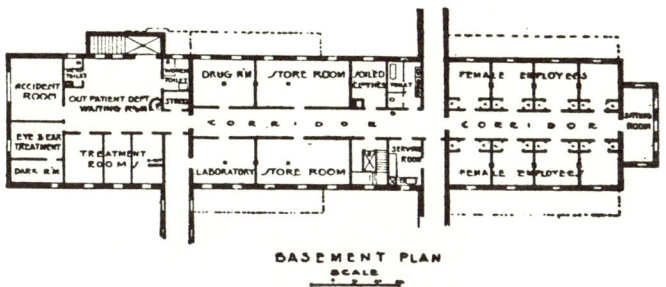

Fig. 26.—Pavilion, basement plan.

Ward Pavilion.—The pavilion is arranged in three sections—a central section containing staircase, elevator, and all dependencies, and at either side wards for patients. This building is planned on the terraced pavilion idea to a limited extent, the roof of the first story forming an airing balcony for the second and a narrower balcony projecting from the third.

Ten rooms are provided on the ground floor (Fig. 26), with closets, and at the south end of the building are four 6-bed wards. This main floor is intended for patients paying private and semi-private ward rates. One of the 4-bed wards may be utilized for the treatment of typhoid fever. The room indicated as an isolating room next the 4-bed ward on this floor should be fitted as a bath room, and the toilet room should be divided, so as to provide for both sexes.

The medical cases (Fig. 28), public ward, may occupy the first story—men in south end, women in the north; and the second story may be devoted to surgery. If desired,

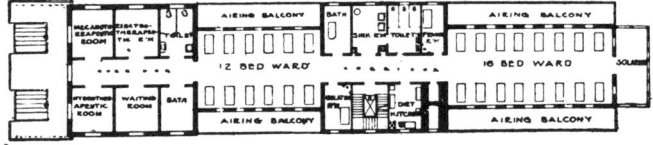

FIRST FLOOR PLAN
SCALE

Fig. 27.—Pavilion, first-floor plan.

the male patients, medical and surgical, may be put on one flat and the female on another.

The dependencies consist of a large sink room containing the sink, slop hopper, sterilizing hopper, utensil holders, etc.; a large bath, with wide door, a toilet, linen room,

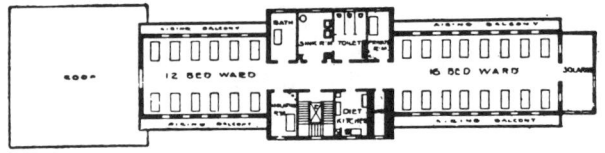

SECOND FLOOR PLAN
SCALE

Fig. 28.—Pavilion, second-floor plan.

diet-kitchen, and isolating rooms, inclosed staircase, and elevator.

The arrangement of all these dependencies is largely suggestive and may be altered to suit the individual idea.

The first and second stories have the dependencies arranged much in the same way as they are on the ground floor. These stories each contain one 12-bed ward and one 16-bed ward on each floor. The third floor is simply the central portion of the pavilion, and consists of small wards with necessary utility rooms for cases requiring special segregation.

To the north of the medical flat (Fig. 27) rooms have been provided for hydrotherapy, electric treatment, and for exercises, this to bear somewhat the same relation to the medical service as the operating suite does to the surgical. This department may be reached from the ward south of the medical dependencies by way of the balcony on the west side of the flat, which would be closed in the winter.

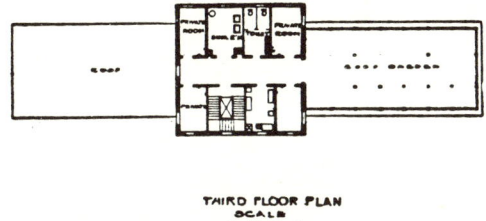

Fig. 29.—Pavilion, third-floor plan.

In the basement (Fig. 26) there are provided toilets, store-rooms, laboratory and drug rooms, room for soiled clothes, and serving room for the wards above. The elevator extends to this floor.

This main pavilion should have walls heavy enough to permit of enlargement by the addition of one or two stories if need be.

The Isolating Building.—The isolating building is planned to be about 60 feet distant from the main pavilion, and is connected with the other group by the basement corridor only. Through this corridor the food for the isolating building will be carried, with basement serving-room, which would only have a lift connection.

In the basement of this building would be the disinfecting rooms, the clothing storage, and such other storage as would be needed for this department.

On the first floor (Fig. 30) would be located, centrally, the main entrance and admitting room, both of which would open to the outside; the general office for the nurse in charge and for consultations; a diet-kitchen and linen room.

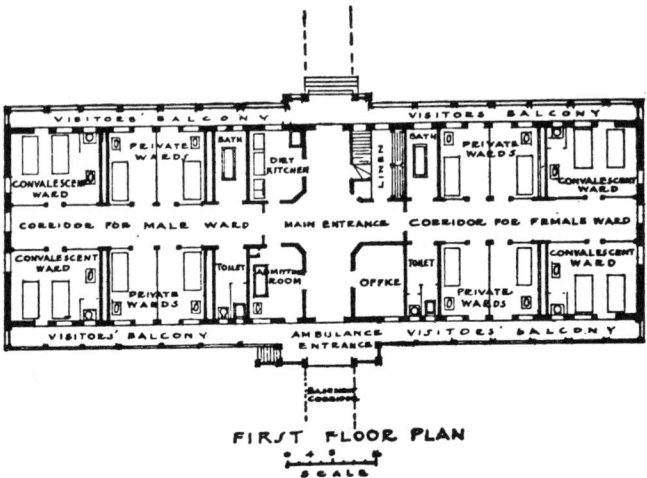

Fig. 30.—Infectious building, first-floor plan.

This building is so planned that any infectious case can be safely cared for without danger of cross infection, being planned on the principle of the Pasteur Hospital at Paris.

The admitting room will answer for *all* patients, giving time to properly disinfect the room between succeeding cases. The patient is relieved of his street clothes, which are dropped into disinfecting solutions in the disinfecting room in the basement. After the bath the hospital clothes are put on, the patient placed on the wheel stretcher, covered with a disinfected sheet, and wheeled into one of the isolating rooms.

These rooms are much like the regular private ward

except that the entire wall toward the corridor is of glass, as well as the partition adjoining the next room. This throws each room into view, the same as if the patients were in an open ward. The nurse can have the same surveillance over the patients, and still they are completely isolated each from the other. Each of these isolation rooms contains a door and a window leading to a balcony, as well as a door to the corridor. This balcony serves two purposes:

First, it enables the parents and friends of the patients to visit their friends and hold communication with them from the outside through the glass, and—

Second, in the case of a particularly malignant disease, the door to the corridor can be sealed and the patient can be approached from the balcony door only.

Besides the bed, each room contains a sink with large faucets from which a portable tub can be filled, and a drain in the floor where the tub can be discharged.

Convalescent wards for three or four beds are provided for the care of convalescents who are recovering from the same disease.

Of course, all food receptacles must be sterilized, all food being brought from the hospital kitchen through the connecting tunnel.

The male patients are placed at one end and the female at the other. One diet-kitchen, one linen closet, and one admitting room suffice for the entire building.

Nurses' quarters are placed directly above this ward for the nurses while on contagious duty. The floors of this building should be of terrazzo or some non-absorbent material; even more than ordinary care should be provided to eliminate ledges or fouling places; all doors should be smooth, and the same care taken about fixtures, hardware, etc., as is taken in other hospital wards.

Pathologic Building.—The pathologic building for this scheme is comparatively small, located as indicated on the lot plan near the operating building (Fig. 31). In this building are located the surgical, pathologic, and bacteriologic laboratories, the autopsy and morgue, and small chapel.

Room is provided on the second story of this building for the male help, consisting of four bed-rooms with accommodations for seven male help, together with bath-room.

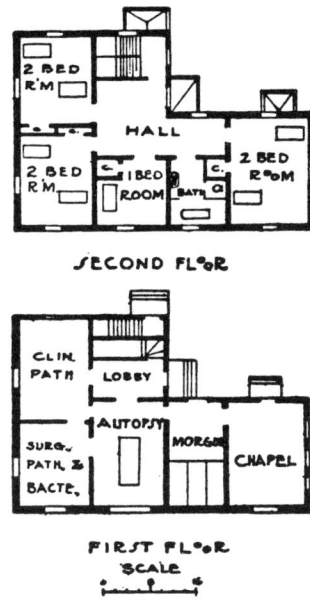

Fig. 31.—Pathologic building.

Boiler House and Laundry.—The boiler house and laundry are placed on ground which is supposed to be somewhat lower, on a line with the infectious and pavilion buildings. In this is provided the heating plant for the building, electric-light plant, if one is contemplated, incinerators, and such other engineering fixtures as would apply. (Fig. 32).

On the second story of this building would be the institution laundry. Here ample provision has been made for washing of all clothing, dressings, and all other material as needed.

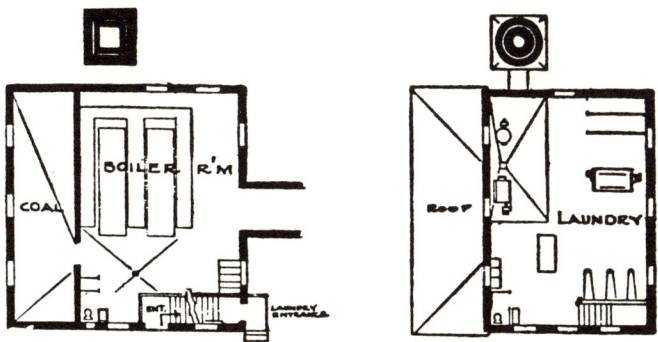

Fig. 32.—Plan of boiler house.

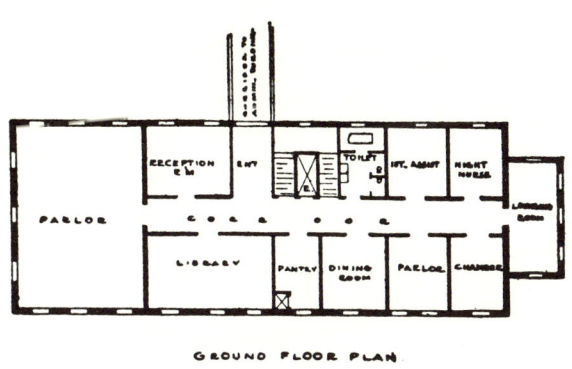

Fig. 33.—Nurses' residence, ground floor plan.

Nurses' Home.—The nurses' home is situated parallel with the main pavilion, flanking the administration building on the west. This provides the housing for 33 nurses.

On the ground floor (Fig. 33) is the main parlor and reception room, a library, a small pantry, or diet-kitchen, the superintendent's dining-room, and suites of rooms for the superintendent, assistant superintendent, and night nurse, with toilets, etc.

On the first floor (Fig. 34) are accommodations for 18 nurses in single rooms, together with toilets, sitting-room, etc.

An isolation department is provided on the second floor (Fig. 34), which occupies only the central portion of the

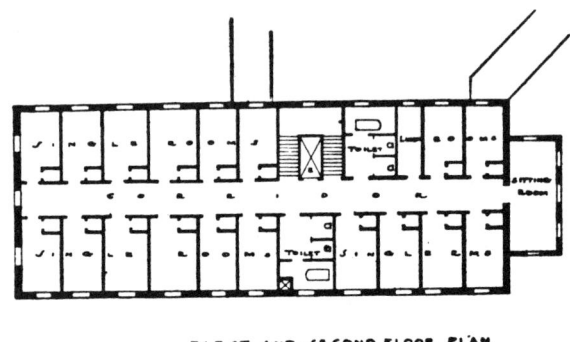

Fig. 34.—Nurses' residence, first- and second-floor plan.

building. From this central portion access is had to the roof-garden on either end of the building.

In the basement (Fig. 35) is located the central nurses' dining-room, the serving room, administration building, class room, petty laundry, housemaid's room, toilets, etc.

From this building a connecting corridor leads to the kitchen.

Alcoholic Ward.—One-story shack wards are provided for the occasional alcoholic and neurasthenic patients, with four private rooms, a nurse's room, serving and toilet rooms.

GENERAL HOSPITAL FOR ONE HUNDRED PATIENTS **143**

Tuberculosis Shacks.—For the care of pulmonary tuberculosis, one or two small "shacks" are provided, each

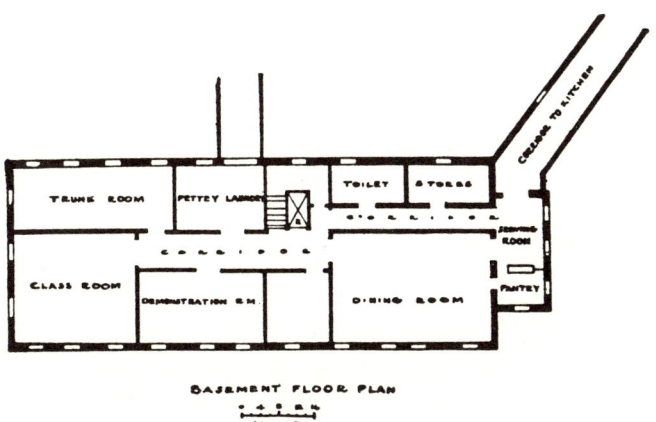

Fig. 35.—Nurses' residence, basement floor plan.

containing from four to six beds. Each of these shacks would contain a dressing-room of sufficient capacity for

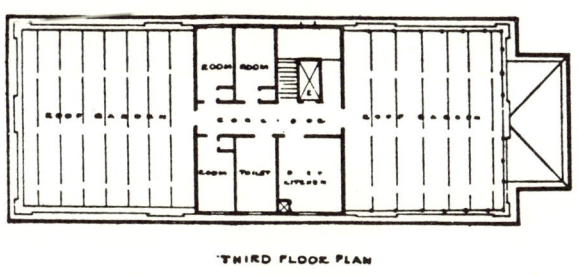

Fig. 36.—Nurses' residence, third-floor plan.

dressing, together with toilet rooms, shower-baths, and a nurses' room, the indoor and outdoor area of the shack being about equal, so that the patients can be kept under the open sky except in stormy weather, when they can be wheeled back under the shelter.

Service Building.—In this hospital the writers have conceived the idea of having on one floor, within easy reach of central ranges and cooking apparatus, all supplies,

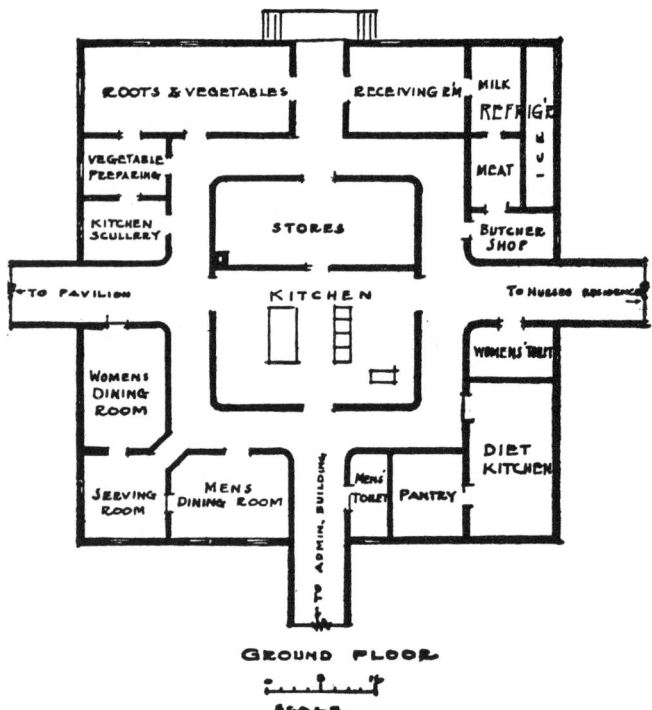

Fig. 37.—Service building, ground floor.

service dining-rooms, serving rooms, pantries, etc. (Fig. 37), and have planned the building approximately 70 feet square.

The main kitchen and main store-room occupy the portion which in a Spanish castle is occupied by the pateo, but in this case the walls of the kitchen are carried some 6 feet above the roof of the outer portion, thus giving a high, airy kitchen, well lighted on all sides, and thoroughly ventilated.

Around this kitchen and store-room is a corridor 6 feet wide, with various rooms in close connection to the main kitchen and service portion. The service entrance is at the south side of the building, the connection to the nurses' home on the west and to the pavilion on the east, while the connection to the administration building is on the north.

It is planned to place this building low, that is, with the connecting corridors from the service building entering the basement of the other buildings. This enables quick service in every direction, so that the greatest possible chance is given for serving patients with hot meals.

Around this kitchen and store-room are located, first, the receiving room, which is at the service entrance, with refrigerators and store-rooms connected, a general diet-kitchen and pantry, the dining-rooms for female and male employees, with serving room to same, kitchen scullery and vegetable room, underneath which is provided root cellar, and such toilets and waiting rooms as a building of this kind would require.

The building being low, only one story in height, it would not cast any shadow or shut off the sunlight from the rooms in the administration building. As only basement corridors connect this building, there is nothing to break the light and air from any of the other buildings.

The floors of this building would naturally be of slate or tile, with the same rounded corners and bases that would occur in the hospital proper.

Electric Work.—It is proposed to light this entire group by electricity, preferably by a private plant in the boiler house, which would show practical economy both in lighting and running of elevators and laundry machinery, and any other mechanical use to which electricity would be put.

For the patients' rooms, reflecting ceiling lights are suggested. This gives a soft, subdued light throughout the room, without any direct rays coming into the patient's eyes. For brighter local light, the bedside light on a flexible cord makes it possible either for examination or for reading, while at the same time it only brightly illuminates around one spot.

For general corridor lighting, ceiling lights are perhaps the most satisfactory, as they light every nook and corner of the walls and ceiling.

For the operating and surgical dressing rooms some form of reflecting lights should be used, the writers preferring some movable fixture which, when not in use, can be swung away from over the operating table by a crane or in some other way.

The use of the intensified arc lamps is coming into more or less favor for operating-room lights.

For nurses' signals, internes' calls, etc., electric lights have been found to be most satisfactory. One of the simplest devices is to have a miniature red electric light over the head of each ward bed and over the door of each private room, duplicate lights being placed in a group at the nurses' headquarters, and if, for any reason, it is wished to have an extra check on the answering of calls, still another set of lights can be placed in the superintendent's office. To signal the nurse, the patient presses the button, which is connected by a flexible cord to the wall plug. Should the nurse be in the ward itself, she is signaled by the appearance of the red light; if in the corridor or in the nurses' room, the lights there give her notice. To extinguish the light, the nurse must go to the point from which the signal is given, pressing another button either in the hand receptacle or in the wall plate, as may be desired. In this way only can the lights be extinguished.

For the calls for the internes, a similar device is arranged and put in conspicuous places in the various corridors of the buildings, the interne being notified by the pressing of a button at the office, the light exposed indicating the interne who is wanted. Seeing his signal, he goes to the nearest telephone and gets his orders from the office.

Both the nurses' and internes' calls are absolutely noiseless, and do not attract the attention of any patient who may be quietly sleeping in private or public wards.

Intercommunicating telephones should be arranged from all nurses' headquarters and working parts of the hospital. For the private rooms it is desirable to put in receptacles where the outside telephones can be connected, for the use of such patients as wish to use the outside telephone. This all passing through the hospital switchboard, calls can be checked off and charged in the ordinary way.

A considerable portion of the main text of the first portion of this article was contributed by one of the writers to the American Hospital Association, and appears in its transactions for the year 1908.

CHAPTER VI

THE FURNISHINGS OF A 100-BED HOSPITAL

By Emma A. Anderson and Louise M. Coleman

While the furnishing of a hospital should be plain and substantial, there is no reason why it should not be attractive as well. In our zeal for asepsis we have almost made a fetich of it. Even in the wards there is room for rather more latitude in favor of pleasing surroundings than was once thought to be the case. The walls are usually painted a soft, neutral color, making a pretty background for growing plants and cut flowers. These are decorative, and far more pleasing to the sick person than even the most beautiful picture, which never changes, but must be looked at day after day.

The Wards.—When we think hospital, we think beds. Indeed, we often speak of a hospital as so many beds. There is no other one article in the whole equipment so deserving of the expenditure of time and money and thought. They should be made of the best welded sheet steel-tubing, the seams brazed with brass to prevent contraction and expansion and the consequent cracking of the enamel. The side rails of the spring should be of tubing of not less than $1\frac{1}{4}$ inches in diameter. The usual size of a hospital bed is 3 feet wide by 6 feet 6 inches long. The height is rather more than that of the home bed. Twenty-six inches to the top of the spring, or, 31 inches to the top of the mattress is a good height. The iron rods at the head should run horizontally rather than vertically. This enables the patient who is sufficiently strong to pull himself up in bed by grasping the rods. The rods should also be close enough together to

THE FURNISHINGS OF A 100-BED HOSPITAL   **149**

prevent the mattress from slipping through at either end. It is a mistake to have the foot of the bed too high—a couple of inches at most above the mattress is enough. The low foot-end facilitates the moving of stretcher patients in and out, and is more convenient if an extension apparatus has to be applied. The National wire spring is best, provided it has a tension of sufficient strength and stiffness. To prevent sagging, the angle ends should be slightly

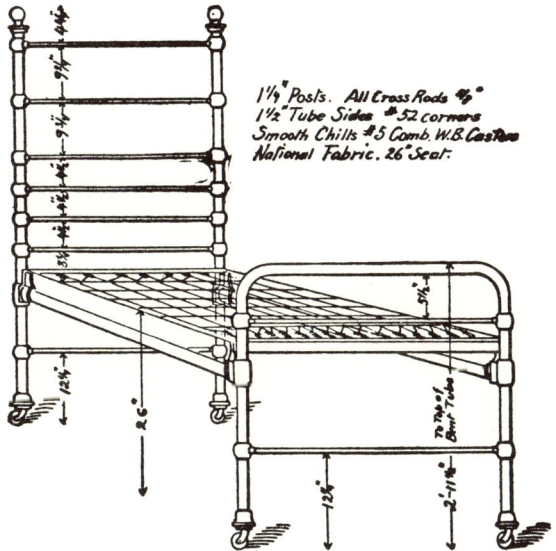

Fig. 38.—A hospital bed.

curved outward, thus increasing the tension gradually from the sides to the center. If the links of the National wire spring are properly closed, there is no danger of their catching and tearing sheets. In these days of outdoor sleeping one must think of the possibility of rust. If the entire spring has been dipped in pure tin after it is completed, it will prevent rusting. Another point worth noting is the proper height of the spring. If it is raised more than 3 or 3½ inches above the bed, it increases the leverage and has a tendency to bow the rails down. The best beds have the side rods cambered or crowned a little to prevent bowing.

Castors.—The question of castors is not an easy one to solve. The rubber tires soon wear out. The wooden castor mars the floor, and so does the leather castor. The glass shoes work very satisfactorily. They can be slipped into the socket in place of the castor, and the bed pushes easily over the hard-wood floor. They break occasionally, but are not expensive to renew.

Mattresses.—There is no satisfactory substitute for a hair mattress, and nothing but the best South American hair cut from live horses' manes should be used. There are various ways of cheapening the initial cost of a hair mattress. For instance, the hair from dead horses is used, but it will not hold the curl and is not resilient. Hair from horses' fetlocks, from cows' tails, goats' hair, and hogs' bristles are used, but these should all be avoided in a hospital mattress.

Another great advantage in using the best material is that the mattress can be remade and the hair picked up and sterilized. About two pounds of new hair will need to be added, making such a mattress absolutely as good as new. As the mattress spreads with use, it should not be quite as large as the bed. For a 3-foot bed, get a mattress 2 feet 11 by 6 feet 3, weighing not less than 28 pounds. For the covering there is nothing better than the old-fashioned blue-and-white striped Amoskeag ticking. It pays to protect a nice hair mattress with a slip-cover of heavy unbleached cotton. This cover should be shrunken before it is made, and the open end tied with tapes, not buttoned.

The frequent and necessary brushing of a hospital mattress with a whisk-broom will eventually pull out the tuftings, allowing the ticking to wrinkle. The slip-cover obviates this.

Every bed must be protected by a rubber sheet. There

THE FURNISHINGS OF A 100-BED HOSPITAL 151

are various kinds, colors, and qualities. But here again the best is none too good. There is a double-faced maroon colored rubber sheeting that has proved, on the whole, satisfactory. It should be at least two feet wider than the bed in order to tuck in smoothly and firm, on either

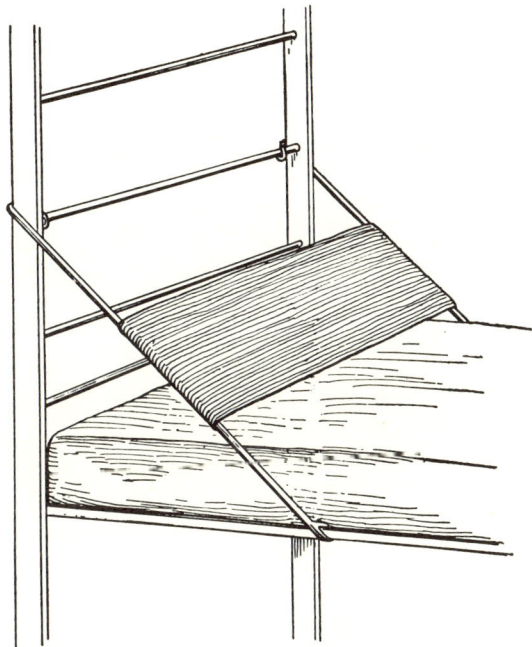

Fig. 39.—Bed-rest.

side, and should extend about 4 feet lengthwise of bed, or from the chin to well below the knees of patient.

Feather pillows are usually about 18 x 20 inches and weigh about 3 pounds. Only the best steam-cleansed live-geese feathers should be used.

Hair pillows are not usually quite as large as the feather pillows. A hair pillow 18 x 28 inches will fit the same pillow-case as the 20 x 30 inch feather pillow. Two and a half pounds of hair is enough.

Every nurse knows how much she can add to the comfort of a patient if she has a number of little pillows to tuck into hollow places. If these are of uniform size all over the hospital they are no trouble. Thirteen by 20 inches is about the size.

Bed-rests.—The illustration (Fig. 39) shows a bed-rest made of iron pipe. The iron hooks should be covered with rubber to save wearing off the enamel of the bed. These

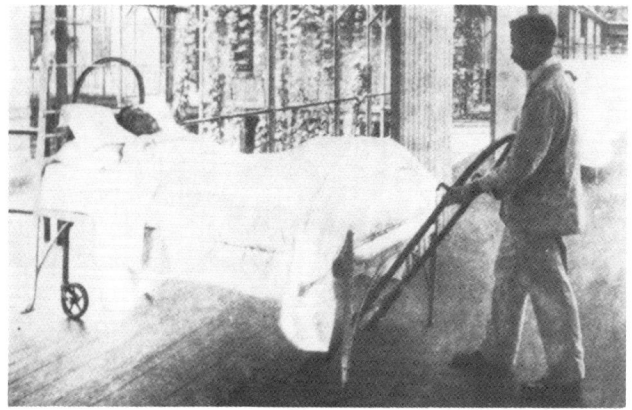

Fig. 40.—Bed-truck in use. Massachusetts General Hospital, Boston, Massachusetts.

hooks engage the horizontal rod of the head-end of the bed and the side rail. The filling is of canvas tightly stretched across. This bed-rest is not on the market, but can be made by any steam-fitter.

Bed-trucks.—The following is taken from the pamphlet which the Massachusetts General Hospital has published on "Home-made Hospital Furniture." The bed-trucks are used for moving the beds any distance—either out on the veranda or from one ward to another. There are two trucks, one with fixed fork to the wheels, the other has

THE FURNISHINGS OF A 100-BED HOSPITAL 153

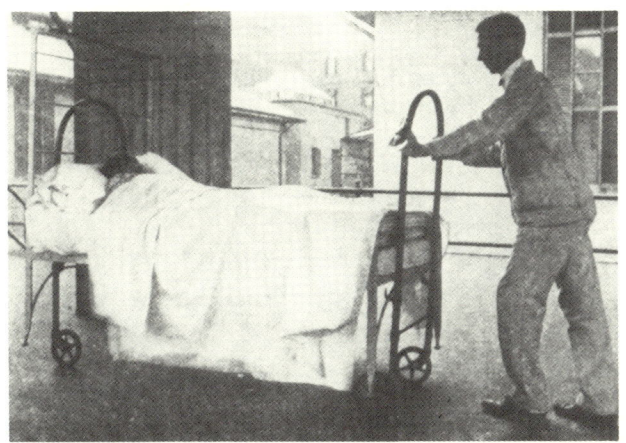

Fig. 41.—Moving a patient to the balcony. Note convenient bed-truck. Massachusetts General Hospital, Boston, Massachusetts.

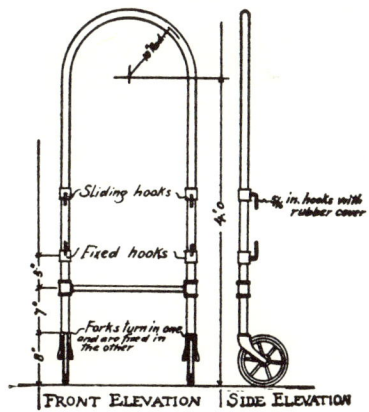

Fig. 42.—Bed-trucks. One truck has fixed forks; the other revolving 1-inch iron pipe; ⅜-inch iron cross-bar, cast-iron wheels, rubber tires.

wheels on pivot. The one with fixed wheels is placed under the lower end of the bed. The other is clamped to the head-end, converting the bed into a truck. The bed is steered from the head-end.

Four of the large-size feather pillows for each bed is not too generous an allowance. Twelve sheets and pillow-slips is a fair number, but if the clean laundry cannot be supplied often, more must be provided. Six blankets for each bed will be required, besides a supply of cotton blankets, to be used in giving bed-baths, and a number of colored blankets for the out-of-doors patients or the con-

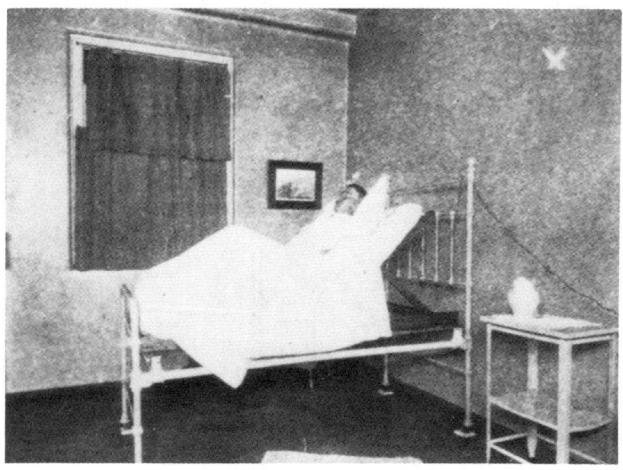

Fig. 43.—Home-made frame, to be used when Fowler position is required. Minnequa Hospital, Pueblo, Colorado.

valescent when he has been ordered chair and blankets in the ward.

Sheets should be two yards by three yards after they are finished, and pillow-slips 22 inches by 38 inches finished.

White dimity spreads dress the beds prettily, are no heavier than a sheet, and not more difficult to wash.

The ward screen is preferably of enameled iron frame with two folding arms. The base must be heavy and provided with castors or the metal or glass shoes that slide

THE FURNISHINGS OF A 100-BED HOSPITAL 155

easily over a polished floor without marring it. The filling or covering of screens should be of white cotton cloth hung upon detachable curtain-rods. These curtains can be easily removed and laundered, and if kept spotlessly clean, are very attractive. More attention should be paid to comfortable bed-side chairs than is usually the case. They should be of wood, with arms, a fairly deep seat, with legs that are not too long. There should be also one or

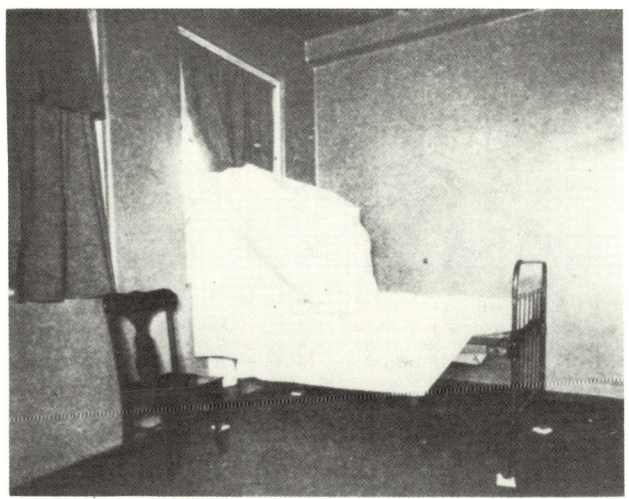

Fig. 44.—Room in ward showing Knopf window-tent. Minnequa Hospital, Pueblo, Colorado.

two reclining chairs with high backs in each ward. A steamer chair is a useful addition. If there is room for one or two wicker lounges, they will prove a great comfort to the weary convalescent. Foot-stools should also be provided. In a surgical ward, a dressing table will be needed where the necessary supply of ward dressings, solutions, instruments, etc., may be kept conveniently at hand.

Chart-holders of white enameled iron are good looking

and easily kept clean. In most hospitals the charts are no longer hung over the patient's bed, but are kept at a convenient place for the physician to scrutinize as he enters the ward.

The bed-side table of enameled iron with glass or enamel top is, on the whole, as satisfactory as any. There are those with a screened shelf which are perhaps preferable to those with a drawer. The objection to the glass shelf is, of course, the certainty of its being broken when a hot

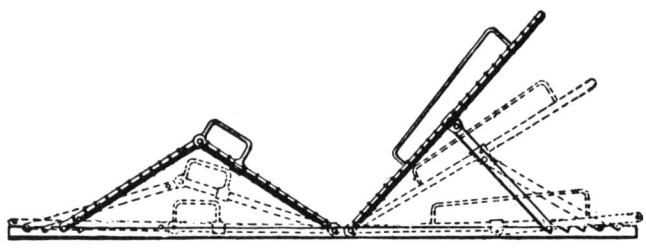

Fig. 45.—Adjustable bed. This device is designed to keep patients in a particular upright or incline sitting position. It is useful especially in the treatment of peritonitis and abdominal cases. The bed is made entirely of metal. It is intended to rest on the springs of a standard ward bed, and any mattress of soft material can be bent and used on this bed, which is 6 feet long and 33 inches wide.

The back-rest is separately adjustable, while the seat and leg-rest are adjustable together; the steel wire is mounted on metal frames, which are adjustable on bed-frame, made of steel angle-bars, enameled white, and is perfectly sanitary. The construction permits the bed and the patient to be laid flat, or to be set to any angle of elevation desired, and the bed holds the patient in a permanent position, without risk of slipping.

poultice-pail or bath-tub is put upon it. Neat-looking asbestos mats covered with flannelette on one side and bound with tape are to be found in the kitchen furnishing stores. If these are provided for the nurses' use, many a polished wood or glass table-top will be saved.

A small three-shelf book-case on castors, filled with good books would take up very little space in a ward. It could be wheeled up to the bedside, and the pleasure that it would give the patient to be able to select his own book would be out of all proportion to the time and trouble it

THE FURNISHINGS OF A 100-BED HOSPITAL 157

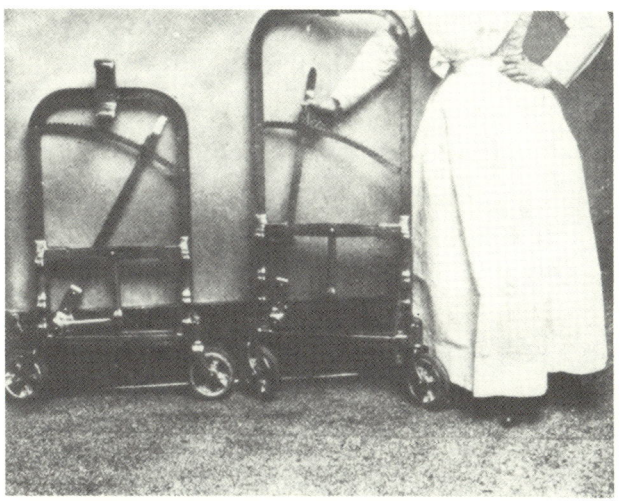

Fig. 46.—Bed-lifters, showing method of movement. Royal Victoria Hospital, Montreal, Canada.

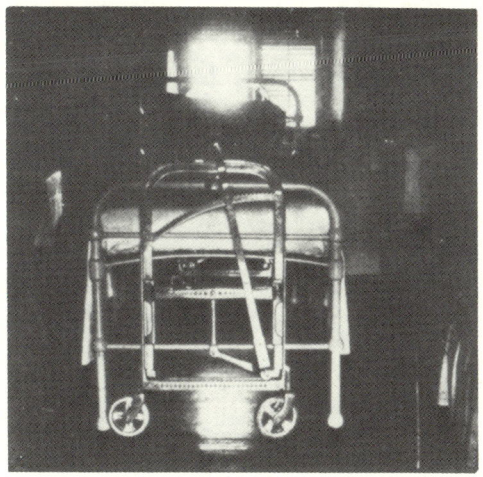

Fig. 47.—Bed-lifters attached to bed. Royal Victoria Hospital.

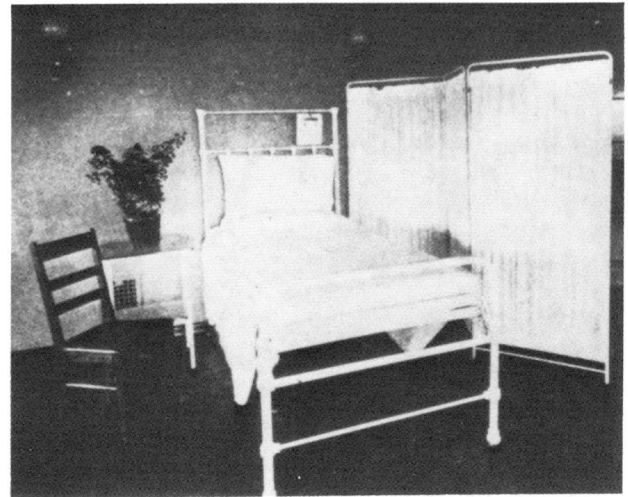

Fig. 48.—Corner of hospital ward, showing bed and screen.

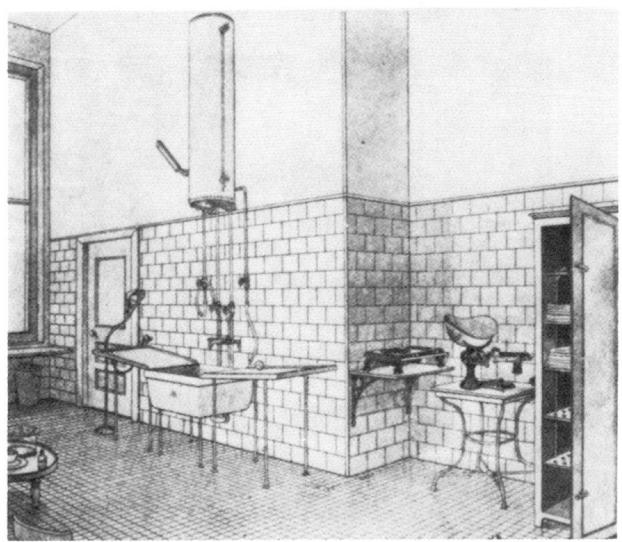

Fig. 49.—Corner of babies' room.   Presbyterian Hospital, New York.

would cost. This is the sort of thing that the Woman's Auxiliary of the hospital would delight in supplying if it were suggested.

Maternity Department.—The furnishings of a ward for maternity cases differ in few respects from those in the general hospital. The private rooms are furnished the same, with the addition of a crib for the baby. There

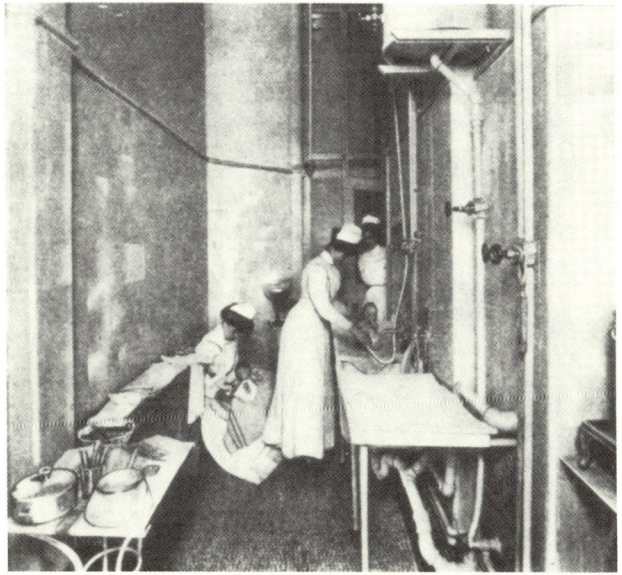

Fig. 50.—Babies' bath-room. Maternity department, Presbyterian Hospital, New York.

should be a nursery in connection with the maternity ward, and in connection with the nursery there should be a linen closet and utility room, where everything used for the babies may be kept entirely separate from those of the patients. The nursery should contain, besides the cribs, only two low chairs and a large table low enough to be serviceable to the nurse when seated. The table should be furnished with scales and trays. The ordinary scoop scales such as are used by grocers are much more accurate than the fanciful basket scales usually provided for babies. The trays contain pins, thermometers (bath and clinical), boric solution and powder, and argyrol. The cut shown is of a crib used at the Wesson Maternity Hospital, Spring-

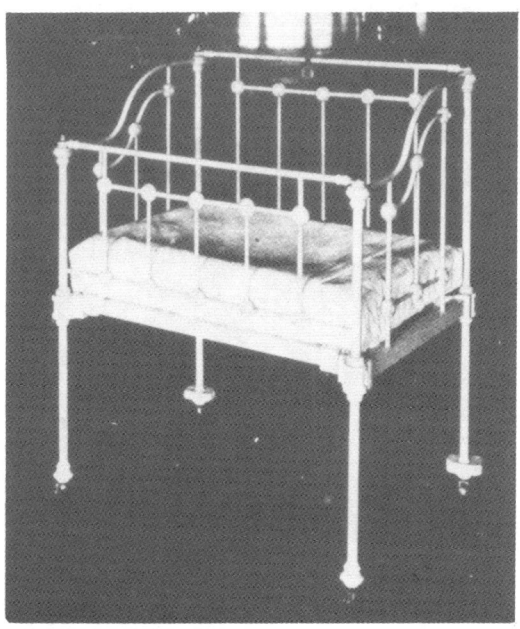

Fig. 51.—Baby's cot. Wesson Maternity Hospital, Springfield, Massachusetts.

field, Massachusetts. It is of enameled iron, and draped with white muslin curtains which are fitted and tied on with tapes.

The delivery room contains a delivery bed. This bed is one made especially for the purpose. It has a slat bottom of strapped iron which does not give, is without castors, and should stand absolutely firm. The mattress

THE FURNISHINGS OF A 100-BED HOSPITAL 161

should be much more solid than that of an ordinary bed, and should be protected its entire length with rubber sheeting. This bed should have the low foot-end. If the head-end is surmounted by a shelf, it will prove of great convenience and may be used for a number of things which it is well to have close at hand during de-

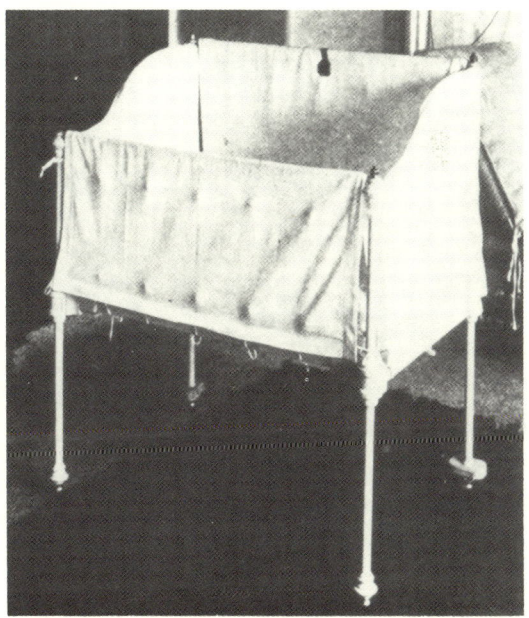

Fig. 52.—Baby's cot, draped. Wesson Maternity Hospital, Springfield, Massachusetts.

livery. This room should contain a chair of white-enameled iron, the feet of which should be rubber tipped. There should be a dressing table which is on castors, and may be moved up to the bed (Fig. 60). Everything needed at time of delivery should be on this table. A glass-topped table for instruments, etc., to be used in case of a forceps delivery, will be needed. The operating-room and sterilizing apparatus of the maternity department differ in no essential respect from those of the general hospital. The instrument case, however, contains only such instruments as are needed in obstetric surgery. The diet-kitchen contains a milk sterilizer and a small ice-box used exclusively for baby's milk. It is well to reserve one room for cases which need to be isolated.

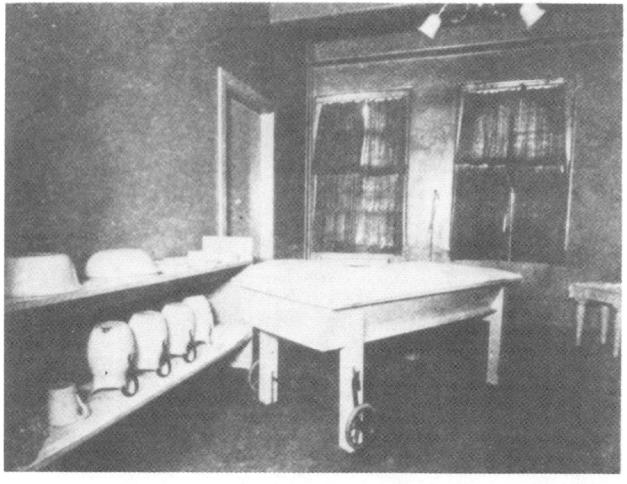

Fig. 53.—Delivery room. Obstetric ward. Shows home-made delivery table with adjustable wheels. Minnequa Hospital, Pueblo Colorado.

Private Room.—The private room should be made as home-like as is compatible with hospital requirements. A rug, if not too large to be taken out each day and swept, is permissible here. White-enameled furniture is, to our mind, the most attractive, as well as most appropriate, for the sick-room. It cannot possibly look clean unless it is clean, and this, to the new-comer to the hospital, must be a satisfaction. A couch bed with a National wire spring and a hair mattress is very desirable in this room. It furnishes a bed at night for the special nurse or the visitor if required, and is also a convenience by day for the patient during convalescence. It may be dressed with a pretty cover and sofa pillows, giving an air of home-likeness to the room. In place of the glass-top bed-side table here we would suggest the old-fashioned somino, which may be found in various sorts of wood in most of the furniture stores. There should be a bureau with a mirror, and good generous drawers. It may be graceful in design, but without filigree. A three-paneled screen with frame of oak, stained

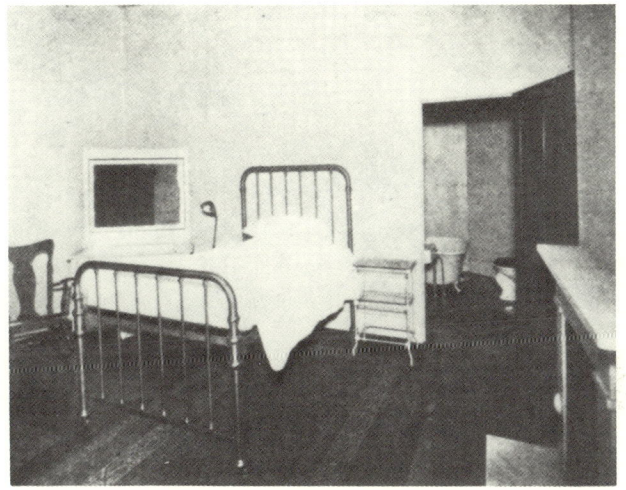

Fig. 54.—Private room, showing furnishings and corner of bath-room.

a dark forest green, with white washable filling, a reclining chair with high back, one other comfortable chair, and an adjustable bed-side table will complete the furnishings of a most attractive room.

The Hopper Room.—This service or utility room, or hopper room, where dressing pails, urinals, bed-pans, and many other homely, but necessary, utensils are kept, is the place where we least like to take our hospital visitors. But if as much attention were paid to fitness, convenience, yes, and asepsis, here, as in the operating-room, we might have reason to take as much pride in it.

A utensil stand is even more essential here than in the operating-room. The accompanying illustration shows the one, with its contents, that is used at the Massachusetts General Hospital. Besides the shelves, which are slatted and of oiled wood, there are hooks at the end for Davidson syringes, douche-bags, etc. The framework is of metal, painted with smoke-stack paint.

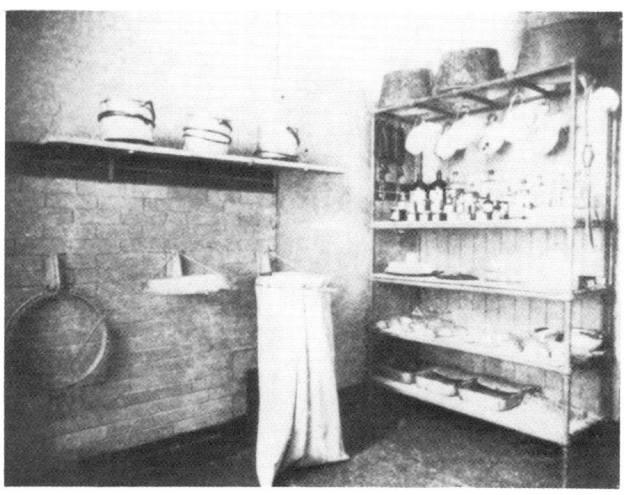

Fig. 55.—Utensil rack and soiled-clothes bag made at Massachusetts General Hospital, Boston, Massachusetts

Note also the holders for soiled-clothes bags shown in this illustration. They fasten against the wall; the bags, which are of bed-ticking and easily washed, are clamped in and out, remaining open while in use. When filled, the linen may be counted, and taken in the bag to the laundry—a much safer way than shooting all the linen through a "chute" as it is removed from the ward. Every one who has had experience with the "shoot" or "chute" method, knows how difficult it is to keep the whisk-brooms, hot-water bottles, instruments, etc., out of the wash, and also to keep any accurate account of the linen from different wards.

A rack for bed-pans and urinals should be fastened to the wall near the hopper. Such a rack may be found described in the catalogues of most of the surgical supply houses, but if the hospital engineer could make one to fit the place

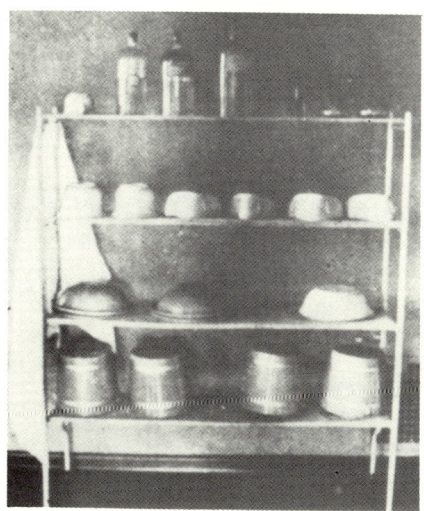

Fig. 56 —Utensil rack.

where it is to go, with the requisite number of pockets of the sizes required, it would be a much more useful article.

A copper hopper is, on the whole, recommended as superior to one of any other material. The only objection we have ever heard is the amount of work required to keep it polished. But it seems to us that it has advantages which make it worth while. It will not chip or crack, as do those of some other materials, and will last almost indefinitely. The sterilizing hopper in use at the Massachusetts General Hospital is far and away the best one that we know of. It disposes of typhoid stools and other infected excreta in the only absolutely safe way, and we think so highly of it that we recommend it for special consideration.

A single soapstone set tub, such as is found in the home laundry, is a most useful and convenient provision for the hopper room. The nurse would find more uses for such a tub than we could take time to enumerate.

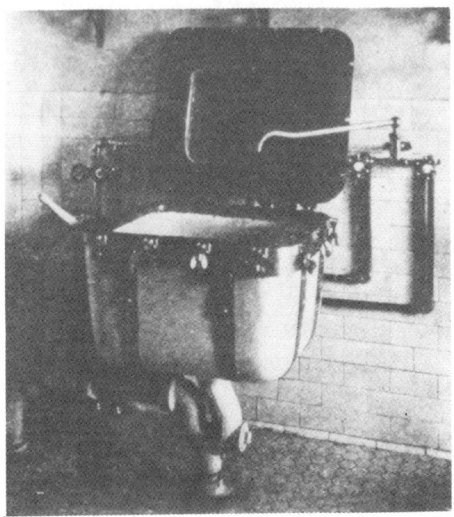

Fig. 57.—Sterilizing typhoid hopper. Royal Victoria Hospital, Montreal, Canada.

There should be shelves for bottles containing solutions here, and pails of white-enameled ware for waste dressings and other refuse.

Provision should be made in this room or elsewhere for shelf space for a good supply of vases for cut flowers. The wood-fiber vases are serviceable, but there is nothing so pretty and so clean as glass, and they may be bought in quantities very cheaply. Be sure to provide vases for long-stemmed flowers, as it is a great disappointment to

THE FURNISHINGS OF A 100-BED HOSPITAL 167

patients to have the stems of their lovely flowers cut down to fit the little vases that the hospital usually supplies.

Ward Serving Room.—A serving room planned for utility and convenience should be large enough to have the steam table placed in the center of the room, the size of which depends upon the number to be served from it. Practical working proves this to be ideal in relieving the hurrying and crowding at dinner time. Stone crocks in which the food will be kept warm are better than agate. The latter chips to such an extent that it soon becomes a source of annoyance, if not real danger. A small built-in ice-chest is preferable to a portable one. It should open from the front and the top should be of the same height and continuous with the stationary serving table. This arrangement, while compact and convenient, adds materially to the table space of the kitchen.

A cupboard for ward china with suitable drawers for silver and also a light and airy one, for saucepans, are necessary. A gas stove should be conveniently placed for the heating of fluids and compulsory light ward-cooking. The best sink for a ward kitchen is copper-lined. Porcelain looks fair at first, but the expense charged up to it in broken china and glass adds materially to the annual cost of supplies.

There are always certain patients whose dishes have to be kept separate. In an institution where there is plenty of live steam it is much simpler and safer to sterilize all the dishes. A dish-sterilizer should, therefore, form a part of the equipment of every modern serving room. The problem of handling a large number of trays in a small diet-kitchen is one that many hospitals are trying to meet, for very rarely does the hospital architect allow space enough for this important part of the work. More grumbles come from patients about cold food than from lack of skill of surgeon or physician, and three times a day the little diet-kitchens are usually overcrowded with nurses struggling with inconveniences that no housekeeper would tolerate for a moment in her own home. Fig. 58 shows a rack of seven shelves which really takes up no more wall space than one shelf. It is made of wood, the shelves are slatted. It is a separate piece of furniture, and does not fasten to the wall, but is on castors, and may be placed wherever most convenient, possibly in the center of the room, where the trays may be reached from either side. It will be noticed that the place for each tray is numbered by a round tag. A corresponding number is painted on

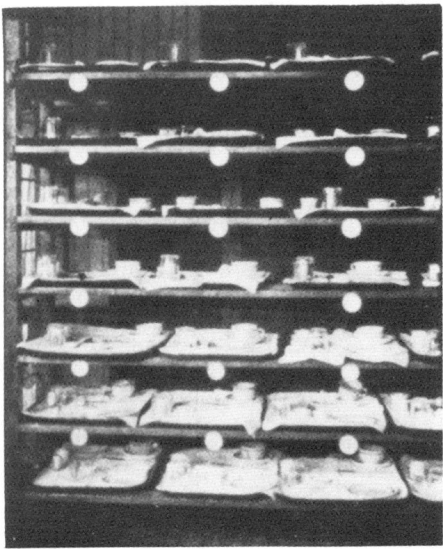

Fig. 58.—Tray rack. N. E. Baptist Hospital, Boston, Massachusetts.

the lower right-hand corner of each tray under the traycloth. This insures each patient his own tray, and facilitates inspection of all trays by the head nurse, not only before they go out, but after they come back. The inspection of the trays returned is greatly worth while, showing at a glance which patients have good appetites, what things are liked, and how to save waste in food by properly gauging amount served.

THE FURNISHINGS OF A 100-BED HOSPITAL 169

Patients' Fruit Closet.—Some provision should be made for caring for the fruit sent in to patients. It is worth while to have a little closet especially for fruit.

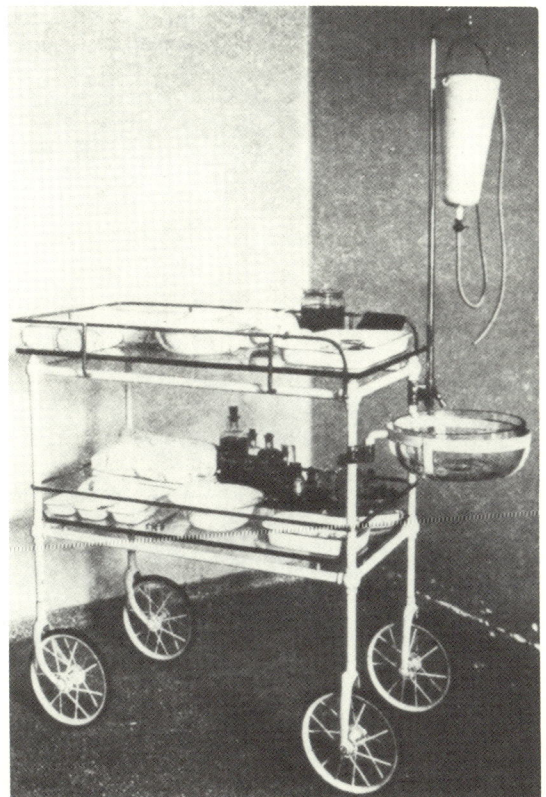

Fig. 59.—Dressing stand, with irrigator and solution bowl. **Wesson Maternity Hospital, Springfield, Massachusetts.**

The back of the closet should be removed a couple of inches from the wall in order that there may be no hiding place for water-bugs. The doors of the closet may be of glass or copper screen wire; the latter is better.

If each patient's fruit is kept in a little wooden grape basket, properly labeled with his name, the closet will look neat, and the fruit can easily be inspected. The cost of providing the baskets is quite insignificant.

Operating-room.—There are so many good operating-tables on the market and so many improvements have been

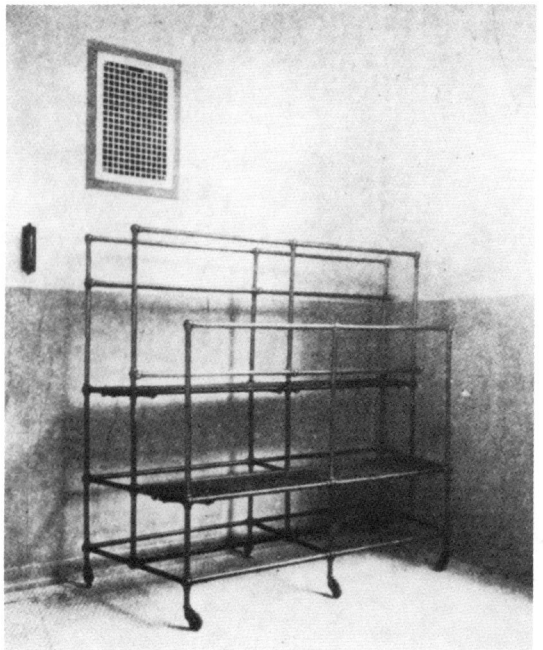

Fig. 61.—Observation stand made at Massachusetts General Hospital.

made to meet new demands of modern surgery that the choice is bewildering. Simplicity is of first importance. A generous provision for drainage is essential, and it is well to have the side gear by which the etherizer may work the Trendelenburg. The frequent use of cocain or spinal anesthesia necessitates a new attachment, an anesthesia

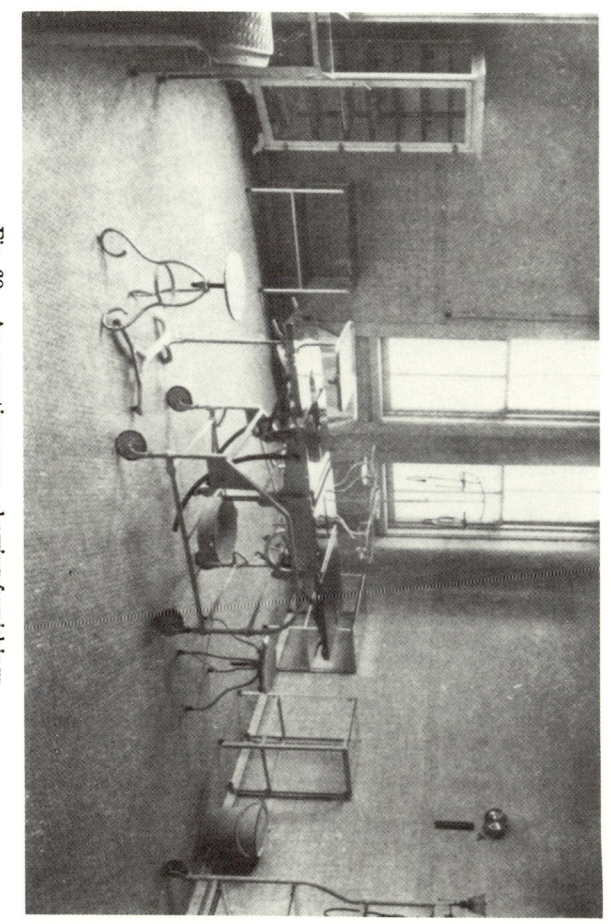

Fig. 60.—An operating-room, showing furnishings.

THE FURNISHINGS OF A 100-BED HOSPITAL 171

screen. This is a low screen with a washable panel, the side rods being attached to either side of the table, and high enough to obstruct the patient's view of the operation.

The instrument or dressing table is about 48 x 20 inches, is of enameled iron frame, with two glass shelves. These need not be necessarily of polished plate glass; sky-light

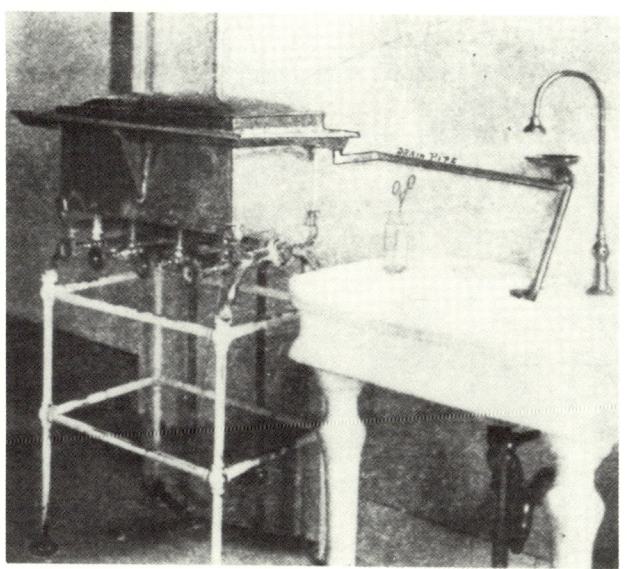

Fig. 62.—Drain put on sterilizer to prevent water dripping on floor when boiling over. Used in Presbyterian Hospital, Chicago, Illinois.

glass answers as well. Many superintendents have discarded the glass tops and substituted enameled iron.

A wall utensil stand with glass or enameled shelves is an indispensable piece of operating-room furniture.

At least two immersion bowl stands will be required. These are of enameled iron frame, with heavy base to prevent tipping when moved, and should be mounted on castors. There should be receptacles for two bowls in each stand, and these may be either of glass or agate—the latter preferably, as they can be boiled.

An irrigator stand is essential, but as it is an awkward piece of furniture and takes up an unnecessary amount of room, we would recommend the combination immersion bowl stand and irrigator shown in most of the catalogues. The Massachusetts General Hospital has made a combination which they think highly of—namely, an irrigator and

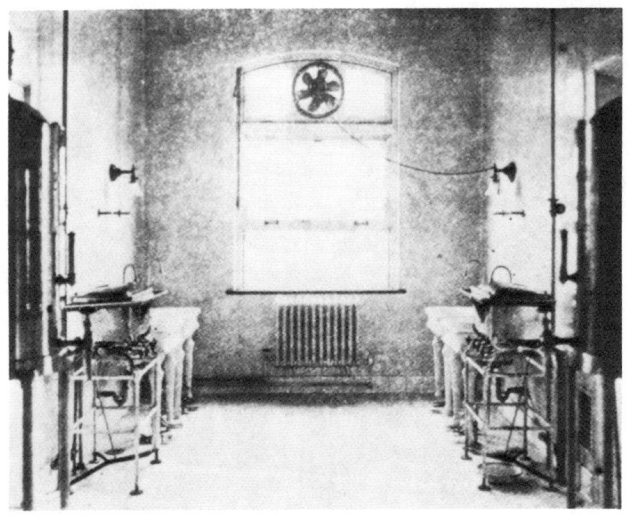

Fig. 63.—Exhaust fan in window to draw out steam from sterilizing room and operating-rooms adjoining. This entirely does away with condensation, dripping walls and ceilings. Total cost, $16.00. Used in Presbyterian Hospital, Chicago, Illinois.

table in one. The table top is of glass with a hole in the center through which is passed a rod of enameled iron and from which the irrigator is suspended. The irrigator is simply an apothecary's percolator.

An observation stand may or may not be necessary, depending entirely upon whether there are clinics or not.

If a corner can be spared either in the operating-room

THE FURNISHINGS OF A 100-BED HOSPITAL 173

or an adjoining room for a blanket-warming closet, it would be quite worth while. Flasks of warm salt solution may also be kept in such a closet.

Agate basins, pails, pitchers, etc., must find a place convenient to the operating-room. Also a salt infusion outfit in case of an emergency requiring hypodermoclysis.

An etherizing room requires very little beyond a wheel truck upon which the ether bed is made, and which should be of the same height as the operating table. A small

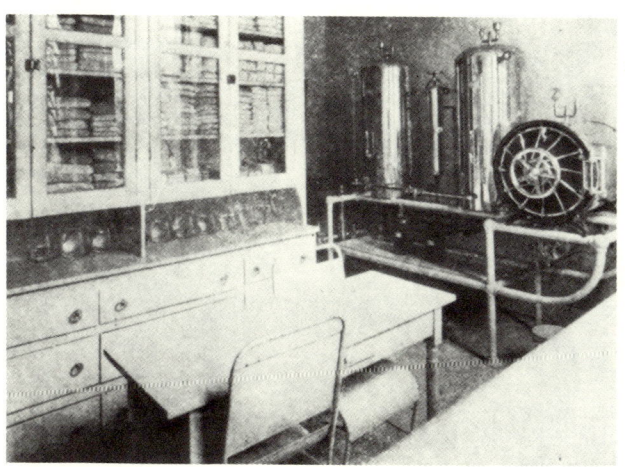

Fig. 64.—Sterilizing room.

cabinet or glass shelves, where ether cones, towels, pus-basins, tongue forceps, gag, a hypodermic outfit, and any other requirement of the etherizer, may find a place in this room.

Sterilizing Room.—The many good sterilizing outfits on the market offer a variety of choice. The simplest apparatus that does the work properly is the one to install. The size can be adapted to the demand of the hospital. A dressing and instrument sterilizer, an apparatus for distilling and sterilizing water, as well as a sterilizer for basins will be the equipment needed. In regard to the basin sterilizer, there is a device whereby the top and tray can be raised by hydraulic pressure, thus doing away with the necessity of touching anything with the hands when ready for operations. A work-table for the nurse and some cabinets in simple design for sterile goods will be necessary also.

Scrubbing-up Room.—Just a word may be said here about the plumbing connecting the set bowls in this room. It should be as simple as possible, and so arranged that

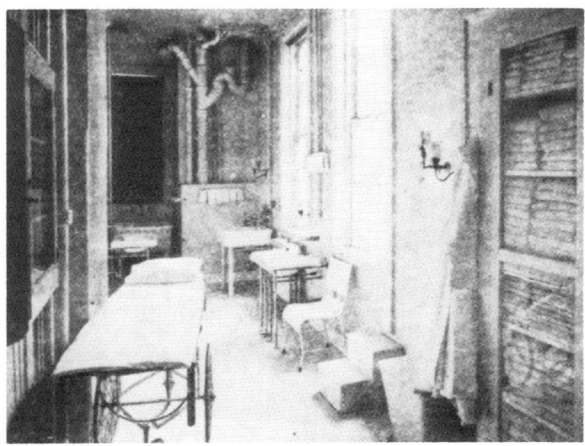

Fig. 65.—Scrubbing-up room.

the water can be turned on and off without using the hand. Perhaps the simplest and most practical device shown is a knee-valve. This is so arranged that either hot or cold water may be obtained, and when desired, the two mixed to the required temperature.

The doctors' dressing-room should contain a toilet, a shower bath, individual lockers, and a table equipped with writing material.

Solarium.—This room, in which convalescent patients spend so much of their time, and which becomes an out-

THE FURNISHINGS OF A 100-BED HOSPITAL 175

of-door sitting-room, should be as home-like as possible. More liberty can be taken in the furnishings of this room than in those of a ward. Cheeriness should abound. Bright chintzes, wicker lounges, easy chairs (no stiff formidable chairs in this room) should be the prevailing tone. Here can be placed a writing-desk and book-cases; also a table for magazines, pictorial and otherwise. Grass rugs add much to the solarium and are easily kept clean. Ferns and flowering plants will cause many a sick patient to take a new interest in life.

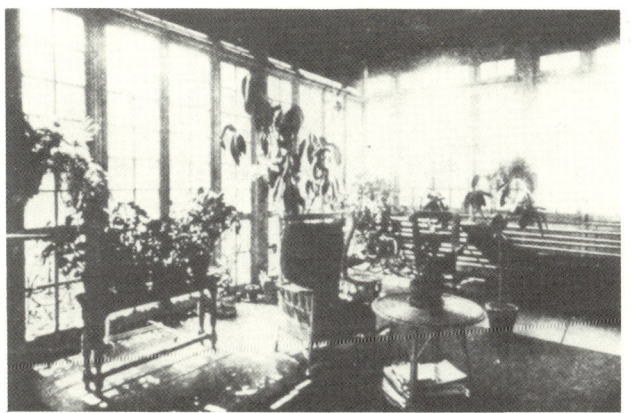

Fig. 66.—Solarium, Hospital of the Good Samaritan, Boston, Massachusetts.

Kitchen.—Certain standard equipment belongs to the kitchen department, and varies in design according to the personal view of the furnisher. The range, broiler, soup kettle, and coffee urns should be placed far enough from the wall to insure cleanliness. Where space permits, it is an advantage to place the range and kettles in the middle of the room. Three sinks are necessary— one of soapstone, with a generous drainer, for washing dishes, and two of iron, for washing pots and pans.

A row of shallow bins along the kitchen wall, each bin

large enough to hold one day's supply of potatoes, onions, carrots, etc., would save as many steps as the kitchen cabinet, with its row of spice boxes, found in the home kitchen. These bins may be of wood lined with zinc, with removable bottoms to facilitate cleaning. They should be high enough to prevent stooping in getting at contents.

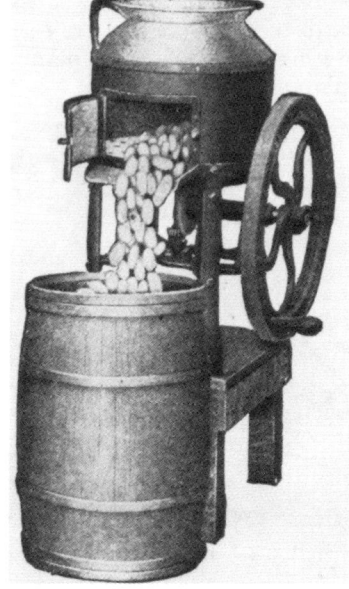

The best kitchen table is made of maple. The top should not be of one solid piece, but of strips running lengthwise and glued. Such a top can be washed and scrubbed indefinitely without warping. Over the table should be a rack where saucepans, spoons, strainers, etc., may be hung. A meat block of the same height as the table, and standing beside it, would be a convenience. This should have "cleats" on the sides with openings for cleaver, meat knives, etc.

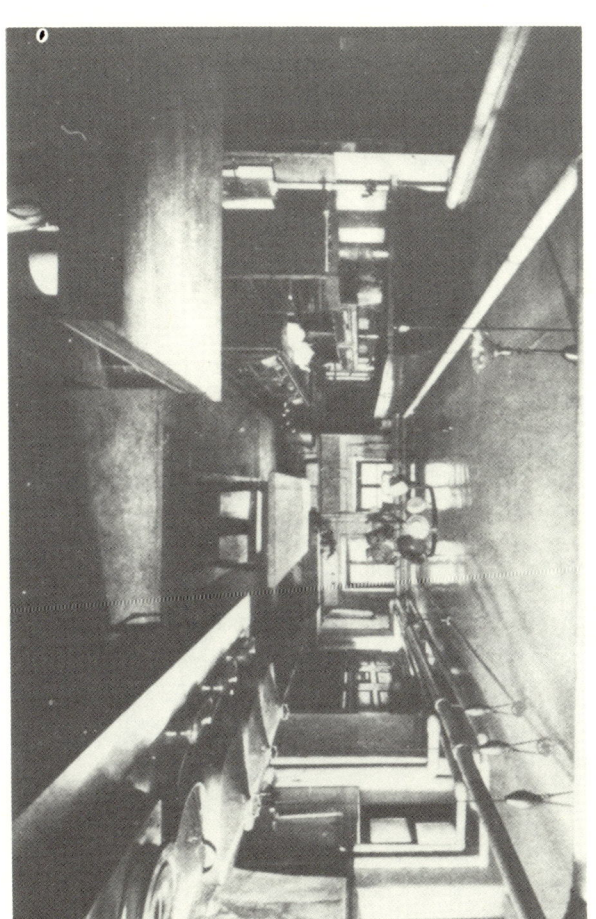

Fig. 67.—A central kitchen.

A kitchen dresser should have copper wire screens in doors instead of glass. This gives a good view of contents, saves the labor of washing glass, and provides better ventilation.

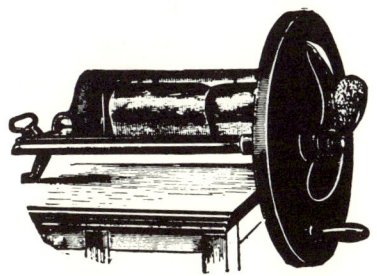

Fig. 69.—Lightning bread-cutter. Bread is fed automatically and knife is guarded to prevent injury to operator.

If possible, use an adjoining room for baking. This relieves congestion in the main kitchen. The baking room should have a brick oven, a bread mixer, and a table.

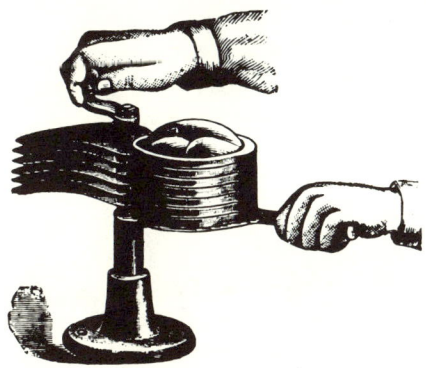

Fig. 70.—Tomato-slicer.

There are a few labor-saving devices that are eminently worth while even in the kitchen of a small hospital. One is a machine for paring potatoes. There is one that rubs the skin off by friction as the cylinder container revolves. A hose is attached to the faucet of the kitchen sink, and while the cylinder is revolving the water runs in and flows out, and with very little labor a peck of potatoes is soon

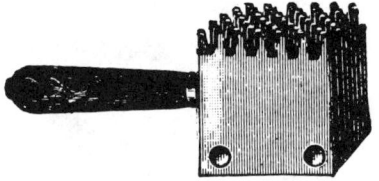

Fig. 71.—Steak masticator. A utensil for making tough steak tender.

pared and washed. Another simple and inexpensive device is a butter cutter. Besides serving neat little patties of butter of uniform size to each individual, it saves

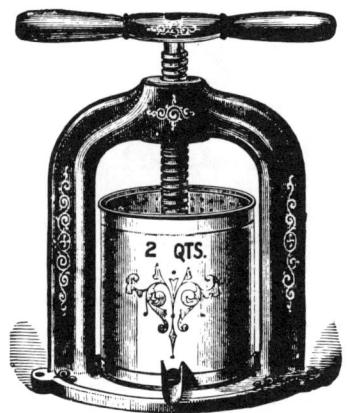

Fig. 72.—Meat-juice press.

in the amount of butter used, as every scrap of tub-butter can be put into this machine, which molds the butter into a brick, and then cuts it up rapidly, and without any waste, into squares of any desired size.

A dish-washer is a labor-saving device that is desirable in every hospital of a hundred beds or more, and many smaller hospitals have installed them. In these days of

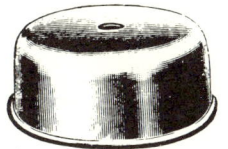

Fig. 73.—Aluminum dish-cover.

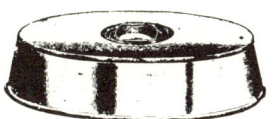

Fig. 74.—Aluminum dish-cover, oval.

uncertainty and perplexity in regard to the help problem, anything that needs to be done as frequently as dish-washing should be done by machinery as far as possible.

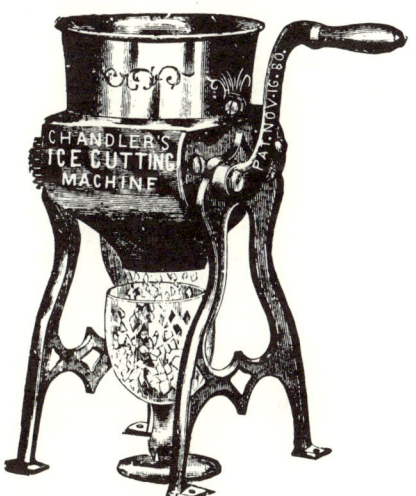

Fig. 75.—Ice-crusher.

Refrigerators.—The question of refrigeration should be considered early in the building of the hospital. Naturally, the variety of materials for refrigerators is great, but the one that, in the writer's experience, has proved the most practical, has sides lined with slate and shelves of same material. The latter should be adjustable so as to be easily removed and cleansed. Where ice is used, it should be put in from the outside, either overhead, or on the end. While provision must be made for an ice-box to supply the wards with ice, yet in the main refrigerators, where the plant is sufficiently large to warrant its installation, artificial refrigeration produces a lower and more even temperature, besides being cleaner than ice. It is also more economic.

The outside of the refrigerators should be absolutely plain, with no moldings of any kind to catch dirt. A door switch for lighting is a great convenience, besides giving the feeling of security that no light is left burning when the door is shut.

Laundry.—The laundry should be equipped with a view to usefulness and service; economy to the point of cheapness should not be practised here. If the best machinery is properly installed, repairs and interruptions of work will be saved later.

Two washing machines should handle the work easily. One of these should be under steam pressure, for sterilizing purposes. The machine can be used as an ordinary washer at any time. The mangle must be sufficiently large to take a sheet opened full width. Two soap kettles should be installed—one for immediate use and the other for "seasoning" soap. By this means it is never necessary to use soap under a week old, thus giving better results, besides a saving in money, as seasoned soap goes farther than new. One extractor, a body mangle, five or six ironing-boards, a folding table of liberal size, three soapstone tubs for hand-washing, three truck clothes-holders for wet clothes, large and small baskets according to the demand,—these, with a generous sized starch kettle, will completely furnish the laundry. Electric irons are recommended by some as being decidedly in favor of economy of help. In addition to being clean, no time is lost in

THE FURNISHINGS OF A 100-BED HOSPITAL 181

changing irons, and the work accomplished fully pays for the extra cost of maintenance.

The steam drying room, in addition to its racks, should have a fan installed to keep the air in circulation. The sorting room, adjoining the laundry, will have pigeonhole sections, each section labeled with the name of the individual to whom it belongs.

Two tables, some pins, and tags are all that are necessary in this room.

Electricity is the cleanest and by far the most satisfactory power for running the laundry machinery.

Hydrotherapeutic Room.—On account of possible leaks, this room should preferably be in the basement. The walls should be constructed of marble or some waterproof material. Over a waterproof floor must be laid a level slat floor, in order to allow the water to run off below. A marble douche table, containing a combination of hot and cold pipes, controls the flow of water by means of regulators, under the care of some one particularly trained to manipulate them. By this means the douche can be given at the prescribed temperature and pressure. A circular douche, consisting of hollow pipe with a series of sprinklers attached, is necessary. The patient stands between these pipes, and the kind of douche ordered is given by the attendant at the douche table.

A hot-air electric cabinet is an important part of the hydrotherapeutic apparatus.

For medicated baths, a porcelain tub is necessary.

With this amount of apparatus practically every prescription for baths may be taken care of.

X-ray Department.—The equipment of an x-ray room is standard, but too much care cannot be given to the installation of the apparatus. A Roentgen apparatus with accessories is all that is necessary. The compression outfit and coil should be in one room, while in the adjoining room, will be the operating-room, containing the table, switches, and an interrupter. These two rooms, for the safety of the operator, should be separated from each other by a lead partition or screen. In the operating-room can be installed the plate storage rack; also the double diagnostic box. This latter, while not a necessity, is a valuable convenience, inasmuch as it allows a series of photographs to be viewed at once in sequence.

A dark room is necessary. The only equipment needed here is a sink with cold running water.

Laboratory.—So much depends nowadays on scientific examination that in a general hospital of 100 beds the laboratory must be equipped with apparatus sufficient for the study of both medical and surgical cases.

A microscope, an oil-immersion lens, a blood-counter, a hemoglobin scale, an incubator, a sterilizer, a centrifugal machine for sediments, a freezing microtome, slides,

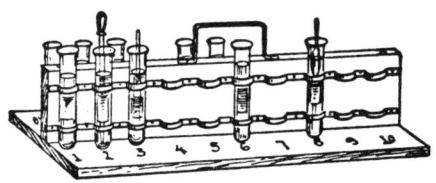

Fig. 76.—A hospital urine tray.

cover-glasses, urinometers, pipets, glass rods, filter-paper, some wine-glasses and test-tubes, glass specimen jars, a Bunsen burner, and graduated glasses, constitute the standard equipment.

On the shelves should be the necessary stains for bacteria and blood; also the reagents for urinary and gastric analyses.

A blackboard is necessary if any teaching is to be done. One painted on the wall takes up no floor space and is out of the way. The best sink for a laboratory is made of soapstone. Revolving stools are better than stationary ones, as they accommodate themselves to the individual height. The working table should be stationary and supplied underneath with drawers.

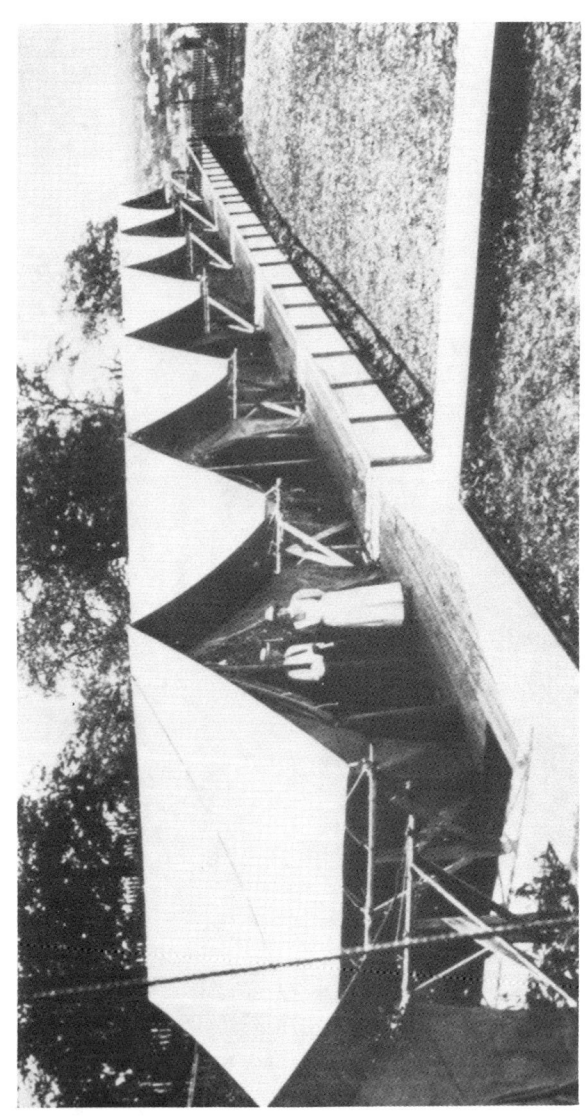

Fig. 77.—Equipment for outdoor work. Baptist Hospital, Boston, Massachusetts.

Equipment for Outdoor Work.—The treatment of patients out-of-doors is now so universally considered a part of modern medicine that the equipment of such a department should be considered. Apart from the unquestioned advantage to the patient living in a tent, there is no other form of hospital construction that brings in such big returns on the money invested. The tents illustrated have formed a part of the equipment of one hospital for from six to eight months of every year for the past nine years. They are of heavy duck, khaki colored, and are about 14 by 14½ feet. The cost is about $95 per tent. The brown color is an important feature, as the glare of a white tent out in the sun would be unbearable. If the location is one exposed to high winds, it will be necessary to have the fly of heavier material than the body of the tent. Twelve-ounce duck is proper for the fly and ten-ounce is sufficient for the body. The fly is raised several inches above the tent, giving sufficient air-space to prevent overheating when the sun is directly overhead. The roof is supplied with several large holes, thus securing ample ventilation even if the sides should be closed. They are the regulation army tent used and approved by the United States Government. A tent of the size described will hold three beds comfortably, but they may be made extremely attractive with two beds or with one bed for a private patient. The platforms are of planed pine boards raised about a foot above the ground. These may be left out-of-doors all winter. The furnishings may be made most attractive at little cost. Brown mission table, chairs, and bureau are pretty with the khaki walls, and a green straw-rug will not be injured by rain, and adds to the attractiveness of the tent. The beds are of the same material as those used in the house, except that the head-end is lower, on account of the sloping walls of the tent. A low screen of one panel, with spreading base, heavy enough to stand up in a wind, will be needed. Unless the house plumbing is accessible, one tent will have to be reserved as a service tent and will be fitted up with all the necessary plumbing and connected with the sewer.

At the hospital where these tents were used during the summer there was such a demand for more out-of-door accommodation in winter that a bungalow, large enough to provide for six private patients and containing bathrooms, service rooms, etc., was constructed at a cost of about $4000. This bungalow faces the south, has a ver-

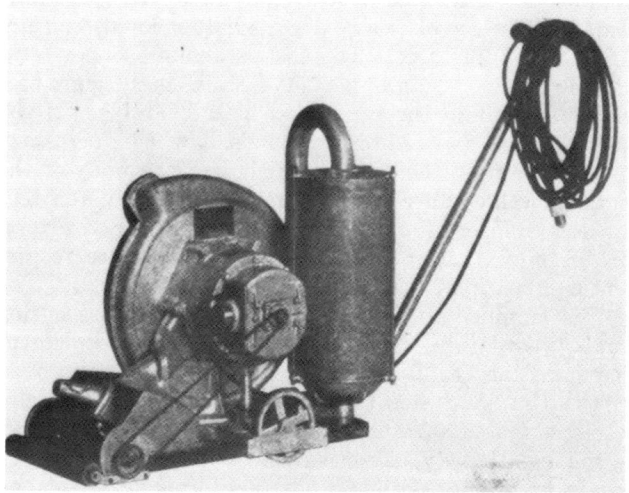

Fig. 79.—"Invincible electric renovator," the vacuum cleaning machine used at Grace Hospital, Detroit.

anda 14 feet wide, and the door of each room is sufficiently wide to admit of wheeling the bed out at any time. The beds move so easily on their five-inch rubber-tired castors that one nurse can handle them. These bungalow rooms are heated by steam; they make a valuable addition to the out-of-door department, both in the summer and winter, and are sufficiently removed from the noise of hospital to give the quiet and rest so greatly coveted and so seldom found in most hospitals.

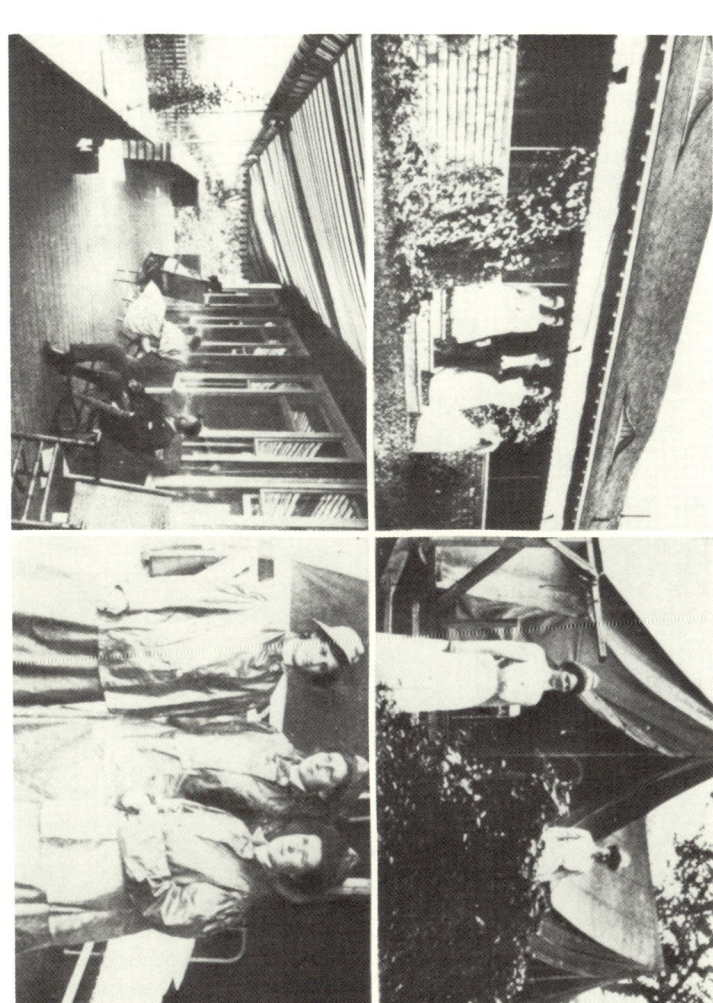

Fig. 78.—Equipment for outdoor work. Baptist Hospital, Boston, Massachusetts.

Incidentals.—The lighting of the hospital, while installed at the time of building, may well be considered as hospital equipment. The most satisfactory but not always

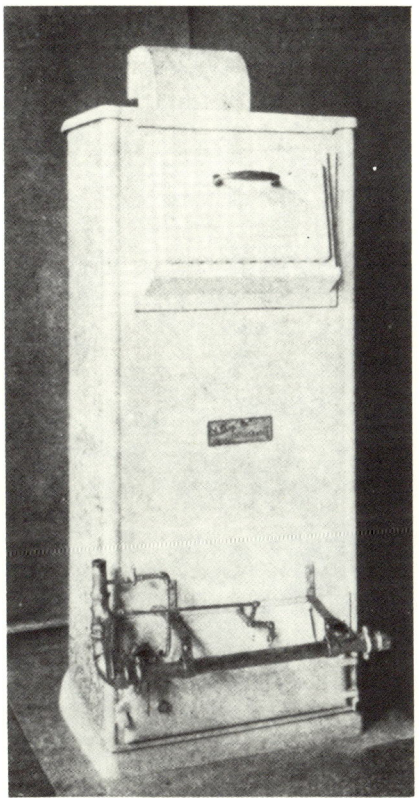

Fig. 80.—Incinerator, Hospital of the Good Samaritan, Boston, Massachusetts.

the most economic, system is electricity. The distribution of lights should be studied in relation to other furnishings of the room. In the wards, the lights should be diffused and come from behind the patient. In private rooms and the administration part of the hospital a great deal of comfort will be obtained from having some wall plugs put in, so that a portable lamp may be used in different parts of the room.

The subject of broom closets is a mooted one, but has to be considered as much a part of the necessary work-

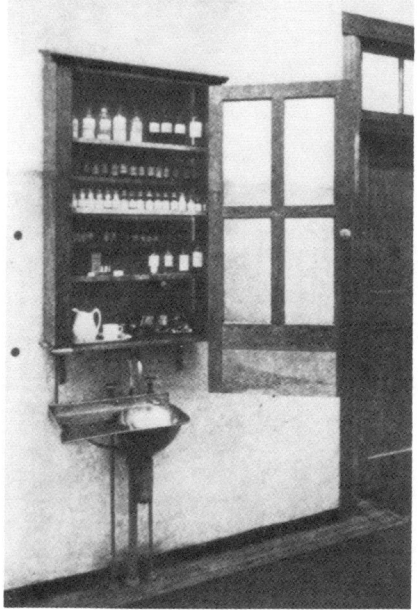

Fig. 81.—Medicine cupboard, Massachusetts General Hospital. Note arrangement of door and faucet.

ings of the average hospital as any other department. Brooms and baskets must be kept somewhere, and why not build a well-ventilated and well-lighted cupboard for that purpose.

The vacuum cleaner has become recently a necessary part of hospital equipment. When the piping has been built in with the hospital and the power comes from an

THE FURNISHINGS OF A 100-BED HOSPITAL 187

engine in the basement, it becomes a simple matter to screw in the machine in different rooms. When provision has not been made for this, there are very good portable machines that can be attached to an ordinary electric light.

The disposition of rubbish requires an incinerator; for that purpose the one shown in Fig. 80 is a good simple

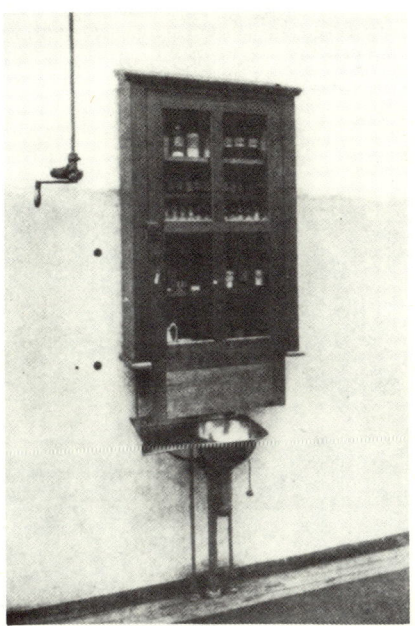

Fig. 82.—Medicine cupboard closed. Massachusetts General Hospital.

type. This is made of the best sheet iron, and having an asbestos jacket, radiates no heat. After having been filled to its capacity the rubbish is ignited by a burning gas-jet. When combustion has taken place, the gas is turned off and the rubbish is consumed in a very little while.

Medicine cupboards should be built in the wall, and so take up no floor space. Glass shelves are easily kept clean.

A set bowl in one end, while not absolutely a necessity, is a great convenience and time-saver. An electric light must be installed to insure safety in measuring out medicine. One with a door switch which turns the light on and off is very desirable for the medicine cupboard.

One of the many good systems of house telephones should be put in when building. Card catalogue cabinets for reference and for the filing of histories will be placed in the office and other departments of the hospital where patients are admitted.

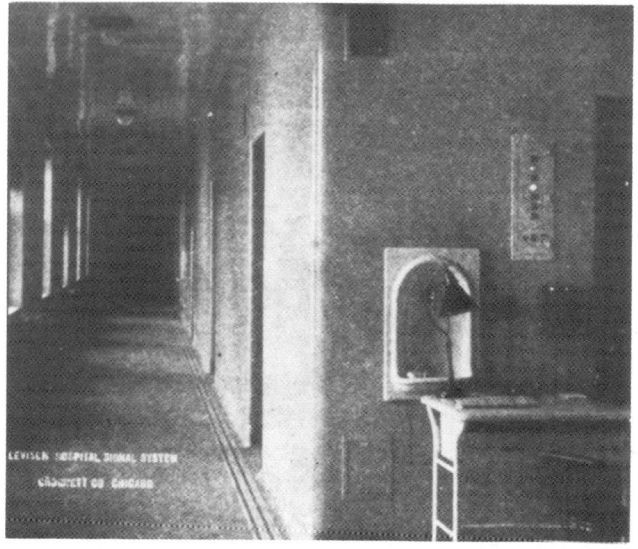

Fig. 83.—Corridor, showing lamps over doors and nurse's station. Signal system used in Presbyterian Hospital, Chicago, Ill.

THE FURNISHINGS OF A 100-BED HOSPITAL 189

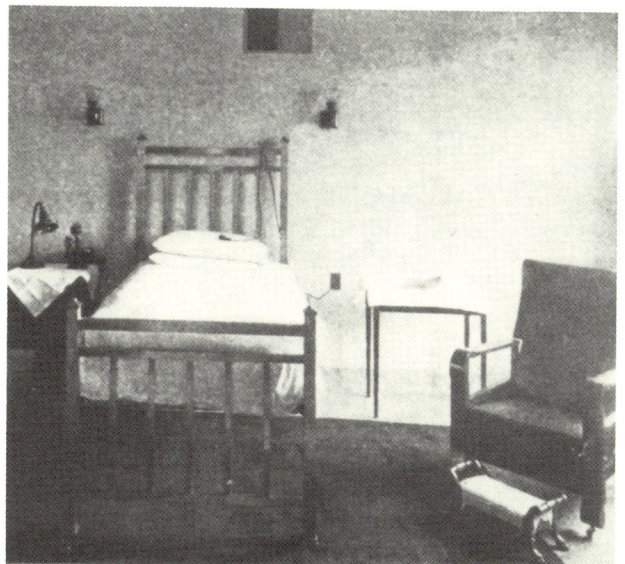

Fig. 84.—Typical room equipment, Levison Signal System.

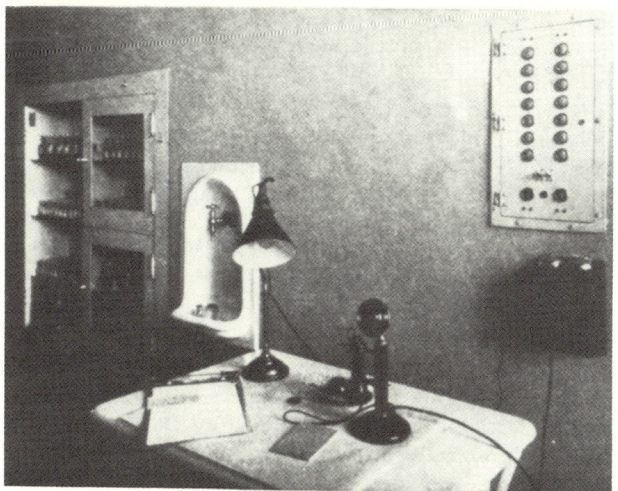

Fig. 85.—A typical nurse's station, showing equipment for Levison Signal System.

CHAPTER VII

THE HOSPITAL INCOME AND MANAGEMENT OF TRUST FUNDS

By Charles A. Gill

The sources of income and the methods of increasing it must necessarily vary considerably according to the social interests and financial resources of the members of the community which the hospital serves.

It is only in highly favored localities that voluntary contributions can be expected, in sufficiently large sums to place the institution at the outset upon a good working basis. By far the large number of hospitals have their beginnings in small buildings donated in whole or in part, and as cottage hospitals, with scarcely sufficient funds to meet the first month's obligations. This is the class of hospital that comes within the intent of the present chapter.

One of the first sources of a hospital's income, usually involved in its organization, is the amount pledged by members of the corporation in the form of annual dues or dues for life memberships. A search through annual reports shows surprisingly few (in relation to the whole number of residents in the district served) who thus from year to year identify themselves with hospital interests. A willingness and desire for such identification may be stimulated by prompt and business-like methods on the part of the management. The hospital's relation with such members as it has should be carefully maintained. Confidence and interest may be increased, for instance, by such a formality as the issuance of annual membership cards or appropriate certificates to life members.

Hospital Organization in Relation to Financial Support.—Managers should be selected, if possible, with a view not only to private integrity, sincere interest, and willingness to work, but also with reference to public opinion. To gain public support, it is desirable that the management shall be widely known and respected.

It may seem advantageous in organizing a hospital to establish, by suggestion or specific regulation, such a precedent or rule as shall bring about the retirement of managers upon reaching a certain age limit. A similar rule is often adopted by large corporations for the retirement of their officers and directors upon reaching such an age as makes responsibility onerous; and many hospitals, too, have found it wise to establish such a rule with regard to members of their medical staff. Such a regulation, by setting up an impersonal bulwark against further active service and responsibility, spares many undeserved pangs which seem, nevertheless, so inevitable to a system which leaves everything to personal experience.

If such regulation for the retirement of hospital managers be adopted, precaution should be taken to reserve for the hospital the privilege of retaining, as honorary members, such of the retiring managers as shall still, by their interest and influence, be competent to give valuable aid to hospital work.

Internal Organization in Relation to Hospital Support.—Too little thought is given to the internal organization, which, if intelligent and able, is a most valuable asset in securing and maintaining public support.

It is highly important that officers, physicians, nurses, and all employees shall be chosen and organized into a body of workers efficient, not only in the various special departments, but in the common human demands made upon them. Any individual act of unkindness or discourtesy may be justly interpreted by the public as a defect in management and efficiency, and a reciprocal detachment of the public from hospital support must be expected.

It must not be forgotten, in the economy of a hospital, that public confidence points the way for endowments, legacies, and contributions, and the most humble patient may prove sometimes to be a powerful index in this confidence.

Employees who come in close contact with the outside world, for instance, the telephone operator and the man who admits visitors at the door, should be chosen with careful reference to intelligence and courteous bearing. These men and women are in a position to do a hospital incalculable good or harm, and their work should be guarded carefully, so that all proper information will be given cheerfully and promptly.

Public Subscriptions and Donations.—Annual subscriptions by charitably disposed men and women constitute by far the most desirable and dignified form of hospital support. This support must of necessity depend largely upon earnest effort on the part of the hospital management.

Every hospital depending on voluntary gifts of the public for its support should seek to build up a permanent endowment fund, and, if possible, place in it all legacies, thank-offerings, memorials, life-membership dues, and similar receipts.

Ways and means of acquainting the public with the needs of the hospital are so numerous as to admit of only the briefest mention.

It is desirable to compile and revise each year a mailing list of all people in the district who have shown an inclination and ability to contribute, special care being taken never to allow the names of deceased persons to remain on the list. A carefully worded letter of appeal may be mailed each year, and an addressed envelope inclosed, making reply comparatively easy. It usually happens that many whose reserve forbids initiative are ready to respond cheerfully and substantially to such an appeal.

Foundries and factories whose employees receive hospital care should be kept in close touch with the work of the hospital. If they are not contributing as their relations with the hospital would seem to warrant, a statement may be presented to them giving such details as cannot fail to arouse their interest. Such details are seldom lacking in the relations of hospital to factory. The number of employees treated during the year should be accurately set forth, together with the nature of the accident or illness calling for such treatment, the number of days each patient was maintained during the year, and the average cost. A comparison of such cost with the amount of annual subscription received from the factory would usually offer an irrefutable argument for the justice of the appeal.

A friendly spirit should exist between hospital, employer, and employees. The hospital should be granted the privilege of organizing among employees Saturday associations which have for their object the furnishing of envelopes and convenient opportunity to employees to contribute their reasonable share toward the support of their hospital.

Women's Aid Societies.—Women's aid societies contribute very largely to the work of securing financial and other aid.

Many hospitals depend almost entirely upon women for securing contributions, managing the annual donation day, organizing auxiliaries, planning entertainments and social gatherings.

Very often too little credit is given the women composing these societies, who give their time and energy and who, as a rule, do not form a part of the board of managers.

It is useless to enumerate in this brief chapter the many means adopted by these societies for obtaining the very large sums that are turned over to the treasurer and board of managers to apply as they see fit. The methods are much better left to individual societies—the more unique the plan, the better the result.

Caution should be taken, however, not to weary the public by too constant solicitation to contribute to the carrying out of specific plans involving the purchase of tickets, etc. Two to four grand efforts each year will yield far better results.

Perhaps it would be interesting to mention in this connection a plan for raising funds carried out very successfully by women interested in the Germantown Hospital. The idea was conceived of repeating in Germantown a plan originating with Pastor von Bodelsechwingh, of the Colony of Mercy in Germany, whereby $4000 was raised in a fortnight for a babies' hospital.

An allusion to this effort appears in Kate Douglass Wiggin's "Marm 'Liza," and furnished the inspiration for the Germantown movement.

Posters were placed in store windows announcing a plan to found a bed in the children's ward as a thank offering from fathers and mothers for their well children. Each parent was asked to contribute a penny or more for every well child; and not only parents, but all lovers of children were asked thus to give evidence of their love. Envelopes for contributions were distributed by business houses. Banking institutions acted as depositories. Not only pennies, but accompanying messages of encouragement flowed in from lovers of children, such as pennies for "four living children," pennies for "our dollies," pennies for "a child in Heaven," pennies "from a child we never had," and pennies "for a happy home."

In a fortnight more than enough was received to endow the bed. The envelopes continued to pour in, however, in such numbers that it became necessary to form a permanent organization known as "The Lovers of Children Thank-Offering Society," for the express purpose of counting the pennies. The ladies elected to the membership roll of this laborious society are, we believe, still counting.

Their receipts in excess of the $2500 necessary for the endowment of the bed have enabled them to donate useful equipment to the children's ward.

Church and Hospital.—It would seem superfluous to urge a spirit of coöperation between church and hospital. No hospital, whether denominational or not, can afford to lose either the moral or financial support of the church. And no hospital can afford to deprive its patients of any desired spiritual aid.

An instance comes to mind of a hospital which lost the support of a very powerful church through lack of tact on the part of an interne, who, unmindful of any but the medical aspect of his patient's needs, informed the minister whose visit was anxiously desired that it was not "visiting day," and, at any rate, that "case" was too sick to receive visitors. It took years for the hospital to overcome the loss sustained through this one act of clumsy and unintelligent discourtesy.

The close connection between church and hospital is inevitably established in the nature of the people whom they serve in common, and any expression of lack of sympathy between them must, therefore, result in the partial frustration of the purposes of each. Churches, on their part, almost without exception, realize this, and show their sympathy by arranging for special collections during the year toward the support of their local hospital, and by encouraging sunday-school interest in hospital work and needs.

Press and Hospital.—A liberal policy should be pursued in giving to the local press news pertaining to the work of the hospital, guarding, of course, the personal rights of the patient, and observing medical ethics.

The press is usually more than willing to publish hospital news, and it is highly important that the public, through this means, should be kept sensitive to the significance of hospital work.

Annual Report.—Publication and liberal distribution of the annual report, in the case of hospitals partially or wholly dependent upon voluntary contribution, cannot be too strongly urged. Through no other, and certainly through no more dignified, medium, can so much accurate and detailed information be given. Here is focused information, not only as to the assets, receipts, expenses, and needs of the hospital, but also as to the diverse sources of the assets. And by bringing together the names of all who have contributed in any way to the support of the hospital,—and this, too, in connection with the particular phase of hospital work in which each is interested,—there is aroused and maintained both a feeling, of common interest and responsibility, and also a more intelligent understanding of individual cases. Such specific information, generously distributed to the public, may very often attract the attention of those whom generalities have consistently failed to interest.

Grants of Public Funds.—The question of the duty of the state or municipality toward privately managed hospitals is one creating a diversity of opinion and not infrequently just adverse criticism.

As a person or corporation or municipality is bound to compensate those who suffer by its action, so the state is responsible in a measure for any imperiling of the public health or safety through conditions which legislation has failed to cover; and the state recognizes this duty by providing certain hospital accommodation at its own cost and under its own management. Many states do not grant public funds to any privately managed institution; others appropriate large amounts to favored institutions in lump sums, almost regardless of the amount of service rendered; while others authorize general hospitals to receive appropriations from counties, cities, towns, and villages, usually on a per capita basis.

One important city is at the present time (1909) paying to private institutions for their needy patients a flat rate of $1.00 per diem for medical cases, and $1.10 for surgical cases; $0.45 per diem for infants under two years of age, and in children's hospitals, under five years of age; $0.80 per diem in hospitals conducted exclusively for consumptives; $0.80 per diem for cancer patients; and $0.40 per diem for chronic, incurable, or infirm patients. Many county councils throughout Canada are now making yearly grants to hospitals, apparently in lump sums. The total appropriations appear to average less than $0.10 on the $1000 assessment.

It is certainly a benefit to the state to have charitably disposed citizens voluntarily contribute to the work of caring for the sick and injured poor. All amounts so contributed and usefully employed relieve the state to that extent, and incidentally make better citizens of the men and women who contribute. "He is truly great that is great in charity."

Many hospitals favorably located will continue to be supported entirely by voluntary contributions, either by charitably disposed citizens or by denominational churches; but others less favored may be compelled to solicit municipal aid; and, assuming that the municipality is responsible, directly or indirectly, for a large proportion of the injured and sick poor, it would seem entirely reasonable to urge legislation tending toward an equitable distribution of public funds through taxation, based upon the extent and character of the service rendered.

It would seem entirely possible for a state or municipality granting appropriations to estimate the amount required, based on the number of hospitals granted aid, the number of free hospital beds, and the average number of such beds occupied each year. There should be a specific rate per patient per diem, payable quarterly, after careful audit by authorized authority.

Such amount within the specific rate per diem as is found to be required should be made by the public treasurer after approval of a Board of Public Charities, unappropriated funds to revert to the public treasury.

In sparsely settled sections, or in communities where the giving power of residents is limited, it may be found necessary for the state or municipality to aid in the purchase of ground and construction of buildings. Institutions so aided should be classed as semi-public and should remain under partial control of authorized authority or Board of Public Charities.

No institution receiving such aid should have power at

any time thereafter to incumber said real estate, buildings, or alterations, to any extent or in any way whatever. If, at any time, after judicial consideration, such semi-public institutions should be found unnecessary to meet local demands, and should become irksome to maintain, it would appear to be for the public interest that the state, county, or municipality should have the right to take possession of the real estate and buildings of such institutions, and operate them thereafter as public charities.

The Physician and the Hospital.—The good will of the physicians of a community is a valuable hospital asset; a hospital's reputation is a part of its capital. Let no hospital be known as any one man's hospital. Make the surgical, medical, and special services alternating instead of continuous, and thus multiply the number of physicians by three or four for each department. Every well-advised addition to the staff, increasing, as it does, the number of physicians personally interested in the work, adds materially to hospital efficiency, and incidentally to revenue. Every physician having a patient in the public ward of the hospital should be made to feel that a friendly visit to his patient is appreciated by the hospital, as well as by the patient. The hospital must recognize and show by its attitude that the interests of its patients are identical with its own, and that whatever makes for the personal pleasure and encouragement of the patients, makes also for the success of the institution. All reputable physicians in the community should share in the privilege of attending their own private patients in the pay department of the hospital. Any alien attitude toward such physicians might result in irrevocable injury to hospital interests.

The Patient and the Hospital.—Patients occupying beds in the public wards should be encouraged to realize their financial responsibility to the hospital.

The ease with which many hospitals admit patients free of charge, and the total disregard in which such hospitals often hold any individual instincts for self-maintenance tend to humiliate and thus pauperize the patients whom misfortune has placed in hospital care. Notwithstanding that many may not feel able to obligate themselves to pay a full weekly ward rate, yet they should be encouraged to pay a part either in weekly payments equivalent to cost of food supplies or in one payment sufficiently large to pay cost of operating-room, appliances, ether, or special medicines. It usually happens that patients are able to pay something, and such part payment, it will be observed, is often the very link which preserves the patients' friendly feeling for the hospital.

A few hospitals have a provident loan fund by which it is possible to arrange for a loan to patients who desire to pay the cost of their care, but are not at the time of the illness financially able to do it. The loan is made without or with a very nominal rate of interest.

It is an observed fact that those who contribute something toward their own maintenance leave the hospital with a higher regard for it than those who have not paid in proportion to their ability. May this not be because the hospital in these cases has not, in preserving the body, killed the spirit of its patients?

Those patients in whom the spirit of pride is already almost non-existent must be admitted, of course, upon the same basis as those whom misfortune alone has placed in the position of drawing entirely upon hospital funds. In spite of the seriousness of the present-day problem involved in helping those who have never shown any inclination to help themselves, and thus putting a premium upon indolence and ignorance, hospitals cannot, of course, take upon themselves the burden of a social problem, but must err always in the direction of the spirit of charity in which they are organized.

Patients Occupying Beds in Semiprivate Wards.—This class of patient (people, for the most part, living on moderate salaries) should not be subjected to the discomfitting conviction that they are a tax on the charity of a hospital. By careful management, accommodations could be provided which, in almost every case, could be adequately met by the financial resources of the patient.

Patients Receiving Treatment in the Public Dispensary.—This department, if properly managed, should be self-supporting.

The multiplicity of abuses from the medical side as well as from that of the patient, should be investigated and eliminated. This involves one of the most difficult details of hospital management.

Patients, except in rare cases, should be required to contribute an amount sufficient to pay cost of medicine and dressings. This would undoubtedly check the many patients acquiring the so-called "dispensary habit," "receiving something for nothing," usually resulting in lack of appreciation of advice received and downright waste of medicine given.

Pay Patients (Able to Pay Fully for Their Care).—The management of this department should be kept separate and distinct. The same business principles should be applied as would be expected in the management of a properly conducted business enterprise. Difficult as it may seem with the private, semiprivate, and free patients blended together, as is usually the case, it is entirely possible, and for many reasons highly desirable, that the managers and contributors should know the cost of maintenance for each.

It is not reasonable to expect the charitably disposed to contribute to the hospital unless they can be assured, through a proper system of bookkeeping, that every dollar given is going to be spent for the care of the sick poor for whom it is given, and is not to be used for the partial payment of those who are able to care for themselves. Neither is it reasonable to expect the hospital managers to fix rates for hospital treatment for the rich, unless some detailed statement of cost is submitted to them as a basis for their schedule of rates.

Consequently all items delivered to the pay department on requisition, properly signed and approved, should be charged up, together with proportion of cost for heat and light, ambulance service, board of resident physician, and salary and board of nurses and employees. Thus an intelligent charge could be made for services, so that the average collections from patients will exceed their cost; for it is entirely reasonable to expect the rich to pay a sum for their hospital treatment sufficient to leave a balance toward the cost of maintaining the free patients. In addition to a charge for room, payment should be required for operating-room appliances, extra nursing, board of special nurses, unusual and expensive medicines, liquors and mineral waters, massage, x-ray treatments, extra trays served to relatives and friends, ambulance service, laundry, and telephone.

Accommodation should be provided for relatives and friends desiring to remain near patients, and a charge should be made analogous to that for similar accommodation in a well-managed hotel.

Many advantages come incidentally to a well-managed hospital receiving pay patients by reason of their influence in increasing its income.

Management of Trust Funds.—This subject has been most adequately treated by Mr. Frank J. Firth, a well-known hospital authority, and printed in the proceedings of the Hospital Association of Philadelphia (1903), as follows:

The Proper Record, Care, and Use by Charitable Institutions of Trust Funds

The proper record, care, and use of trust funds is a subject thought worthy of careful consideration. It is well known that institutions receive large sums from the charitably disposed, either during life or in bequests by will. Certain amounts are so received free from any special conditions, and are therefore available to meet current operating expenses or any other institution need. Other amounts are received with a variety of accompanying conditions and directions, sometimes as to the investment and care of the principal, and sometimes as to the use of the income. Gifts and bequests are most useful when unrestricted. Institutional needs change with time. These needs are best known to the management, and it is often very discouraging to find a welcome gift so burdened with conditions and limitations as to make its use impossible in directions where it would do the greatest amount of good. Gifts that call for the erection of buildings not needed, and that do not provide through proper endowments for their operation and maintenance, are often a burden rather than a benefit.

It is quite a common and natural desire on the part of donors that their gifts shall constitute permanent funds, to be kept separate and designated by the name of the donor. Very often gifts are made for the purpose of providing for the permanent endowment of beds, memorial or otherwise. Such gifts are always welcome and sure to be beneficial.

It is a growing and commendable institutional practice to place in permanent funds, voluntarily created by their boards for the purpose, all important gifts received (not intended to meet current expenses), and particularly all bequests by will, so that the principal of such gifts and bequests may be kept intact and the income, only, used to meet necessary expenses. This represents a safe and conservative financial management of charitable institutions, that it is *believed will meet with the approval of the charitably disposed and attract further gifts.* Institutions should recognize it to be a moral obligation of the most binding description that every possible effort shall be made to safeguard the principal and the income of all such gifts, and to strictly conform, for all time, to the wishes of the donor in connection therewith. It is easy to grow careless in these matters. Institutions managed by boards of active business men are often willing to commit to the care of an associated member acting as treasurer without pay, or of a finance committee, practically its chairman, securities representing large amounts, and to accept thereafter with approval formal reports of receipts and expenditures, including investments and reinvestments, without giving said reports due investigation and consideration. The result of these lax methods is seen in occasional losses of institutional funds through inefficient or defaulting clerks or officers. That these losses do not occur more frequently is a tribute to the honest intentions of trusted men, rather than to the efficiency of the systems under which their work is conducted.

Then, again, with the passing of years and of men, knowledge may be lost or lost sight of with respect to the exact conditions under which gifts are held. The result may be a failure to keep separate funds intact and properly designated, or a use of their principal or income for purposes other than those desired by the donor. Managers must not forget that the donor's conditions should govern, whether the managers approve of them or not. The managers are merely trustees to carry out the known will of the donor; it is not their function to act as critics, or to attempt any improvement thereon, no matter how pressing may be the apparent need.

It is thought that an illustrative reference may, with propriety, be here introduced to the practice in an institution with the methods of which the writer is familiar.

Some years since an institution received a liberal gift to which no restrictions were attached, but which came to the institution under conditions that made its custody and use a peculiarly sacred trust. It was seen to be at least possible that needs for enlargement or to meet deficiencies in current expenses might at some time tempt the management to divert more or less of the principal of this valued gift to the care of such needs, and that it would then cease to exist in its entirety. The consideration given to this case by the board resulted in the adoption of a policy that, while it may be capable of improvement, is thought to be worthy of presentation. The board voluntarily created, by unanimous action, a permanent fund, and placed its securities in the custody of a committee of three consisting of those holding for the time being the offices of president, treasurer, and chairman of the finance committee. As the by-laws of the institution now stand, gifts and bequests by will calling for the permanent investment of the hospital principal and use of income only, go at once into this permanent fund. Further appropriations are made to the fund from time to time, of unconditional gifts or bequests received, when so ordered by a vote of not less than twelve of the fifteen members of the board. Amounts once voluntarily placed by the board in the permanent fund may not be thereafter removed therefrom except by the order of twelve or more members of the board. This guards the permanent fund from possible hasty and ill-considered action on the part of the board at times when, it may be, new buildings appear to be so badly needed as to justify the depletion of permanent funds on the income of which the institution may largely depend to meet its current expenses. Investments and reinvestments for the permanent fund are made with the approval of the finance committee and board. Securities are kept in a trust company box, which is held in the names of the committee of three members, and may not be opened at any time by less than two of them. A written and signed book record is kept by the committee in the box, showing the date and purpose of every visit made. The permanent fund committee reports to the board monthly, and its accounts and securities are audited annually by a special committee of the board. All income is paid over to the treasurer as it falls due.

Another rule of this institution appears to be of sufficient interest to mention. It is the duty of the treasurer to keep a complete record, in the language of the donors, of all legacies and gifts, in a book specially prepared for the purpose, and to submit this record book to the board once in each year, for its information. This affords an opportunity at least once in every year to consider the latest facts with reference to contingent bequests not yet due. It also enables members of the board to know what gifts or bequests are held subject to conditions or restrictions imposed by the donors, and that they are currently complied with.

The by-laws of this institution also require, and this is regarded an essential condition in the safe management of any trust funds in the care of a board, that all receipts shall be deposited with a depository approved by the board and in an account to be kept in the name of "The............................Hospital, by ....Treasurer."

It is not thought just or wise for the board to attempt to relieve itself of the responsibility of selecting or approving depositories used, by transferring this responsibility to a treasurer or a finance committee. Nor should it be possible for any treasurer to deposit, or in any way confuse, the funds of an institution with his own personal funds, or with any other trust funds in his custody; nor should the claims of family or of friendship be permitted to influence in any way the selection of depositories, or the loaning or use of trust funds. These pitfalls should be most certainly avoided by relying upon the united wisdom of an entire board to justly decide all such questions, rather than by vesting undue authority in any one individual, treasurer, or other party.

1. Each institution receiving bequests by will, or other important gifts, should provide clear methods for their care, principal, and income, not allowing this care to depend for its efficiency upon any one man or woman.

2. Conditions attached to each gift should be made the subject of a clear permanent record in the exact language of the donor, and this record should be submitted periodically to the members of the board and to the officials of the institution, so that there may be a continuing knowledge of the obligations thus imposed.

3. It may be found advantageous for each institution to formally create a permanent fund and to set forth in its reports the rules governing such fund and the safe method of its management, so that the charitably disposed may be attracted by the care and security offered and may be induced to increase their gifts with a reasonable certainty that such gifts will be properly cared for and used.

4. It may be well to consider the advantage and additional security that would result from having permanent funds cared for by joint trustees, consisting of a committee of the board of the institution and a designated trust company of known reputation. Provision could be made for a prompt change of trust company, for cause, through court proceedings or otherwise.

5. All such funds should be audited periodically by some disinterested public accountant, not relying, as is now too often done, upon an auditing committee of the board, who would be naturally averse to appearing as critics of their friends, and would be more likely to give a superficial examination and a worthless approval.

CHAPTER VIII

HOSPITAL BOOKKEEPING

DESCRIPTION OF BOOKS AND SYSTEMS OF ACCOUNTS FOR THE USE OF GENERAL HOSPITALS

By W. L. Babcock, M.D.

THE general principles underlying all correct systems of bookkeeping are applicable to hospital accounts as well as those of any other business. Certain features of hospital work, however, render it imperative that special business forms and bookkeeping side lines be introduced. Any system of bookkeeping, arranged for hospital work, should take into consideration the following:

1. The necessity of making a monthly financial and statistical report to the board of trustees or directors.

2. That each department of the hospital be charged with its earnings and expenditures. This is to enable the superintendent to keep a daily check on the income and expenditures of the various departments.

3. That material stock on hand be inventoried on the last day of the month. By material stock we mean the sundries, contents, or new goods in the general storeroom or the individual storerooms. In other words, everything that is issued as provisions, supplies, etc., for consumption or use in the daily work of the hospital.

4. That an annual financial and statistical report be furnished the board of trustees or the proper accounting authorities on December 31st of each year.

5. That the bookkeeping system be of sufficient detail to permit the cost of all items or groups of items, *per*

patient per day, to be drawn off at the end of each month, for the purpose of checking up on expenditures.

It is well known that superintendents of small hospitals are obliged, in many instances, to keep the hospital books without the assistance of a trained bookkeeper. This has often been a bugbear to institutional nurses who contemplate taking charge of small hospitals. A little preparation should obviate any difficulty in this direction. A few months' course in bookkeeping in a business college, or one month's study or training with the bookkeeper of any hospital, will usually prove sufficient preparation for the office management of a small institution.

CARD SYSTEMS IN HOSPITALS

All simplified methods of bookkeeping will make use of as many card systems as possible, thereby permitting easy

DISCHARGE CARD.

| | Ward |
| | Room |

Admission Date	19	No.
Discharge Date	19	No.
Sex	Age	Civil Cond.
Occupation		
Physician		
How Discharged		Time
Diagnosis		Signed

THE GRACE HOSPITAL

Fig. 86.—Discharge card.

and quick reference. In the general hospital office, cards can be used for patients' index, patients' ledger cards, patients' history cards, patients' discharge cards, bill register, etc. They can be used in the storeroom as receipt cards, bill cards, or inventory cards. They can be used in the pharmacy and other departments of the hospital for the same purpose. It is an admirable plan to furnish each nurse in charge of a ward or corridor, and each head of a department, with a small box of cards in an alphabetic thumb index, to use as stock cards. By means of these cards she can keep a record of all supplies on hand for which she is responsible, and on it she enters each article issued, lost, worn out, or replaced. In the general office and stockrooms 5- by 8-inch cards will be found the most useful. In the other departments of the hospital a 3- by 5-inch card is sufficient, unless the department is a large one.

GENERAL BOOKS

The following books in use in all double-entry systems are usually considered necessary: Cash blotter or day book, cash book, journal, general ledger, voucher record, and board book.

The following forms are necessary: vouchers or voucher checks, pay-rolls, ledger cards for patients' accounts, inventory sheets, and monthly report blanks.

Cash Blotter.—This is a day book or a desk blotter and is used for the entry of cash receipts. This should be manifolded with the second page perforated for removal. The second page should contain a blank for a cash balance. Both pages should be double ruled. The credit column in this cash blotter is to be used for cash rebates and for cash paid for the collection of old accounts, etc. The second page can be left on the superintendent's desk each morning by the bookkeeper, thereby giving the superintendent a complete itemized record of the cash receipts of the previous day, together with a cash balance. Distribution to the cash book. (See Figs. 87 and 88.)

Journal.—Many bookkeeping systems attempt to discard the journal, but my experience has shown it to be an exceedingly useful book as an intermediary for transactions which do not pass through the cash book or day book. Expenditures for special purposes, profit and loss items, investments, etc., should be entered in the journal and then transferred to the general ledger. The items that are entered in the journal give greater

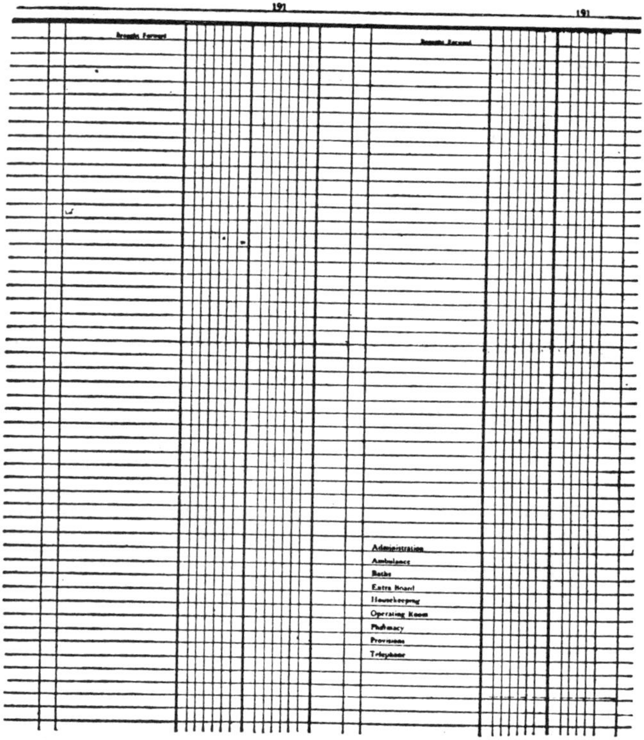

Fig. 87.—Cash blotter.

detail than the bare footings carried to the ledger, and permit easy references to investments, miscellaneous transactions, etc. Distribution to the general ledger.

Cash Book.—This book is well known and needs little comment. Summarized cash items are transferred to this book daily from the cash blotter in greater or less detail. Distribution to the general ledger.

Voucher Record.—This book is for the entry of invoices and the classification of expense items under their

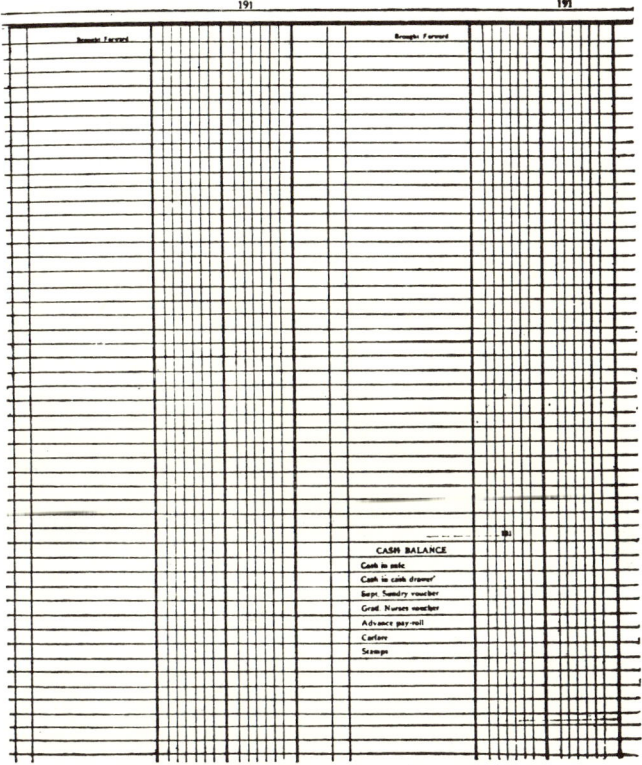

Fig. 88.—Cash blotter for carbon copy.

various headings. Distribution to the material stock book and general ledger. (See Figs. 89, 90, 91.)

Patients' Board Book or Register.—This is one of the important records of the hospital, and is arranged on the same lines as a hotel board book. This book should have

THE GRACE HOSPITAL VOUCHER REGISTER, 19

	Voucher Number	In Favor of	Amount	Date Paid	Material Stock			Pharmacy
					Provisions	Pharmacy	Soap and Starch	
1		Forward						
2								
3								
4								
5								
6								
7								
8								
9								
10								
11								
12								
13								
14								
15								
16								
17								
18								
19								
20								
21								
22								
23								
24								
25								
26								
27								
28								
29								
30								
31								
32								
33								
34								
35								
36								
37								
38								
39								
40								
41								
42								
43								
44								
45								
		Forward						

Fig. 89.—Voucher record.

HOSPITAL BOOKKEEPING

The Grace Hospital Voucher Register,

Superintendence	Laboratory						MISCELLANEOUS		
							Ledger F	Accounts	Amount

Fig. 90.—Voucher record, continued.

a 11- by 16-inch page, and contain the following headings: consecutive number, name of patient, where located; date of admission; date of discharge; rate per week; number of days in hospital; amount due, and diagnosis. The distribution of the total board earnings is to the journal and thence to the general ledger.

THE GRACE HOSPITAL *material Stock*										
Voucher No.	In Favor of	Description of Voucher	Amount	SUPPLIES			D Pharmacy	E	F Fuel and Light	
					A Provisions	B Pharmacy	C Soap and Starch			

| G Ambulance | H Hospital Nursing | I House-keeping | J Laundry | K Stationery | L Training School | M Laboratory | N Current Repairs | | | L. F. | Miscel. | Unpaid Vouchers |

Fig. 91.—Voucher register headings.

General Ledger.—This book should be the repository and record of all hospital investments, endowment funds, income funds, department receipts and expenditures, etc. Distribution of footings to trial balance each month when making monthly report.

Patients' History and Ledger Cards.—Each patient should have an individual card, ruled on one side as a history card, and on the reverse as a ledger card. These should be consecutively numbered and filed. Index according to consecutive numbers with a Graves' index.

HOSPITAL BOOKKEEPING 215

The card history is made out from the history taken by the nurse. Distribution is to the board book. As pay-

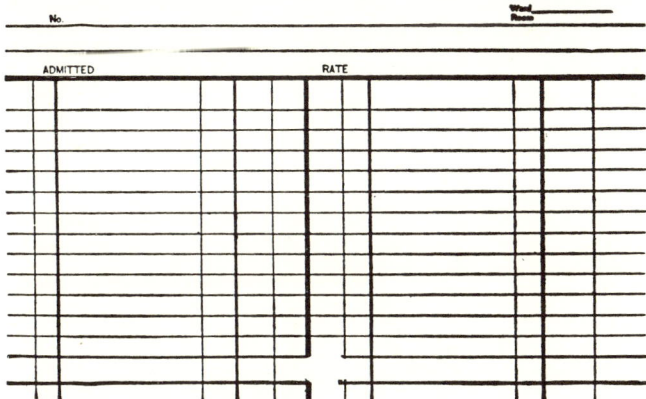

Fig. 92.—Patient's history card.

ments are made the patient is credited on the ledger card. (See Figs. 92 and 93.) With individual ledger cards it

Fig. 93.—Patient's ledger card, printed on reverse of history card.

is not necessary to open a patients' ledger, and their use will avoid duplication of much book work.

Vouchers and Checks.—Combination vouchers and checks are coming into general use in hospital work. (See

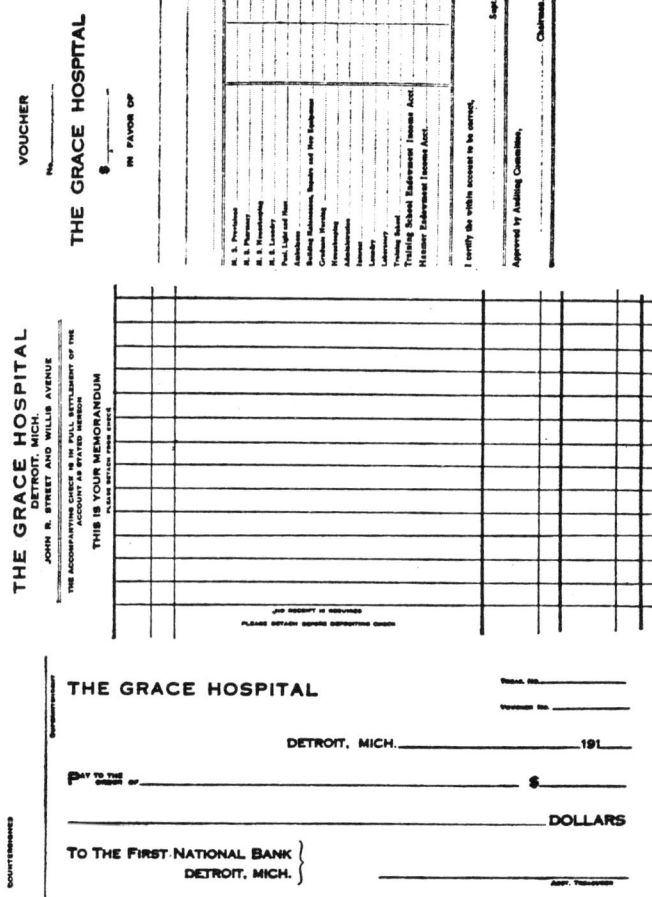

Fig. 94.—Combined voucher and check.

Figs. 94 and 95). This form is self-explanatory. They should preferably be typewritten, and, after being checked and countersigned by the superintendent, are entered in the voucher record, and forwarded to the treasurer's office.

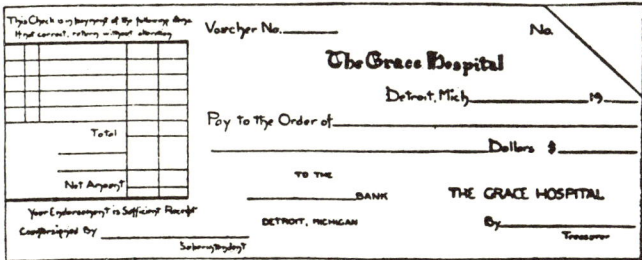

Fig. 95.—Combined voucher and check.

Another form of combined voucher and check is illustrated in Fig. 95. With either of these forms it is not necessary to have receipts from the payees.

Fig. 96.—Form of pay-roll.

Pay-rolls.—Each department in a hospital of 100 beds or more should have a separate pay-roll, so that employees in one department will not become too familiar with the wages paid in another department. The pay-roll distribution is to the voucher book the same as expense accounts. (See Fig. 96.)

Material Stock or Inventory Book.—The storekeeper's inventory, previously described, and the expenses as classified in the voucher register are transferred on the first of each month to the material stock and inventory book, under the proper headings, such as provisions, housekeeping, pharmacy, etc. This book has a four-column ruling as follows:

First column, inventory, December 31st.

Second column, January purchases.

Third column, storekeeper's issues for January.

Fourth column, inventory, January 31st.

For example, the provisions may be subdivided, as shown in the material stock account (p. 225). The issues in the third column of the material stock book are found by adding the inventory for the preceding month to the purchases during the month and subtracting the inventory at the end of the month. This will give the book issues, which can be compared with the storekeeper's requisition issues after they are totaled, and a check kept on the storeroom issues in this way.

PURCHASING DEPARTMENT

As this department furnishes most of the items for the bookkeeping system, it seems wise to consider it somewhat in detail.[1]

Storekeeper's Books and Forms.—(1) Storekeeper's purchase order blank. (See Fig. 97.)

(2) Storekeeper's receipt sheets, cards, or book. (See Fig. 98.)

(3) Storekeeper's bill book, for entry of invoices.

(4) Storekeeper's issue sheets. (See Figs. 99 and 100.)

(5) Storekeeper's inventory sheets or cards.

[1] See chapter on "The Hospital Store," by Dr. J. Lyman Belknap, elsewhere in this manual.

The order blank should be made out in triplicate.

THE GRACE-HOSPITAL. Order No._____
JOHN R STREET AND WILLIS AVENUE.
PURCHASE ORDER BLANK.

W. L. BABCOCK, M. D.
SUPERINTENDENT

Detroit, Mich. _____ 19____

To _____

Please deliver to The Grace Hospital the following supplies:

_____
Superintendent.

Enter order number on invoice.
This order is contingent on immediate delivery of above articles in good condition. Invoice must accompany all goods delivered and *itemized* Statement should be rendered promptly on last day of month.
All bills will be paid on or before the 15th of month.
Keep within the specified order both as to quantity and price.

(Form 5)

Fig. 97.—Form for storekeeper's purchase order blank.

Though the majority of orders in most hospitals are given over the telephone, it is recommended that these blanks be made out for telephone orders, as well as mail or personal orders. The second copy should be sent to the book-

THE GRACE HOSPITAL
STOREKEEPER'S DEPARTMENT

The following goods were received at this department, in good condition, with exceptions stated, on

_____ 19___

Storekeeper_____

AMOUNT	ARTICLE	CONVEYOR	CONDITION

Fig. 98.—Form for storekeeper's receipt sheets.

keeper's office, and the third copy retained in the storeroom.

The head storekeeper should be responsible for the receipt of all supplies, even though several storerooms be

HOSPITAL BOOKKEEPING 221

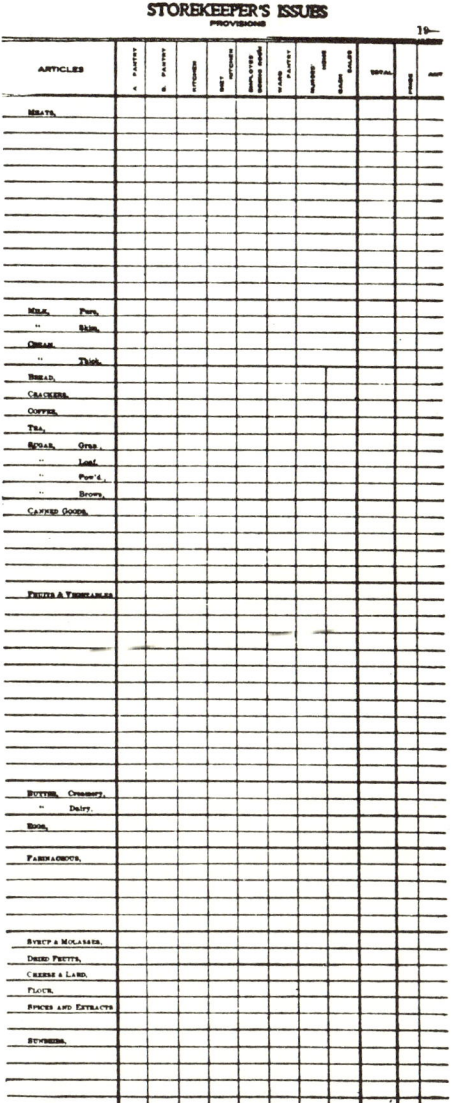

Fig. 99.—Form for storekeeper's issue sheet.

maintained. In other words, kitchen supplies, housekeeping supplies, drugs, liquors, etc., and even flowers and gifts for patients, should be receipted for and entered in the general storeroom, and thence forwarded or distrib-

STOREKEEPER'S ISSUES. _____ 19__
HOUSEKEEPING, LAUNDRY, PHARMACY AND TRAINING SCHOOL

	HOUSE-KEEPING.	LAUNDRY.	PHARMACY.	TRAINING SCHOOL.		CASH SALES.	TOTAL	PRICE	AMT.
SOAP, CHIP.									
SODA, WYANDOTTE									
STARCH, WHEAT									
STARCH, CORN									
SOAP, WHITE									
" BROWN.									
" OIL.									
" SCOURING.									
SAL SODA.									
FLOOR OIL.									

Fig. 100.—Form for storekeeper's issue sheet.

uted to the proper destination or placed in stock as the case may be.

The storekeeper's receipt sheets should be in duplicate, the original being forwarded to the bookkeeper's office, where it can be checked with the bills as to quantity and prices and the duplicate retained in the storeroom. The bills and invoices, after being checked and compared with purchase orders and quotations, are to be signed by the storekeeper, and sent to the general office for filing in the voucher covers.

The Grace Hospital Requisition.

Furnish the following supplies to_____

_____Supt.

Received the above supplies_____191 __

Signed_____

Fig. 101.—Requisition blank.

The storekeeper's issue sheets should have headings to correspond with the various departments of the hospital, and the goods issued charged to the department making the requisition. Each department to which goods are issued, such as housekeeping, pharmacy, training-school, engineer's, ambulance, laundry departments, etc., should keep an account of *their* receipts and issues on printed index cards arranged for that purpose. The card should be headed with the name of each article used in that particular department and should show date, kind and quantity received, amount used or distributed, and how distributed. This system may seem complicated and cumbersome to those who have not tried it, but its simplicity will soon be apparent if it is given a trial.

Issue of Supplies.—No supplies should be issued from the general storeroom, except on a requisition prepared and signed by the head of department and countersigned by the superintendent. (See Fig. 101.)

Material Stock Inventory.—On the last day of each month a complete inventory of the goods in stock should be furnished to the chief bookkeeper by the storekeeper. This inventory should state the amount and cost of each article in stock, and should be arranged under proper stock headings. It is advisable to keep a separate heading for provisions, even though the provisions may be distributed under various department heads, in the record of distribution of expenses. Personally, I do not believe that the cost of provisions can be distributed throughout the various departments of a general hospital so that each department is properly charged with its use of provisions. It is true that this can be approximated, but as it depends on the individual equations of clerks, it is far from accurate. This difficulty in charging supplies is due largely to the intimate associations of one department with another, especially in kitchens, dining-rooms, etc.

It has been found in practice that the following classification of provisions, pharmacy, and housekeeping supplies is simple and adequate. The division illustrated below is a method that can be carried throughout all departments, such as training-school, engineer's department, laundry, etc.

In small hospitals it is not necessary that all departments have a material stock account, owing to the fact that few supplies are kept in stock for them, and are issued or used immediately on receipt.

Material Stock Account.
(Division.)

Provisions, material stock:

Bread and crackers.	Fruits and vegetables.
Butter.	Ice.
Canned goods.	Meat.
Cheese and lard.	Milk.
Coffee.	Spices and extracts.
Dried fruits.	Sugar.
Eggs.	Sundries.
Farinaceous foods.	Syrup and molasses.
Flour.	Tea.

Housekeeping, material stock:

Brushes, mops, and brooms.	Soap and sal soda.
Crockery.	Sundries.
Dry goods.	Tin, wood, and iron utensils.
Paper and paper bags.	

Pharmacy, material stock:

Drugs.	Surgical dressings.
Instruments.	Surgical supplies.
Liquors.	

The material stock inventory should classify all goods in stock under the above and such other headings as may be used. On completion the priced inventory should be checked with the bills by clerks in the main office, not connected with the storeroom, to make sure that the cost prices carried out are correct. The inventory is then entered on the material stock book.

Purchase Ledger.—A good business man will discount bills for cash within ten or thirty days. Where such bills are discounted, a purchase ledger should be opened. All cash discounts of the preceding month are totaled

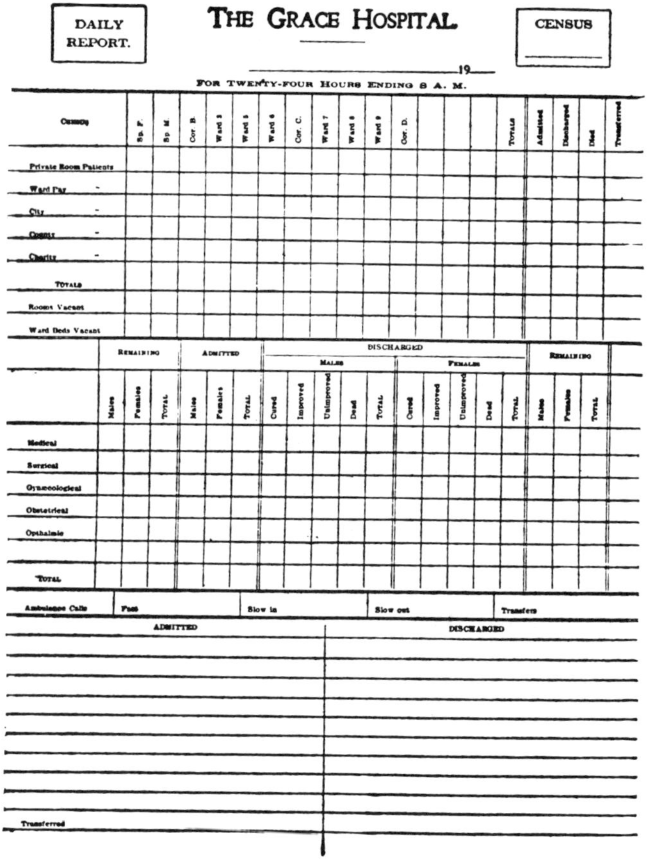

Fig. 102.—Form for daily report

from the treasurer's report or the vouchers, and entered in the following month's transactions as discount earnings.

HOSPITAL BOOKKEEPING

THE GRACE HOSPITAL.   Report for Month of _____ 19__

PATIENTS TREATED IN HOSPITAL.

	Remaining On			Admitted In			Discharged In											Remaining On		
							Males					Females								
	Males	Females	Total	Males	Females	Total	Cured	Improved	Unimproved	Dead	Total	Cured	Improved	Unimproved	Dead	Total		Males	Females	Total
Medical																				
Surgical																				
Gynæcological																				
Obstetrical																				
Ophthalmic																				
TOTAL																				
GRAND TOTAL						Treated					Discharged									

OUT-DOOR DEPARTMENT POLYCLINIC

	New Cases			Visits		
	Male	Fem.	Total	Male	Fem.	Total
Medical						
Surgical						
Gynæcological						
Ophthalmic						
Dermatological						
Laryngological						
Diseases of Children						
Neurological						
TOTAL						
GRAND TOTAL						
PRESCRIPTIONS						

AMBULANCE

	Brought In	Taken Home	No Case	Total
Emergency Calls				
Sick Calls				
Transfers				
TOTAL				

MAINTENANCE

Day's Maintenance—Staff, Nurses and Employes	
" Patients	
Total Days of Maintenance	
Total Meals Furnished	
Average Cost of Food per Person per Meal	
Average Cost of Maintenance per Person per Day	
Average cost per patient per day.	

MISCELLANEOUS

Number Officers and Employes	
Administration Dept.	
Ambulance "	
Fuel, Light and Heat Dept.	
Housekeeping "	
Laundry "	
Medical "	
Repair and Building Maintenance Dept.	
Training School, Officers	
" " Nurses	
" " Orderlies	
" " Employees.	
Average Daily Population	
Total Number Treated	
Number of Deaths	

Fig. 103.—Form for cover of monthly report sheets.

Monthly Report.—The monthly report should contain a general report of all earnings and expenditures. The earnings should include the regular hospital earnings and the income from the endowment fund, which it may be necessary to prorate for twelve months. The interest earnings, insurance, and interest charges are also generally prorated, and carried into the expense account in the ledger until the end of the year. The monthly and annual reports, when presented to the board of trustees, are generally faced with a statistical summary, more or less varied, such as is illustrated in Fig. 103.

Training-school Ledger.—This should be kept in the clerk's office, from the daily records of the superintendent of nurses. It should include charges made for graduate and pupil special nursing. The following headings are necessary: consecutive number and name of patient, name of graduate or pupil, date of assignment and relief from case, total number of days of special nursing, and total amount earned. Distribution to journal and thence to general ledger, to the credit of graduate nursing or training-school, as the case may be.

COST SYSTEMS

All hospital authorities should attempt to maintain some kind of check on expenditures. This is done by classifying the various expenditures from day to day, and month to month, and charging them to the department in which they originate. By this arrangement of expenditures, the cost of items of service, per patient *per day*, can be ascertained. This is the unit upon which all expenditures should be based and finally reduced. A cost system enables the superintendent, at any time, to ascertain the exact cost per patient per day of any given item in use in the hospital. After a few months' use of this system, any fluctuation in the *per diem per patient* cost will show the superintendent that the particular article under investigation was used in greater quantity, was wasted, or was increased in cost price. The scope of this article does not include a detailed discussion of cost accounting.[1]

```
                                          No. _____
                    AMBULANCE
                The Grace Hospital
                          ———
                    VISITING TICKET
                          ———

                    _____ 191___
                    Time _____
        Dr. _____
                Please_____ by ambulance.
        Name _____
        Address _____
                                        Room
        Directions _____ Ward _____
        Left _____ Arrived _____ Ret'd _____
                    _____ M. D.
---------------------------------------------------
                                          No. _____
                    AMBULANCE
                          ———
                    _____ 191___
        CLERK:
                    Charge M _____
        Room
        Ward _____
        
        For ambulance service. $ _____
                    Signed _____
```

Fig. 104.

Methods of Charging Sundry Items.—Most hospitals make a charge for ambulance services, operating-room

[1] In this connection readers are referred to an excellent article by Dr. Thomas Howell, Supt., The New York Hospital, published in the Eleventh Annual Report of the American Hospital Association.

services, patent medicines, wines, liquors, hot-air baths, telephones, etc. The head of each department rendering service for which a charge is made is furnished printed double charge slips, perforated between, in pad form.

BATHS: No. 1692

The Grace Hospital

_____ 191___

BATH ATTENDANT:

Please give _____ Room Ward _____

One _____ Bath.

_____
Principal.

....

BATHS: No. 1692.

_____ 191___

CLERK:

Charge _____ Room Ward _____

one_____ bath $ _____

_____
Bath Attendant.

Fig. 105.

The first or upper half orders the service and the second makes the charge. The first slip goes to the employee who carries out the service, such as the ambulance surgeon or bath attendant, and the second slip is filed with the

HOSPITAL BOOKKEEPING

No._____

EXTRA BOARD

GUEST MEALS

The Grace Hospital

_____M. _____191____

DIETIST:

Please serve_____meal

for_____in Room_____

_____
Principal.

No._____

EXTRA BOARD

_____M. _____191____

CLERK:

Please charge_____Room_____

_____Tray.

_____
Principal.

Fig. 106.

The Grace Hospital.

..................M

..............................191...

Pharmacy

  Please supply...

for.................................... m. ....

_____
                    NURSE.

..............................191...

Office:

  Charge .... $

for.. supplied

to..

_____
                PHARMACIST.

Fig. 107.

TELEPHONES: No..........

THE GRACE HOSPITAL.

..............................191...

..............................M.

CLERK.

Charge .... Room / Ward ....

for telephone service............call............cts.

_____
           Telephone Operator.

Fig. 108.

bookkeeper daily. These slips should be of a different color, in each department, and numbered consecutively, so that no error will occur in their final distribution.

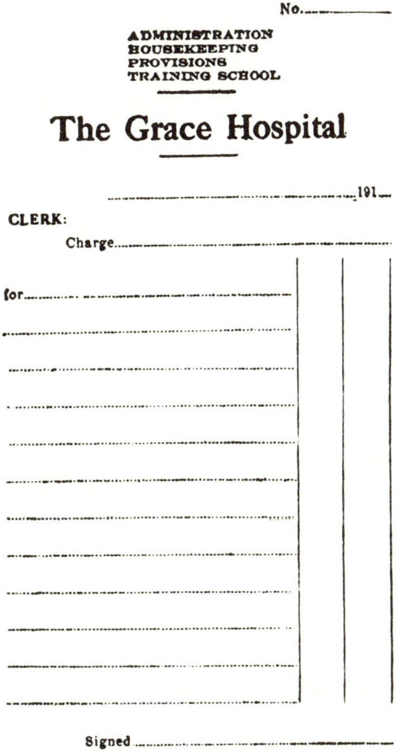

No._____

ADMINISTRATION
HOUSEKEEPING
PROVISIONS
TRAINING SCHOOL

The Grace Hospital

_____191__

CLERK:

Charge_____

for_____

Signed _____

Fig. 109.

They are charged daily by the bookkeeper on the ledger card of the patient receiving the service, and are credited in the earnings to the department furnishing the service or supplies.

ESTIMATES

In state and public institutions it is necessary for the executive to prepare monthly, quarterly, or annual estimates for the maintenance of the institution. These estimates are usually subdivided under headings for the

No._____

BOOKKEEPER'S REBATE
AND
COLLECTION ACCOUNT

The Grace Hospital

_____ 191___

CLERK:

Please charge rebate account of _____

Room
Ward_____ $_____

Charge same to _____ account

_____

_____

_____

_____
Superintendent.

Fig. 110.

respective departments of the institution. In addition estimates are prepared for any special or extraordinary repairs or expenditures that may be necessary, such as the erection of new buildings, the purchase of additional real estate, etc.

HOSPITAL BOOKKEEPING

Estimates for the maintenance of institutions of this character are based on the cost of operation of the institutions on a *per capita* basis. No fixed rule can be laid

```
                                          No._____
              OPERATING ROOM

             The Grace Hospital
                         _____ 191___
    CLERK:
                                    Room
              Charge_____       Ward _____

    for operating room services.  $_____

                     Signed_____
                                      Resident Physician.
```
Fig. 111.

down for the preparation of such estimates, owing to the fact that they are required in more or less detail, in accordance with the recommendations laid down by the board, commission, or municipality in charge of the institution.

CHAPTER IX

THE HOSPITAL STORE

By J. Lyman Belknap, M.D.

The hospital store or storeroom should be something more than a mere room where supplies are kept until needed; it should be a store in every sense of the word, run with systematic, business-like methods, the only difference being that money is not handled. In order to do this, all supplies must be taken up by making a careful and complete stock inventory at least once a year, usually January 1st; then all stock added should be entered in a book known as the receiving book. Nothing should leave the store except by requisition, which will act as a receipt for the article issued. If this plan is carried out, one can easily know the stock on hand by keeping a perpetual stock inventory.

Stock Inventory.—A simple and accurate method of taking a stock inventory is that used by the library bureau. Cheap cards of any shape desired are numbered serially to take up the entire stock. The stock-room is divided into sections for convenience, and two persons, if possible, take the inventory of each section. Each person or party is given inventory cards, and the first and last numbers given out are noted by the person in charge of the inventory taking. When two people are working together, one calls off the name of each article and the number in stock, as brooms, corn, 10; the other writes the card and leaves it on the article. In this way they go through the stock. Unused cards are returned by a party and reissued. A person who has not taken the inventory of a certain section collects the cards of that section, counting the stock and checking each card as he picks it up; his card numbers should be the same as those who took the inventory, as inventory taker, cards 125 to 277; checker, cards 125 to 277. After all the cards have been collected, they are sorted into groups, as bedding, furniture, stationery, and each group arranged alphabetically if a permanent stock inventory is to be made and valuations taken. When a perpetual stock inventory alone is wanted, the cards are arranged alphabetically, and checked again as the amounts are transferred to the stock cards.

Receiving Book.—The receiving book should be kept in the store, and the storekeeper should be responsible for it. A good form is one kept in duplicate by using a carbon copy. The original sheets are torn out and have holes for filing; they are sent to the person in charge of the perpetual stock inventory every day, best in the evening, and filed in a binder; the carbon copy remains in the receiving book. The original sheets and carbon copies are numbered alike, and the numbers continue throughout the year. The receiving clerk begins a new sheet every morning, and as the goods received are examined and weighed, if necessary, the quantity, style of package, as barrel, box, bag, the proper name of the article, and the name of the shipper are entered. If weights are made they are entered after the article. (See sample sheet of receiving book.) The store receipts should be posted in the perpetual stock inventory daily, and each article checked on the receiving sheet when posted.

There should be a column on the original sheets for checking bills, and bills as soon as received go to the stock clerk, who verifies them, writes the date of receiving the bill opposite the article, and puts his mark on the bill. Thus, incorrect weights or charges are easily detected and second bills recognized.

Requisitions.—The variety of requisitions used depends on the number of articles carried and the issues made, as daily, weekly, monthly, emergency. If the store is a large one there should be at least weekly and emergency requisitions. If the articles usually called for on the

Massachusetts General Hospital

..................191

Please deliver for use in .... *a WEEKLY SUPPLY of the following articles:*

On Hand	Returned	Wanted	Delivered				On Hand	Returned	Wanted	Delivered			
				Compress, piece							Paper, toilet, bundles		
				Cotton, absorbent, lbs.							Paper, wrapping, quires		
				Cotton, picked, lbs.							Polish, brass box		
				Gauze, new, lbs.							Soap, Bon Ami		
				Gauze, washed, lbs.							Soap, hard		
				Sheet wadding, doz. sh.							Soap, toilet		
				Straps, perineal, doz.							Soap, powder, lbs.		
				Blotters, large							Soap, sand		
				Books, order							Bowls		
				Charts, tempt., clinical							Butter chips		
				Charts, tempt., 4 hourly							Cups		
				Envelopes, manila, pkg.							Plates		
				Pads, scribbling, large							Saucers, preserve		
				Pads, scribbling, small							Saucers, tea		
				Paper, history							Tumblers		
				Pens, stub							Bedpans		
				Pens, fine							Cups, sputum		
				Pencils							Glasses, specimen		
				Matches, boxes							Mugs, medicine		
				Pins, common, papers							Urinals		
				Pins, safety, large, gross							Brooms, corn		
				Pins, safety, small, gross							Brooms, hair		
				Twine, balls							Brooms, whisk		
				Bags, paper, B. H. doz							Brushes, nail		
				Bags, paper, plain, doz.							Brushes, scrub		

Write in below unlisted articles needed

Requested by ....

Approved by .... *Res. Phys.*

Delivered by ....

Received by ....

Fig. 112.—Weekly supply requisition.

weekly requisition, as soap, gauze, pens, pins, matches, and the like are printed on the requisition in groups, as stationery and dressing supplies, and the units issued, as dozen, boxes, pounds (Fig. 112), the requisitions will be

Massachusetts General Hospital

DAILY REQUISITION

Store................   Ward................

	Oz. Butter		
	Doz. Eggs		
	" Lemons		
	Lbs. Sugar		
	" Crackers		

.... *Head Nurse*

Approved..
.... *Resident Physician*

Date,................................*191*

Fig. 113.—Form for daily requisitions.

more easily handled because the same article will always appear in the same place. Blank spaces should be left on the requisition to write in articles not commonly called for. A daily requisition may be used for supplies issued daily, as butter, eggs, fruit; a monthly requisition for linen and an emergency requisition for anything needed between the times of filling the regular requisitions. Different colors make the requisitions easy to separate, as daily, pink, and

REQUISITION.
FOR EMERGENCIES ONLY

Mass. Gen. Hospital, January 3 1911

The following articles were delivered from Store, Dept.) to Kitchen, (Dept.)

Please use a separate blank for each Department, and place all blanks on file at office daily.

Quantity.	DESCRIPTION OF ARTICLES.		
1 bbl	Sugar, granulated		

Requested by .... M. C. Cody.
Approved by .... L. C. B. .... Supt.
Delivered by .... T. S.
Received by .... M. C. Cody

Fig. 114.—Form for emergency requisitions.

emergency, white. (See Figs. 113 and 114). The requisition may be made out singly, in duplicate or in triplicate, but the single form properly signed will meet the usual needs. The signature should be: (1) The nurse or person requesting the articles; (2) the superintendent approving the requisition; (3) the storekeeper delivering the articles requested and approved; (4) the nurse or person receiving the articles delivered. The requisition should then be returned to the storekeeper to go on file, as his receipt for goods expended.

Perpetual Stock Inventory.—The perpetual stock inventory is kept on stock cards or sheets filed in a binder; the former is more easily handled. One card is kept for each article; or if several sizes of an article are carried, one card for each size. These cards are kept in a tray, ordinarily arranged in alphabetic order by name of article and by sizes under each article. They may be arranged numerically by catalogue number, if there is a complete catalogue classification. An alphabetic or numeric guide is inserted about every twenty cards. The exact form of stock-card is determined by the conditions existing in the store in which it is to be used. A good form is a light-weight 5 by 8 inch card, without holes for tray rod and printed on both sides. Space is provided at the top of the card for the name of the article; the catalogue number or size of the article; where stored, and section; the unit of measure, as pound, box, dozen, and for maximum and minimum limits between which stock on hand must be kept. The columns below are for the date and amount of each receipt and disbursement, and for the balance on hand after each receipt or delivery. Each side of the card has space for 64 entries; these 128 entries are usually enough unless stock moves very actively.[1] When both sides of a card have been filled, a new card is inserted in the file directly in front of the old card, and the balance on the old card carried forward to the new. The old card is taken from the file as soon as its record is of no more interest and either stored or destroyed. As new articles are put into stock, new cards are made out and inserted in their exact place in the file; if articles are dropped from stock, their cards are removed. If this inventory is to be of any value, it must be posted daily; in this way, the inventory is always one day behind, but never more; the receipts and deliveries of Monday are entered on Tuesday. When this

[1] See sample stock card, Fig. 115.

is done, it is a perpetual record, practically up to date, and keeps the person in charge of supplies informed concerning the important facts of the store or storeroom, as—(1) it shows the balance on hand of each article at any time, thus aiding purchases to be made at the right time and to the best advantage; (2) it shows how fast any article is being used and the amount used in any given time; (3) it makes it possible to find out if there is any leakage of stock, and places the responsibility of careful honest work on the storekeeper; (4) if the maximum and minimum amounts

Article: Sugar, granulated					No. or Size: —	Where Stored: 1st flor. Sec. 6	Unit: 8 lb	Max. 20 Min. 2		
DATE	RECEIVED	DATE	DELIVERED	BALANCE	DATE	RECEIVED	DATE	DELIVERED	BALANCE
		Dec 31-09	1	3					
Jan 1-10				3					
		Jan 1-10	1	2					
Jan 3-10	20			22					
		Jan 3-10	1	21					
		Jan 4-10	1	20					

Fig. 115.—Sample stock card.

are used, it shows just when to order, so that the fresh supply will arrive before all the old has been issued; also makes it possible to work with a small supply of stock which is always kept moving, thus saving the interest on dead or slowly moving stock, and preventing the storeroom from being filled with articles not needed for immediate use.

In a hospital where the store or storeroom is not large, and there is no storekeeper or clerk to post the receipts and deliveries, a perpetual stock inventory card may be made, about 10 by 4 inches, of medium weight cardboard, printed on both sides, and hung on a hook above or beside each compartment containing an article. The words article, number or size, unit, maximum and minimum, should be at the top of the card; the columns below being the same as on the 5- by 8-inch card. The balance is set down when the inventory is taken; then one person should look after the storeroom, and as an article is issued or received, the date and amount are put on the stock-card and the balance drawn. An order is made when the minimum amount is reached, the order bringing the stock on hand to the maximum amount. In this way a check as to the amount of stock and when to order may be kept without much bookkeeping. A receiving book should not be required, and written requisitions could be used or not as desired. In the case of a large store, the question of where shall the perpetual stock inventory be kept, is an important one. The ideal method is to have it in the hands of a clerk or cashier who is not interested in the store; this makes the bookkeeping done by one department while the store-keeping is done by another. The storekeeper simply receives and delivers goods, without keeping track of them, and is not concerned with the supply on hand, amounts ordered, or bills. Of course, his supply of any article should equal that on the balance of the stock-card, and if it does not, he alone (barring incorrect clerical work) is responsible for the error and has to account for it. The ordering should be done by an authorized person, and the bills paid by the same person, after they have been checked up from the receiving book by the inventory keeper.

Example of Perpetual Stock Inventory.—The following is an example of the method of keeping the perpetual stock inventory. The stock-card for sugar, granulated, showed a balance of 3 barrels after the delivery of December 31, 1909, and the same balance on January 1, 1910, when the annual inventory was taken. After the delivery of January 1st was made, the minimum amount, or 2 barrels, was reached; therefore an order for the maximum of 20 barrels was placed with J. C. Brown Co. by the person in charge of the purchasing. The reason for these maximum and minimum figures is that the average rate of issuing granulated sugar is 1 barrel a day and an order is filled and delivered the same day or the morning of the next day; this prompt delivery allows the low minimum and lessens the maximum, as a 20-barrel order is the smallest on which the wholesale discount can be obtained; 20 is used as the maximum and orders are placed about once in three weeks, instead of ordering larger quantities less often. This method saves storage space, interest on stock, and lessens the chances of loss or deterioration. When the storekeeper receives this order, he posts the quantity—20; style of package—barrels; article—sugar, granulated, and shipper—J. C. Brown Co., on the original sheet of his receiving book for the date January 3, 1911. (See Plate I.) This original sheet is detached from his receiving book when he closes the store in the evening, and sent to the stock-keeper, the carbon copy remaining in the receiving book of the storekeeper. On January 4th the stock-keeper posts the stock-card sugar, granulated, as is shown, and draws the balance, 22; at the same time the receiving sheet is checked in the column as marked; on January 3, 1910, the kitchen has sent a requisition to the storekeeper for one barrel sugar, granulated. (See Fig. 114.) This issue was made and the requisition turned over to the stock-keeper with the receiving sheet of January 3, 1910. The sample stockcard shows that this has been posted and the balance of 21 drawn; a similar requisition dated January 4th is posted on January 5th. On January 5, 1910, the bill from J. C. Brown Co. reached the stock-keeper; it was found to be correct, so the date of receiving it is posted on the receiving sheet in the column—check for bills—opposite the sugar entry. The bill is initialed by the stock-keeper, to show that the sugar was received and that it is correct, and sent to the person in charge of the purchasing or first to the cashier if payment is made by check. In this case

PLATE I

January 3-1911

Check for posting	Check for bills	Quantity	Size of package	Article	Shipper
✓	Jan 5-11	20	Bbls	Sugar, granulated Wt 6500 lbs	J. C. Brown Co.

Sample receiving book sheet.

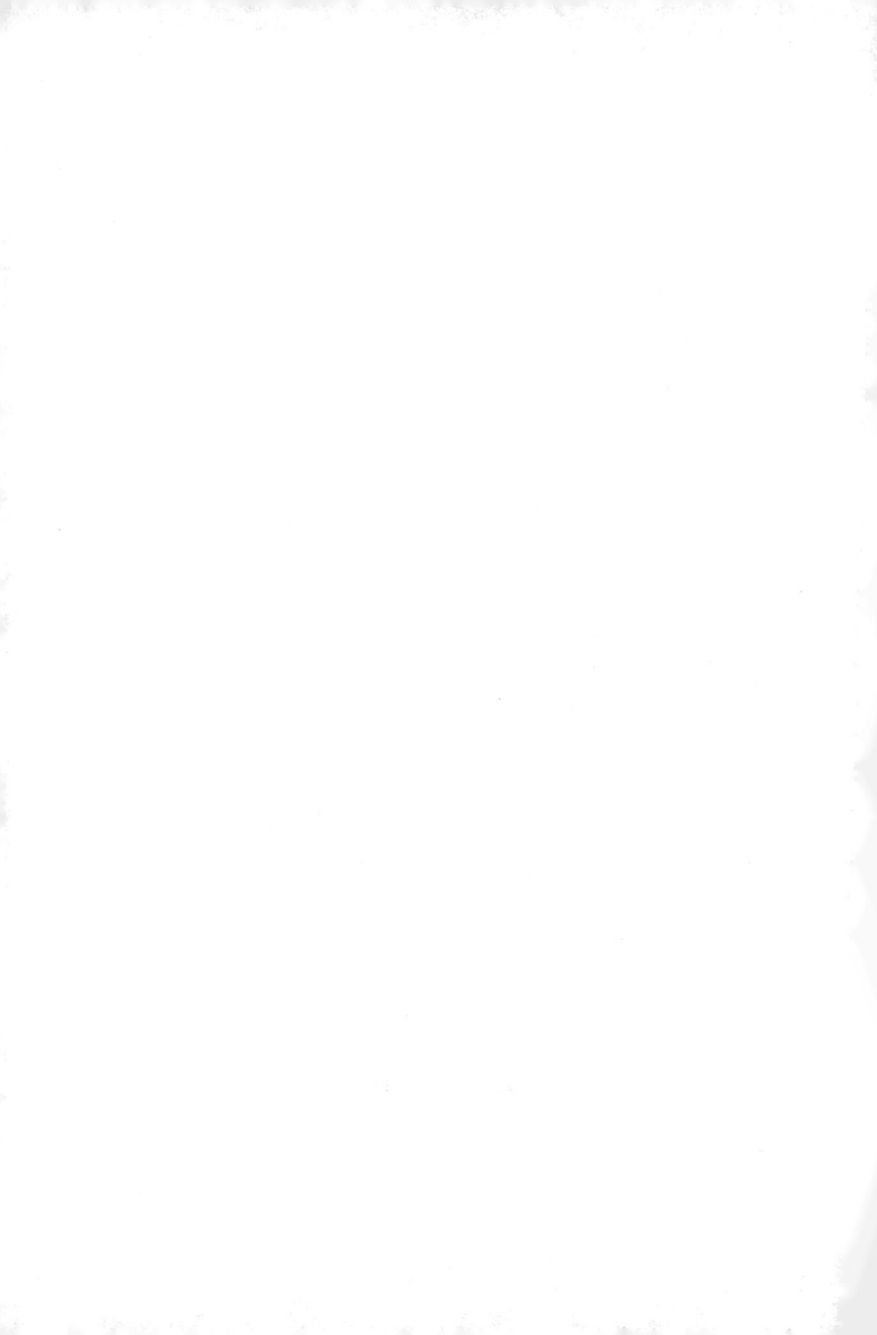

the stock-card heading shows that No. or Size is not used because there are no numbers or sizes; also the unit is bbls. and not lbs., because the amount of granulated sugar used in issuing is an unopened barrel instead of pounds. Here the sugar is stored in section 6 on the first floor. The maximum of 22 and the minimum of 2 have been explained.

Selection of Articles for Perpetual Stock Inventory. —It can be readily seen that certain articles of a class cannot be posted on a perpetual stock inventory with accuracy, while others can. In the main meat, vegetables, and fruit are not suited for it; beef, pork, lamb, and the like, purchased in bulk, would not give the same weights when cut up for the kitchen, while bacon, ham, sausages and corned beef would. Cabbages and cauliflower purchased by the box and issued singly could not be carried, while potatoes bought and issued by the pound could be; bananas purchased by the bunch could not be issued accurately by the dozen or fraction of dozen; also apples received by the barrel; oranges might be carried if the number contained in the box is stamped on it. Certain articles passing through the store the date of receipt are best not inventoried, as fish, bread, milk, and cream. All canned goods and sealed packages, as cereals, crackers, and vegetables, are easily carried. Hospital furnishings, dressing materials, toilet articles, crockery and glassware, linen, blankets, and certain articles of stationery are important articles for the perpetual stock inventory, while small stationery articles, as pens, are hardly worth the trouble. Where a hospital has a large number of forms, these do not seem suitable for the stock inventory; also small inexpensive articles are best omitted.

If all the store receipts, including those not carried on the perpetual stock inventory, are entered in the receiving book, the stock-keeper can check the bills accurately; as the receiving book is not dependent on the perpetual stock inventory, while the latter is dependent on the former.

CHAPTER X

THE KITCHEN

By Renwick R. Ross, M.D.

Any discussion of the kitchen and food question of a hospital is necessarily a difficult task, for a plan has yet to be devised which will at all times give a satisfactory service to all people. Hospitals are run on the table-dehôte plan, and with the varying tastes which must necessarily exist both among patients and employees, it is a difficult problem to serve a meal which will be satisfactory to all. The best that can be done is to have food well prepared and satisfactory to the greatest number possible.

In order to approach the question in a logical way, it is best that the kind of building required and service it is expected to fulfil be first taken up. For some years there have been held conflicting views as to the best location for a kitchen. Some prefer the basement or first floor, some the top floor, and still others a separate building. To the writer it seems impossible to give any definite answer without knowing something of the plant to be constructed; circumstances must control the location of this important branch of hospital work. If the hospital is in a crowded district where land is high, the building will probably be many storied, and not occupying a large amount of ground space. In buildings of this character the kitchen had better be placed on the top floor, where the odors from cooking will not be carried through the building. This seems the only logical reason for such a location being chosen. The objections are many. First that part of the building which should be devoted to patients is taken up. If the ranges and ovens are heated by coal, the elevating of the coal and bringing down the

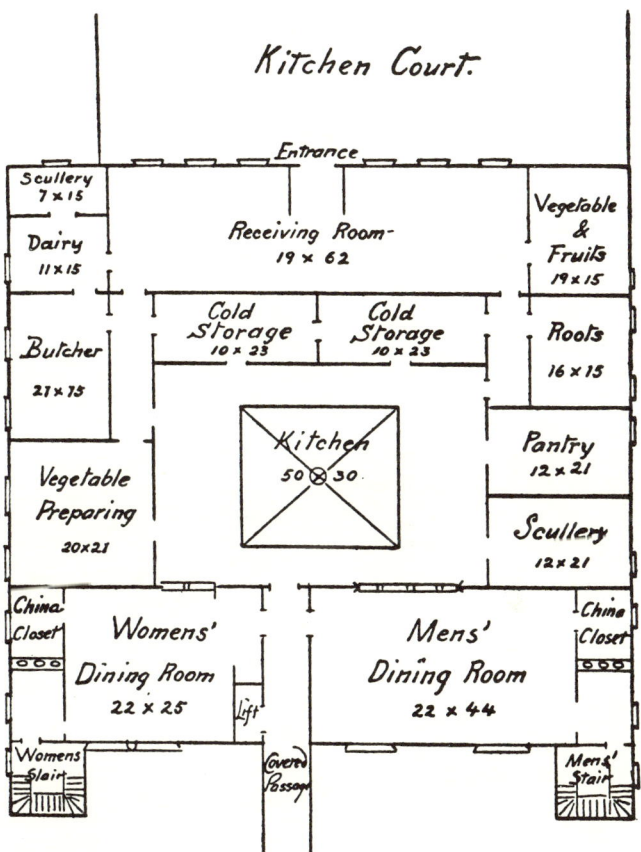

Fig. 116.—Basement plan of kitchen building suggested for new Toronto General Hospital.

ashes produces a large amount of dirt; steam-cookers are a long distance from the boilers or source of heat. To serve a top floor kitchen properly an elevator must be installed, kept in repairs and properly manned; the delivery and checking-in rooms must necessarily be near the ground level, and hence a long distance from where the goods are to be used. To elevate all food to the top floor is a greater task than it at first seems. There is also the question of the disposal of the garbage. This must be sent down, and its handling is always an unpleasant task. The sculleryman is not likely to be a man of intelligence or great care, who will always do his work in a satisfactory manner. About the kitchen there is more or less slopping and spilling, and no matter how tight the floors of large rooms are laid, there is likely to be some cracking. This is more likely to take place on the top floor of a high building than in a low one, and as a result of these seams or cracks ceilings underneath are sometimes stained. The great objection to the kitchen being in the basement or first floor is the odor of cooking. None of the objections which I have mentioned above apply to a kitchen of this location; on the contrary, it has some advantages not possessed by the room higher up. It is near the receiving room, near the checking-in room and store-rooms, near the ice supply, and many times occupies a space which cannot be advantageously used for patients. My preference is for a separate building, but closely connected to the main building by a covered way. It has all the advantages of the first floor kitchen, and does not permit of odors being carried through the main building. Many of us, however, are not so fortunate as to be able to start with a vacant plot and construct "de novo." We have a plant constructed perhaps some years ago, and the kitchen so located that there is no choice as to whether it shall be on the roof, on the first floor, or in a separate building. All too frequently we find it tucked away in some dark basement with bad light, poor ventilation, and unsanitary surroundings, a place in which no thought has been given to the comfort and health of those who must spend fourteen hours a day for every day in the year in it. In planning for the kitchen service of a hospital thought must be given to many things

THE KITCHEN

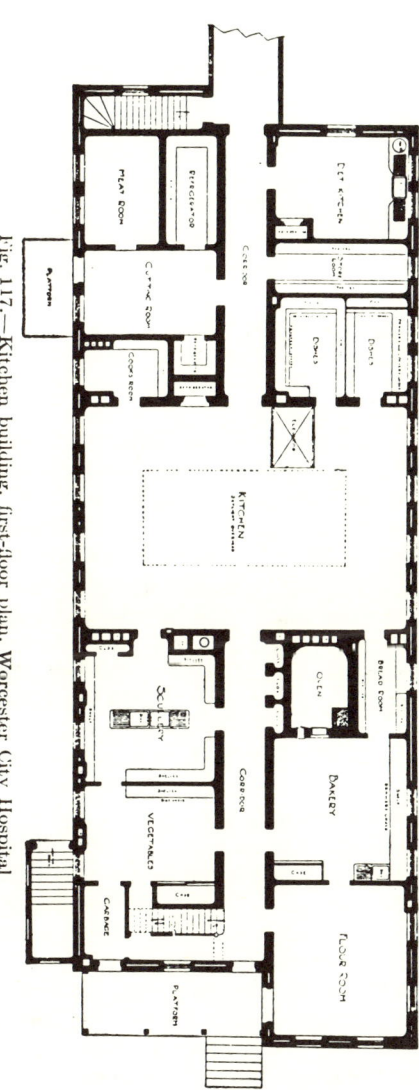

Fig. 117.—Kitchen building, first-floor plan, Worcester City Hospital

besides that of providing a room for the cooking of foods. It should be of such a size as to permit of future growth of the hospital; care should, however, be taken to see that it is not too large. When oversized, distances between sinks, ranges, etc., are great, and steps are unnecessarily multiplied. In construction, convenience and adaptability should be the chief aim.

Store-rooms should be so placed that supplies can be easily reached, but other features must be taken into consideration when locating this room. They will probably be entered as many times for the purpose of distributing goods to other parts of the hospital as they will be to give out supplies for the kitchen; the location should, therefore, be such that the kitchen will not be entered in getting to the store-rooms. It is to these rooms that all goods must be delivered, and this makes it necessary to have them so placed that delivery-wagons may easily approach them and dispose of their goods in a quick and convenient way. In placing the receiving scales, this should be taken into consideration. I have seen storerooms so remotely placed that much time and labor have been consumed in wheeling goods through corridors.

Were it possible to carry out a complete plan of refrigeration, I would attempt more than is usually done in hospitals, I would devote much more space than is usually allowed for this department, and feel confident that it would pay a good rate of interest on the investment, Hospitals have little or no space devoted to storage and, as a result, goods are bought in small quantities and on daily orders. With good storage it is frequently possible to take advantage of gluts in the market and thus materially reduce the cost. Artificial refrigeration has reached such a stage of perfection that even the smaller hospitals will find it advantageous to use it, especially those institutions which maintain power plants. The space for refrigeration should be divided into several rooms—a meat room, a milk and butter room, vegetable room, and cooked-food room. I have said enough, I believe, on the question of storage to stimulate those who contemplate building kitchens to give this subject further study.

Rooms for the preparation of vegetables, baking, etc., must all be taken into consideration when planning the kitchen work. In connection with the kitchen, or adjacent to it, should be placed the dining-room for employees, where food can be served with the minimum of expense consistent with good service.

For the nurses and doctors, many hospitals still have to rely on the main kitchen, but in many of the newer institutions, kitchens are being maintained in the nurses' residences with uniformly satisfactory results.

In hospitals having both a private room and a ward service it is best that the food for the private-room patients be cooked in a separate kitchen. The service required is so different that one kitchen does not give satisfactory results.

It has been the custom for many years to build serving kitchens in connection with the ward and room service. The equipment of these, however, appeals to me most strongly. The hospital with which the writer is connected is discarding steam tables, and is using gas plates and stoves, which have proved much more satisfactory. Articles of food, such as toast, zwieback, crackers, etc., do not become toughened by escaping steam, as happens when steam tables are used. The gas-stoves are more cleanly and have the distinct advantage of giving the nurse facilities for preparing any special article of diet desired.

Much trouble has been experienced by hospitals in keeping food hot until it is served to the patient, part of which has been due to the carelessness in the distribution from the main kitchen to the serving kitchens. Various carriers have been devised and put on the market. The institution with which the writer is connected is using one constructed after its own ideas, and which has given more satisfactory results than any yet tried. Some have been heated by compressed fuel, some by hot water, none of which have been entirely satisfactory. The one the Buffalo General Hospital is using is briefly as follows: One heavy tin box is placed within another with a space between of one inch, both on the bottom and on the sides; this is thoroughly packed with asbestos, and the space between the edges of the two boxes covered over. To fit the bottom of the inner box there are two plates—the two cover the entire bottom. These plates are made of asbestos one inch thick, and covered with black iron. Before the food is to be distributed these plates are laid for a few minutes on the top of the ranges, then placed in the bottom of the boxes. The food boxes are placed on these, and the whole covered with a tight-fitting cover. We have been able to keep food hot in this carrier for several hours. It is mounted on a suitable truck, which is easily wheeled to any part of the buildings or disconnected buildings.

It would be an ideal thing if all dish-washing could be done in one place where machinery for this purpose could be installed. This plan, however, does not seem practicable for hospitals, and the best plan is to make provision for this class of work in connection with each serving kitchen.

Psychologists tell us that persons employed about furnaces, kitchen ranges, or any place where they have to work in a high temperature, are likely to become unstable in disposition and intemperate in habits. If this be true, it is an explanation of the trouble so often experienced in this department. It is probably true that institutions, hotels, etc., have not given sufficient thought to the comfort of those who are expected to do this difficult and exacting work. The stokers and engineers of the great ocean ships, until recent years, have been given scant consideration. It is now beginning to be recognized that they are the ones who supply the power, and their skilful handling of the vessel many times wins the battle. Have the culinary department well handled, and much has been done to satisfy patients and to make employees contented and happy.

The organization of each plant will depend largely on its size and resources. In the smaller hospitals the superintendent frequently does the purchasing and issuing of supplies. In still others this work is relegated to the head cook—a plan not to be advised. The ideal arrangement is to have an efficient person, whether it be a man or a woman, in charge, and the minor positions as cooks, helpers, butchers, etc., under his control.

The person preparing the ménus should have control of the ordering, especially such articles as green goods, etc., otherwise it is difficult to have a harmonious ménu, or to practise the greatest economy in working up "left overs." Appetizing dishes can be prepared from unused foods if sufficient latitude is given to those in immediate charge.

Requisitions for the purchase of supplies should be brought to the superintendent's office, where duplicate orders are made out, one copy being retained by the institution to be used in checking deliveries and bills. All deliveries should be weighed, counted, or measured. If the stock on hand in the storerooms is added to the purchases and from this is subtracted the daily distribution, the balance will always show a perfect inventory of the amounts of each article. The distributions should always be made on written orders; the storekeeper will then have proper data from which to make his entries.

It is difficult to here lay out any definite plan for the organization of kitchen help. When the size of the institution permits, it is advisable that a dietitian be employed, with the necessary meat, vegetable cooks, and baker. Just what each institution requires is an individual problem, and must be solved to suit its needs. It is essential that intelligent help be secured and that a spirit of harmony and mutual help prevails. All too often unintelligent, disinterested, negligent, and dishonest persons are found in the kitchen, who give a correspondingly bad service. The writer knows of an institution which a short time ago had a cook who could neither read nor write.

With such a degree of unintelligence as this it is impossible for a person to have any knowledge of the chemistry of food or its proper preparation.

Menus.—It is a mistake to have a regular fixed ménu for each day in the week, and made out for weeks and months in advance. The articles which the market supplies at the various seasons and also conditions of the market should be important considerations, and, besides, any arrangement of meals which permits those who are to partake of them to know in advance what the meal is going to be is a bad plan. For patients it is best that some classification of diets be made, such as a nitrogenous diet, farinaceous diet, milk diet, soft diet, etc. No hospital, however, should feel that any classification will meet the needs of all patients. Many patients have idiosyncrasies. These and the orders of the attending physicians must control. Too little attention in many hospitals has been paid to the likes and dislikes of the patients. I have seen patients go without a meal because an article of food was served for which they had always had a dislike. If the idiosyncrasies of the patients are studied, it is possible to serve practically the same elements in another form—one which would be agreeable to him. For doctors, nurses, and employees the individual does not have to be so carefully watched nor is it possible to do so. A good wholesome meal, well cooked, must answer. There will be complaints when a large number are served with the same article at the same time, but if the article is wholesome and well prepared, these can properly be ignored.

Waste.—The conservation of food supplies appeals to a hospital as it has never before. The unprecedented high prices of all foods have been keenly felt by benevolent institutions. The rates charged patients remain about the same, but supplies are from 10 to 50 per cent. higher. In many hospitals the ménu cannot be cut down, but waste can be eliminated. Experience teaches that food is more frequently wasted in the serving than in the kitchen. Poorly cooked food is unappetizing and is likely to be thrown out. Every care should be exercised in the kitchen, but it is a mistake to cut off such adjuncts as will make any article cooked appetizing and appealing to the eye. A little flavoring or coloring will sometimes work wonders. Nurses should be instructed that to feed a large number of patients is an expensive item, and that if each one wastes but a little, the aggregate is considerable. I once watched some bread being cut, and noticed the thick ends of the loaf which were discarded; these I had weighed and found that they equaled 14 per cent. of the weight of the entire loaf. The individual was surprised when her attention was called to the fact. It is, however, a practical example of the waste going on every day. The overloading of trays is a common thing. If thought was given to the condition of each patient, the person serving would discover that one patient wants a full meal, and the next only a small quantity of one or two articles. To serve the latter a full tray many times creates a disgust for food, besides being a waste.

The plan I once saw practised at the Johns Hopkins Hospital seemed in every way practical. The tray with the empty dishes was passed to each patient, then the food, each patient being served with such articles and in such quantities as he desired. The result was that there was little to be thrown into the garbage pail.

In trying to practise economy the pendulum must not be allowed to swing too far. There are certain expenditures which must not be regarded as extravagance. A sick man reduced in vitality is to be fed, and at times the more expensive articles are the cheapest.

CHAPTER XI

THE DIETITIAN'S PROVINCE AND ITS MANAGEMENT

By Elizabeth Hinchman

A WOMAN's work is too often written of from an idealized outlook. She begins it frequently with an ideal which she would be glad to attain, but for which she is unwilling and unable to pay the price—an ideal of success toward which she has no right to dream until she has lived up to it.

A woman of forty-five was talking to a senior student of domestic economy as to her future ambitions. The senior said she expected on graduation to have some such positions as the elder woman was then holding—a case of the conceit of twenty-two *vs.* the experience of forty-five. A number of superintendents and trustees have told me that domestic science graduates—many of them—seem to have the idea that to teach nurses is to be their chief work. They would like to conduct marketing tours with nurses, teach the theory of buying and the theory and practice of cookery; but when they are told they are to be responsible for getting out three meals a day and special diets for 40 or 50 or 100 patients, they either retire in dismay or make a trial and failure of the job. Half of those who apply for such positions are too young, and superintendents are beginning to prefer a good practical woman without special training, who has had some experience with life and its problems, and who could command the respect of nurses and servants, rather than intrust the department to the fully trained domestic science graduate who is young and without experience. Yet, in spite of this, the schools are unable to meet the demand made upon them for trained workers, thus proving that there is the desire, greater than the discouragement, to have the hospital dietaries and the institutional kitchen presided over by some one who understands the chemistry and functions of food, as well as its proper preparation. The chief reason that the schools are unable to supply the demand seems to be that so few women deliberately plan to take up the work of a practical dietitian. Not that the task itself is so difficult, but it looks and sounds so appalling when she thinks of the years stretching beyond, with her highest ambition the serving of three meals a day, and the hiring and management of from ten to seventy-five servants, she is inclined to hesitate and think that she would prefer to teach or do something else. She thinks, like the senior before mentioned, that she ought to begin with a position which only a woman of not only training but of broad experience would be capable of managing. If she could be trained to think and to know that after graduation she must serve an apprenticeship in a very small, humble position, aspiring to her ideal through many days and months and perhaps years of service, there would not be so many superintendents hiring dietitians in good faith, only to find them unwilling to stand the burden they have assumed or making the effort and a failure.

A woman enters a standard school of domestic economics to make a study of institutional management. The school of its kind may be perfectly arranged, where she may study the planning of ménus as to the points of hygiene and science, the cooking of the prescribed dishes, going through a course of cookery from soups to black coffee, a course in buying, a course in the diet-kitchen, but it is done under practically ideal conditions. The students themselves act as servants in regular turn, each as anxious of success as the acting manager. The sweeping and dusting, the cooking and serving, are done with an intention of perfection. The waste is small, since the cooking is done by pounds and ounces, and each one concerned is as deeply interested in that side of the problem as the other one. Things go on thus smoothly and pleasantly for a year or two, according to the length of the course. She graduates with a great deal of self-assurance, applies for and accepts a moderately large position, say, in a hospital of 100 beds. Here the servants may have been in institutional work for some time, or they may not. Be that·as it may, the work moves on for a while of its own momentum; but there comes a morning when the dishwasher is drunk, the coffee-maker overslept, the milk sour, the cream turned, and the superintendent "jolly cross." Now, unless the dietitian has met several of these difficulties alone or in combination before this time, and even if she has, unless she be a woman ready for emergency, with a good head for management, full of resources, and, above all, the absolute assurance of knowing that she knows she can meet and overcome these difficulties, she will think she is killed or greatly abused and want to run away. If there are added to the above-mentioned troubles poor coal and a surly chef, she very likely will run away. Suppose she be able to tide over this, but another morning finds the cold storages all leaking, a shortage of vegetables on account of their not getting in on time from the market, therefore a cross vegetable cook. How prosy, even small, these things sound, but how vital to the serenity of the dietitian and the smooth running of the household! Perhaps the night of the same day just at supper dish-washing time all the electric lights go out and the work must be finished by candle or lamplight. There is the dreariness, the discouragement, that one has not been prepared for in any school of domestic economy. She perhaps telegraphs the school which sent her that she will not stay in the position. The school withdraws her and she is sent to another hospital, where, with this minimum of experience gained at the other hospital's expense, she may tide along, finding that her troubles are but as other people's in like situations. But supposing, on graduating, she had served an appren-

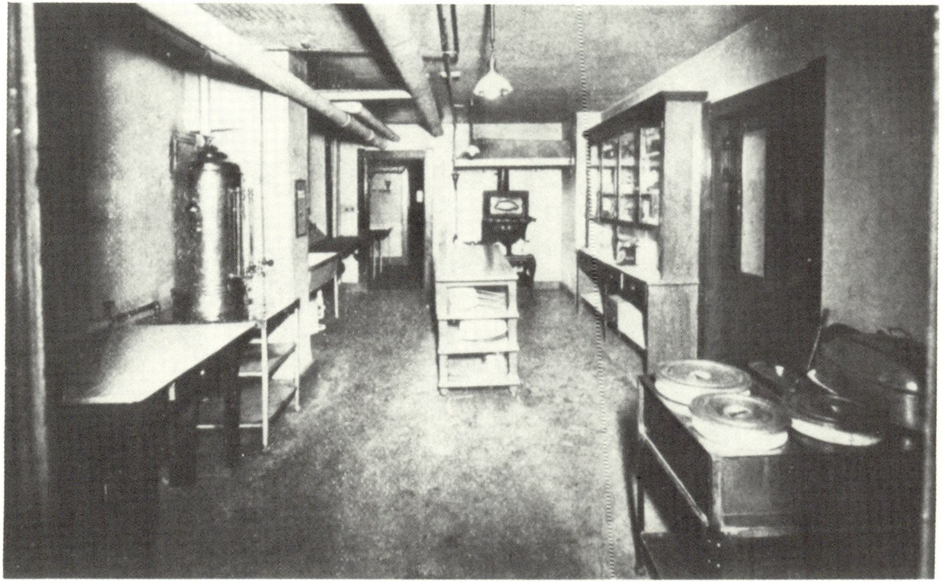

Fig. 118.—Dietitian's kitchen.

ticeship of three or six months in some large general or private hospital, working with and taking observations from a dietitian already experienced in a multiplicity of petty details. The problems to be met in actual work cannot be duplicated elsewhere. The solution depends upon the dietitian's judgment, which can be had only by training and experience. Only experience in addition to training will enable her to act wisely in the necessary disciplining which arises in her department among her servants. Only by experience can she make proper use of the theories involved in the forming of dietaries and the regulation of expenditures for supplies. These are vital questions in an institution, and the dietitian's work stands or falls by their proper management. If she gains this experience, she then has a working basis upon which she may stand firmly and with assurance, and wherewith she can meet and make demands.

The demands made upon a dietitian vary with every hospital she may enter. Two years ago Simmons College wrote to many of its former graduates who were holding hospital positions to send an outline of the work required of each in her particular position, and it was discovered that almost everything, from helping in the kitchen to executive work, had been exacted. There seems to be no definite line of work prescribed for a dietitian—a teacher of cookery, an executive, and a housekeeper seem to be mingled in one. There seems to be a sort of mist or haze over the name "dietitian"—no one seems to know exactly who or what she is. Her social position is also a variable quantity. In one famous hospital in New York you will find her eating her meals as head of one of the nurses' tables. In one hospital in Boston, equally as famous, she belongs to the official staff, and has her meals in a private dining-room. In some instances she has her meals served on a tray in her office, or in her diet-kitchen, as she is neither an official, a nurse, nor a servant. Since to hold successfully the position of a practical dietitian she must be an educated woman, and an educated woman is more frequently than otherwise a gentlewoman, she has the right to demand a social footing, not a tolerance, and should be rated as a member of the official family. She has the right to demand hours of regular work or regular hours of work, as far as possible, a resting or relaxing time, a holiday as a man has it, a recognition of her ability, a respect for her labor, and a competent salary. I have in mind an infirmary in one of the Southern States which has a diet-kitchen on each of its four floors—not a serving diet-kitchen, but one in which the special diets are actually prepared. In each one of these four kitchens are two nurses on continuous duty, also a maid. These kitchens send out the diets simultaneously to about 1500 patients, and until three years ago had been under the supervision of the superintendent of nurses and an under-housekeeper. At that time it was decided to employ a dietitian, both as to practical ability and teaching qualifications. A graduate from Boston was interviewed—a woman of training and experience. On conversation with the board of trustees it was made known that nothing short of a paragon of perfection was desired, and to this paragon was to be offered the munificent sum of $60 per month—this for managing four diet-kitchens that were sending out meals at the same time on separate floors—$60 per month to buy a dietitian's training, her experience, and her loyalty. If they had been offering a position of necessity of the same training and experience to a man, they would in all probability have offered him a salary of $1200 a year as a beginning. When the dietitian refused, and said she would undertake the work on a beginning salary of $1000, with a possible one of $1500, they were, as they thought, righteously indignant, and with some bit of promptness showed her the door. This illustration is, I think, an unusual thing in the North. A beginner may demand only a beginner's salary, but a woman of good training and experience is usually paid a salary commensurate to her ability. More and more the schools of economics themselves, rather than the students and institutions employing

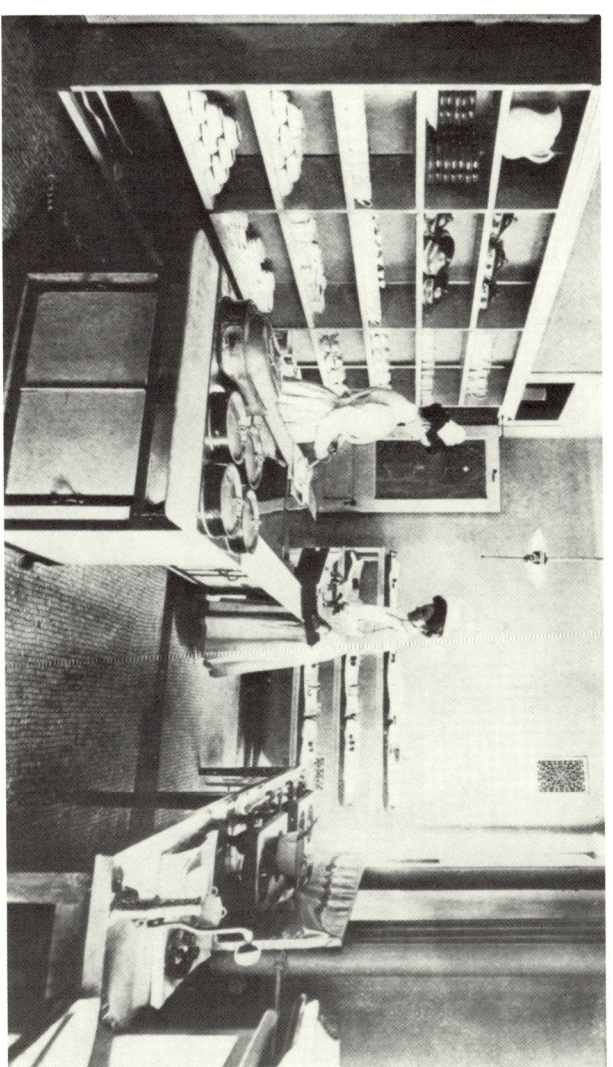

Fig. 119.—Serving kitchen for private patients. Presbyterian Hospital, New York.

these graduate students, are setting the standard salary. If, by reason of her superior excellence, she be worth more to her institution than a standard wage, that may be safely left to herself and her superior officer. It is a matter beyond the authority of any school from which she may have graduated.

If she be an executive dietitian, as she would be as a matter of course, in a large hospital, she will be allowed to make her own office hours, trusting that she have wisdom enough to be near by when she is needed, having at her command an assistant who looks after the diet-kitchen and teaches the nurse and an under-housekeeper, who is held responsible for the time and labor of the workers in the main kitchen. This executive dietitian may or may not do the buying, but she most certainly should have the ability to buy in large or small quantities. She should know the different cuts and qualities of meats, and fish, fresh and seasonable fruit and vegetables in their season, the grades of flour, and a good bargain when she finds it. If she does not buy, she must be held responsible for the ordering, and the quantities and qualities of the materials received. She has a right to demand, and insist upon her demand, that the qualities be above reproach, and of as high a grade as the institution can afford. This point having been gained, she should assume entirely the burden of the dietaries, and in no degree should the superintendent be held responsible for unsatisfactorily fed people. Food complaints are by far the most trying things that befall a dietitian, but if she have good support from the medical staff and the consciousness of feeding the best for the money sums at hand, she has nothing whereby she may reproach herself.

But she should know without fail the money sums at hand—for instance, whether she may run a dietary costing 30 or 40 or 50 cents per person per day. If she feels that, on the sums allowed her, she is not able to manage her part in accordance with the good management of other parts of the institution, it is her business to make this fact known to her superior officer. In doing this she should have dignity and poise enough and be sufficiently backed by facts to carry her point.

It is the custom in many hospitals when the need of economy is felt to begin with the food. This may be true economy many times, but often it is not. Many times the excessive cost of food is due to waste, and this matter should receive the most careful and faithful attention. If the serving is done from one serving room, the question of waste is not so large a one as the individual service can have personal supervision from the dietitian in charge. She sees or should see the return waste, and can govern her service accordingly. If the serving be on different wards, especially in different houses, she has a larger, more difficult, task, one that will take more thought and time and attention. The only thing that can then be done is to give as close supervision to the service as possible and daily attention to the various garbage pails. This latter is not a pleasant task. It does not appeal to a woman of fine breeding, but it is a matter of business. It goes with the position, and must be as conscientiously attended to as looking after the ice-cream, bread, and cake. It is true here, as elsewhere, that one equal to the greatest task may often find herself required to perform the humblest. If she be really capable, she will turn from one phase of her work to the other, finding advantage in the whole experience.

If she be able to get good qualities of supplies in sufficient abundance; if she be able to keep down extravagant serving and excessive waste; if she have the good will of the house physicians—her battle is won, save at one point. She must have the ability to get and to keep good help and to get good service from them. This writes easy, but is a hard thing to accomplish—one of the very hardest things —and has caused more discouragement than all the other things combined. Theories may be advanced, but fail on application. Only experience and a knowledge of people are of much avail, and it takes time and opportunity

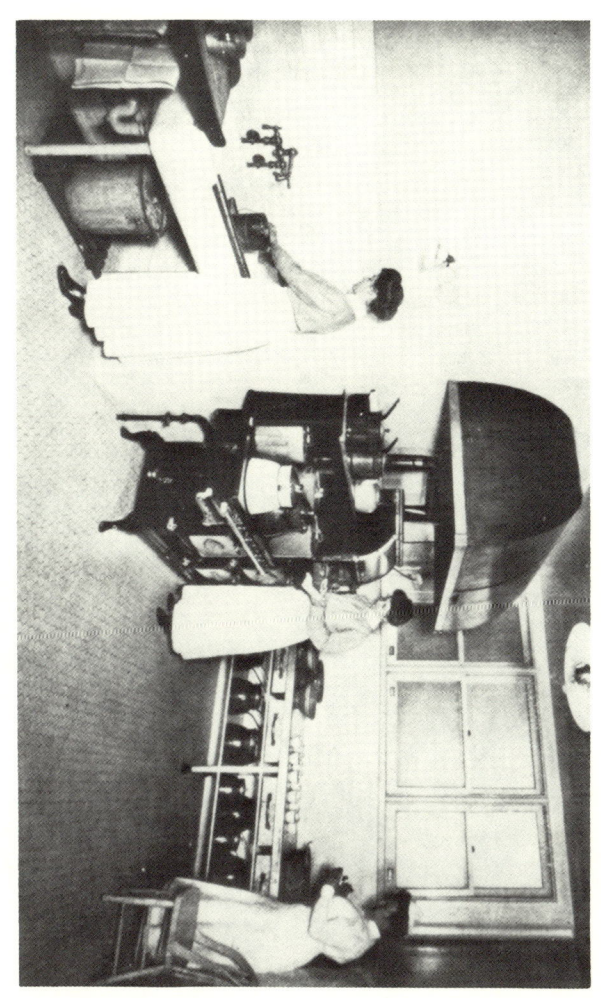

Fig. 120.—Kitchen for private patients' diets. Presbyterian Hospital, New York.

McLEAN HOSPITAL.

DIET ORDERS *Central* KITCHEN.

WARD W B 2 nd DATE July 5 tho 1907

Patients 16 Nurses 1 Night Nurses 1 Maids 1 Cooks — TOTAL 19

BREAKFAST.	No.	DINNER.	No.	SUPPER.	No.
Fish		Soup	18	Beef Juice ....oz.	
Meat	4	Fish		Chicken Broth "	5
Beef Juice ....oz.		Meat	18	Mutton Broth "	
Chicken Broth "		Entree		Beef Tea "	
Oysters		Beef Juice ....oz.		Oysters	
Milk ....pts.	1 Can	Chicken Broth "		Milk ....pts.	70
Cream "		Mutton Broth "		Cold Meats	
Bread, white loaves	6	Beef Tea "			
" graham "	2	Oysters			
Fruit for day	19	Milk ....pts.			
Lemons "	12	Ice Cream		L. Chop	1
Oranges	4	Fruit			
		B. Steak	1		
		S. of beef	1		
Entree		*L. Chop*	1	Entree	19
Eggs, raw	20			Oyster Stew	
" poached				Eggs, poached	
" boiled		Oyster Stew		" boiled	
Potatoes	18	Eggs, poached		Potatoes	
Rolls		" boiled		Rolls	
Biscuit		Potatoes	17	Biscuit	
Muffins		Vegetables		Muffins	
Corn Cake		Pudding	17	Toast	
Toast	18	Pie		Cake	19
Mush		Cake		Sauce	19
Malted Milk		Toast		Malted Milk	10
Horlick's Food		Malted Milk		Horlick's Food	
		Horlick's Food			

House Kitchen.

Milk ....pts.   Bread ....loaves.

☞ Articles printed in this type will be cooked or issued from the Center Kitchen.
☞ Articles printed in this type will be cooked or issued from the House Kitchen.
These orders must be made out before 4 P. M., on the previous day, and sent to House Kitchen.
After they are issued, this blank, signed by the Cook, must be sent to the Storekeeper.

I hereby certify that the above order is correct, and not in excess of the written orders given me this day.

M. J. Dehon,
Head Nurse.

I certify that I have correctly filled the above order,

Cook.

Fig. 121.

to gain these. Not long since the pot-washer in the chef's kitchen came into my office and said: "I go home;

work too hard. I go home in two days at 3.30." I said to him, "If you go home, who will wash the dishes?" "I don't know, I don't care; I go home Thursday 3.30." On the following morning he came to my assistant and said, "Where's the lady? I go home now." On being told he could not go, would not get his pay until 3.30 according to his notice, he went away apparently contented. But on the following morning he came again to the office and finding me, said, "I go home now?" "No, not until 3.30"; and he did stay until 3.30, coming then for his money.

Another instance: Saturday is usually a hard day, as many things are done to make the Sunday an easy, restful day. On this particular Saturday a carload of flour was expected in to be unloaded about 4 P. M. Three of the porters decided among themselves that they would strike, thinking, I suppose, as it would be Saturday evening and the next day Sunday, I would be frightened into a bit of submission. One of the loyal boys reported the whisperings to the head porter, and he brought the trouble to me. Instead of being frightened, as it was desired I should be, I said "we will let them strike. Better a good blaze than a continual smoldering." I therefore telephoned to a reliable employment bureau and told the facts—that I expected a strike and requested them to have two men ready to come by 4 o'clock if they should be needed. Sure enough, the three boys refused to unload the flour, and came with fire in their eyes to the office. They lined up outside the door, and the leader came in to talk. And talk he did: but when he found it of no avail, he gave up, showing it was but a "bluff." Nevertheless, the leader was discharged. The man came from the city to take his place, and the work of the hospital went on as if nothing had happened. I think both of these cases of discipline would have seemed overwhelming to a young, inexperienced woman. If the dietitian can keep her poise of spirit and let her workers understand that she can and that she knows what she is doing and going to do, test emergencies, such as those mentioned, will soon cease, and the help will keep on at their work as smoothly as the machinery part.

Another instance: The under-housekeeper was ill and I had put in her place, with a limited amount of authority, a maid who had been with us for three years. Her undermaid had been with us but a few days, and her work was so new that she was decidedly timid about assuming duties alone. One morning the temporary housekeeper came to me and said: "This is my afternoon off, but Kate seems so timid that I think I had better stay and help her for a while, so that she will not have to get along alone very long." Just a few days ago the vegetable cook came to me and said "I won't take my afternoon off this week—too much to do." This shows a loyal spirit among the help which is worth a good deal. It is usually not difficult to bring into line new, rather incompetent employees when the old ones are full of the idea of lending a helping hand. When you can walk down a corridor and say to a porter, "What are you doing?" If he says "Nothing, just now, Miss," and you can say "Come, lend a hand at peeling potatoes," without fear of hearing the remark "that is not my work," you may feel sure you have learned something, and accomplished something worth while in regard to managing help. When working with people who are hard to manage, I often recall an incident which has helped me over difficulties many times. When I was but a child, a playmate told me to pull a certain weed. I undertook to do so, but found it stung my hands. A man who was looking on said to me "Grasp it hard and quickly." I did so, and found the sting was gone. Many times I have found if a misdemeanor arose and I took hold of it quickly and firmly, the sting which I had in a degree feared was not there. I have no hesitation about speaking sharply to my help, and just as little about praising them. They are human, like the rest of us. They get tired and sick and cross. So do we, and a little encouragement helps a lot.

Working with nurses in the diet-kitchen is quite a different matter. They know that beyond you, in a case requiring discipline, is the superintendent of nurses, and back of her is the superintendent of the hospital, if need be. So but little friction is encountered in this part of the work. More frequently than otherwise, they bring to their work a degree of pride in learning and accomplishing something. They are securing a training and experience which will add to efficiency and culture in after years, and they appreciate this fact.

It is customary to have two nurses on continuous duty for two months, changing one each month, so that there is always in the diet-kitchen a nurse with some experience in preparing and sending out the diets. The class of nurses come in at specified hours for their two or three hours' lesson or lecture and practical work in cookery. The following is a suggestive outline which may be helpful in arranging for such classes:

COURSE IN COOKERY AND DIETETICS

WOMEN NURSES

Twenty-four lessons, one hour lectures, two hours' practical work.

1. *Food.*
   Definition of.
   Classification.
   Source, composition, and use of.
   Nutrients.
   Cookery, reasons for.
   Fuels and their uses.

   Show kitchen refrigerator and everything in connection with the cooking of food.
   Class rules.

2. *Care and Preservation of Food.*
   Utilization of left-over food.
   Tables of weights and measurements.
   Suggestions as to saving of time, labor, and utensils when cooking.
   Beverages: Kinds, their value and dietetic use.
   Methods of serving hot, cold, and iced beverages.

   Preparation of acid, albuminous beverages, and fruit.
   Egg-nogs.

3. *Selection of Food as Regards:*
   Age, occupation, climate, season of year.
   Digestibility.
   Economy.
   Individual taste.
   Standard dietaries.
   Dietaries for the sick.
   Explanation of charts and dietary systems.
   Making out of diet sheets.

   Preparation of wheys.
   Starchy beverages.
   Syrups.

4. *Serving.*
   Selection of linen.
   Selection of dishes.
   Laying of trays and tables for individual and family serving.

   Preparation of combination beverages.
   Tea, coffee, chocolate, cocoa.

5. *Milk as Food.*
   Composition.
   Care.
   Food value.
   Specific gravity.
   Adulteration.
   Cause of souring.
   Methods of preservation:
   (1) Sterilizing.
   (2) Pasteurizing.
   (3) Condensing.

   Simple desserts made of milk with rice, oat flour, moss, gelatin, custards.

6. *Milk—Its Products.*
   Cheese, buttermilk, koumiss.
   Modified milk, method.
   Butterines and butter.

   Cream, butter. Simple desserts.
   Toasts: dry, milk.
   French, etc. Cream.

7. *Fruits and their Cookery.*
   Composition, digestibility, and dietetic value of fresh cooked and dried fruits.
   Nuts, fungi.

   Methods of serving raw fruit, *i. e.*, orange, grape-fruit, bananas.
   Cooking dried fruits, as figs, prunes.

8. *Starch and Starch Cookery.*
   Starch, dextrin, cellulose.
   Vegetables.
   Division of vegetable foods.
   Composition, digestibility, nutritive value.
   Preservation.

   Cooking of cereals, potatoes in various ways, other vegetables.

9. *Preparation of Meat.*
   Vegetables and fruits for salads.
   Value of salads in diet.
   Salad dressings.

   French, boiled, mayonnaise dressings prepared.

10. *Sandwiches.*
11. *Eggs.*
    (1) Composition.   Cooking of eggs in various ways.
    (2) Signs of fresh eggs.
    (3) Preservation.
    (4) Digestibility.
    (5) Nutritive value.
12. *Soups.*
    Broths, beef-tea, beef juice.   Preparation of cream of vegetable soup.
    Comparative food value.
    Digestibility.   Lamb, chicken, beef broths.
    Beef juice.
13. *Meat.*
    (1) Composition.   Broiling of chops, steak, chicken, squab.
    (2) Factors influencing value of meat.
    (3) Nutritive value.
    (4) Digestibility.
    (5) Objects of cooking.
14. *Fish.*
    (1) Classes of.   Broiling and boiling fish.
    (2) Means of distinguishing kinds.   Cooking of oysters.
    (3) Signs of fresh fish.
    (4) Preservation.
    (5) Nutritive value.
    ((6) Digestibility.
15. *Bread and Bread-making.*

    Each nurse before the course is completed makes and bakes some bread.

16. *Frozen Dishes.*
    Nutritive value and use in a diet.   Preparation of ice-cream, sherbet, water-ice, mousse if possible.
17. *Biscuit, Muffins, Cookies.*
18. *Predigested Foods.*
    Junkets.
    Peptonized milk.
    Peptonized gruel.
    Peptonized beef-broth.
19. *Candy-making.*
20. *Serving of a Luncheon.*
    Four courses.
    Menus prepared by nurses and the best one selected.

The other four lessons are devoted to the making of cake, work in the ward, and care of serving room and dining-room after a meal has been served.

If the dietitian be but a teacher of cookery, she should be able to have two classes each day, each session three hours in length; but if she is both teacher and practical dietitian, one class will be all she can manage in one day, and that one but two hours in length. Her plans regarding her work should give her leisure to think and plan for the hospital, and a little leisure or rest time for herself, lest, growing overweary, she finds herself using irritability when dignity would serve the purpose better.

There is no field open to woman that is more important than that of dietetics. A woman who takes up this work needs native ability, education, dignity, tact in meeting and handling people, and good health. With these, if she finds the work a strain, she is either not well upheld by those in authority, or is not playing at the right game in life for one of her make-up and temperament.

SUGGESTIVE MENUS

Wednesday, June 1st.

BREAKFAST.	DINNER.	SUPPER.
Grape-fruit.	Oxtail soup.	Cold tongue.
Wheatlet and cream.	Meat pie. Radishes.	Hashed brown potatoes. Rolls.
Fried fish.	Boiled potatoes.	Sliced pineapple.
Baked potatoes.	Mashed new turnips.	Citron cake.
Graham muffins.	Pistachio ice-cream.	Tea. Coffee.
Parker house rolls.	Cake. Coffee.	
Coffee.		

Thursday, June 2d.

Cantaloupe.	Consommé.	Cold chicken.
Oatmeal and cream.	Broiled steak.	Escalloped tomatoes.
Pork chops.	Mushroom sauce.	Rolls.
Hot apple sauce.	French fried potatoes.	Strawberries.
Baked potato.	Baked Bermudas.	Doughnuts. Cheese.
Biscuits.	Lettuce.	Tea. Coffee.
Parker house rolls.	Quince Bavarian cream.	
Coffee.	Rhubarb pie. Coffee.	

Friday, June 3d.

Oranges.	Purée of split peas.	Cold ham.
Hominy and cream.	Fried fish.	Spaghetti and cheese.
Omelet.	Tartar sauce.	Rolls.
Baked potato.	Boiled potatoes.	Strawberries.
Corn cake.	Baked tomatoes.	Plum jelly.
Parker house rolls.	Cucumbers.	Chocolate cake.
Coffee.	Steamed fruit pudding.	Tea. Coffee.
	Whipped cream.	
	Fruit salad.	
	Coffee.	

270   HOSPITAL MANAGEMENT

BREAKFAST.	*Saturday, June 4th.* DINNER.	SUPPER.
Apples. Bananas. Wheatlet and cream. Liver and onions. Baked potato. Rye muffins. Parker house rolls. Coffee.	Vegetable soup. Roast stuffed veal. Tomato sauce. Mashed potatoes. Creamed cabbage. Rice custard. Apple pie. Cheese. Coffee.	Cold meat. Lyonnaise potatoes. Biscuit. Sliced pineapple. Gingerbread. Tea. Coffee.

Sunday, June 5th.

Grape-fruit. Oatmeal and cream. Baked beans. Piccalilli. Fish cakes. Brown bread. Rolls. Coffee.	Clear tomato soup. Roast lamb. Mint sauce. Riced potatoes. Peas. Tomato and lettuce. Salad. Chocolate ice-cream. Drop cakes. Coffee.	Creamed chicken on toast. Preserved pears. White cake. Tea. Cocoa.

Monday, June 6th.

Oranges. Cream of wheat and cream. Bacon and fried eggs. Baked potato. Muffins. Parker house rolls. Coffee.	Bouillon. Roast beef. Olives. Franconia potatoes. Wax beans. Cocoanut blanc mange. Custard pie. Coffee.	Cold meat. Baked beans. Brown bread. Watermelon. Pickles. Sliced pineapple. Orange cake. Tea. Coffee.

Tuesday, June 7th.

Apples and bananas. Oatmeal and cream. Lamb chops. Baked potatoes. Rolls. Muffins. Coffee.	Clear soup with croutons. Roast pork. Apple sauce. Boiled potatoes. Spinach. Lettuce. Snow pudding. Custard sauce. Strawberry shortcake. Whipped cream. Coffee.	Potato salad with chives. Rolls. Baked rhubarb and lemons. Molasses cookies. Cocoanut cake. Tea. Cocoa.

Wednesday, June 8th.

Grape-fruit. Wheatlet and cream. Tripe in batter. Boiled eggs. Baked potato. Biscuit. Rolls. Coffee.	Okra soup. Roast stuffed chicken. Olives. Cranberry jelly. Mashed potatoes. Wax beans. Lettuce and tomato salad. Vanilla ice-cream.	Baked hash with green peppers. Biscuit. Quince marmalade. Cake. Tea. Coffee.

Thursday, June 9th.

Grape-fruit. Cornmeal mush and cream. Fried fish. Baked potato. Rolls. Graham muffins. Coffee.	Consommé. Boiled dinner. Boiled potatoes. Beets. Cabbage. Turnips. Gingerbread. Whipped cream. Fruit salad. Coffee.	Cold meat. Potato au gratin. Strawberries. Doughnuts. Cheese. Tea. Cocoa.

DIETITIAN'S PROVINCE AND ITS MANAGEMENT 271

Friday, June 10th.

BREAKFAST.
Cantaloupe.
Wheatlet and cream.
Bacon. Fried eggs.
Baked potatoes.
Corn cake. Rolls.
Coffee.

DINNER.
Tomato bisque croutons.
Cold turkey.
Boiled fish.
Egg sauce.
Boiled potato.
Cabbage salad.
Lima beans.
Strawberries. Apple pie.
Cheese. Coffee.

SUPPER.
Egg salad.
Rolls.
Sliced pineapple.
Raisin cake.
Tea. Cocoa.

Saturday, June 11th.

Oranges. Apples.
Oatmeal and cream.
Broiled ham.
Baked potatoes.
Biscuits. Rolls.
Coffee.

Vegetable soup.
Veal cutlets. Tomato sauce.
Mashed turnips.
Cucumbers.
Cottage pudding.
Brandy sauce.
Rhubarb pie. Coffee.

Cold meat.
Hashed brown potatoes.
Baked rhubarb.
Spice cake.
Tea. Coffee.

Sunday, June 12th.

Grape-fruit.
Cream of wheat and cream.
Baked beans.
Fish cakes.
Brown bread. Rolls.
Coffee.

Mock turtle soup.
Roast beef.
Horseradish.
Watermelon pickle.
Franconia potatoes.
Summer squash.
Ginger ice-cream.
Cake. Coffee.

Lobster salad.
Rolls.
Strawberries.
White cake.
Tea. Cocoa.

Monday, June 13th.

Cantaloupe.
Lamb chops.
Baked potatoes.
Rye muffins. Rolls.
Coffee.

Clear soup.
Roast pork.
Spiced rhubarb.
Boiled potatoes.
Fried parsnips.
Leeks on toast.
Lemon pie.
Bread pudding.
Coffee.

Cold meat.
Baked beans. Brown bread.
Piccalilli.
Sliced pineapple.
Cake. Tea. Cocoa.

Tuesday, June 14th.

Grape-fruit.
Oatmeal and cream.
Fried fish.
Baked potatoes.
Rolls. Muffins.
Coffee.

Mulligatawney soup.
Roast duck.
Spiced jelly.
Boiled potatoes.
Green peas.
Tomato and lettuce salad.
Coffee.

Cold tongue.
Escalloped tomatoes.
Rolls.
Strawberries. Cookies.
Cake.
Tea. Cocoa.

Wednesday, June 15th.

Cantaloupe.
Hominy and cream.
Sausage pats.
Baked potato.
White muffins. Rolls.
Coffee.

Clear soup with barley.
Lamb chops.
Mint jelly.
Riced potatoes.
Spinach.
Vanilla ice-cream.
Strawberry sauce.
Cake. Coffee.

Potato salad.
Rolls.
Baked apples.
Whipped cream.
Citron cake.
Tea. Cocoa.

Thursday, June 16th.

BREAKFAST.
Oranges. Bananas.
Wheatlet and cream.
Omelet.
Baked potatoes.
Biscuit. Rolls.

DINNER.
Okra soup.
Maryland chicken.
Cranberry jelly.
Mashed potato.
Green beans. Lettuce.
Baked rice pudding.
Lemon jelly with Maraschino.

SUPPER.
Baked hash
with green peppers.
Buttered toast.
Sliced pineapple.
Doughnuts. Cheese.
Tea. Cocoa.

Friday, June 17th.

Cantaloupe.
Oatmeal and cream.
Bacon. Fried eggs.
Baked potatoes.
Graham muffins. Rolls.
Coffee.

Black bean soup.
Boiled salmon.
Egg sauce.
Boiled potatoes.
Green peas.
Cucumbers.
Cocoanut blanc mange.
Jelly tarts.
Coffee.

Cold meat.
Egg salad. Rolls.
Strawberries.
Caramel cake.
Tea. Cocoa.

Saturday, June 18th.

Grape-fruit.
Wheatlet and cream.
Broiled ham.
Baked potato. Muffins.
Rolls. Coffee.

Bouillon.
Broiled steak. Olives.
Mushroom sauce.
French fried potatoes.
Baked Bermudas.
Rhubarb pie. Fruit jelly.
Coffee.

Fish chowder.
Toasted crackers.
Stuffed peppers.
Preserved plums.
Gingerbread.
Cake. Tea. Cocoa.

Sunday, June 19th.

Cantaloupe.
Hominy and cream.
Baked beans.
Fish cakes.
Brown bread. Rolls.
Coffee.

Oxtail soup.
Roast lamb. Mint sauce.
Radishes.
Mashed potatoes.
String-beans.
Sliced tomatoes.
Frozen pudding. Cake.

Fresh asparagus
on toast.
Hot biscuit.
Strawberries.
Drop cakes.
Tea. Cocoa.

Monday, June 20th.

Cherries.
Wheatlet and cream.
Hamburg steak.
Baked potatoes.
Corn muffins. Rolls.
Coffee.

Vegetable soup.
Roast stuffed turkey.
Cranberry marmalade.
Boiled potatoes.
Summer squash.
Asparagus in cream.
Steamed rice.
Caramel sauce.
Jelly tarts. Coffee.

Lobster salad.
Rolls.
Preserved pears.
Cake.
Tea. Cocoa.

Tuesday, June 21st.

Cantaloupe.
Cornmeal mush and
cream.
Fried fish.
Baked potatoes.
Biscuit. Rolls.
Coffee.

Scotch broth.
Roast ham.
Spiced rhubarb.
Riced potatoes.
New turnips.
Green peppers and okra.
Strawberry shortcake.
Junket. Coffee.

Cold tongue.
Potato au gratin.
Strawberries.
Cookies. Cake.
Tea. Cocoa.

CHAPTER XII

THE ENGINEERING DEPARTMENT

By Clarence W. Williams

The trained nurse who has been appointed superintendent of a 50- or a 100-bed hospital has, as a rule, received sufficient training in matters pertaining to the care and handling of the sick and injured. She knows well what is required of her along these lines before she assumes the responsibilities of a superintendent. As a rule, she enters into her work with great enthusiasm, and soon has the work in the operating-room, the wards, the diet- and main kitchens, etc., in good working order. Because she has been trained along these lines, the work becomes a pleasure. Of the numerous details entering into the successful management of the kitchen, laundry, engineer's, and other important departments, she is frequently wofully ignorant, and a large part of the problems of the new superintendent are very apt to center around those departments.

Before long perhaps there comes a complaint from the linen department that the flat work is not well done, and the clothes have greasy or yellow streaks. The laundry matron is called; she states that she cannot give any assistance, for the steam was not sufficient to properly heat the mangle, or the trap was not working, and therefore the mangle did not do good work; also that the hot water that was drawn from the pipes was oily or full of something that colored the clothes. While attempting to solve this problem, perchance, the house telephone rings and the kitchen matron reports that there is no steam in the vegetable cooker, or the warming table is cold, so that dinner will be served late, or, if served at all, it will be cold.

Her perplexity increases as another call on the house telephone reports that the operating-room temperature is down to 60° F., and that an operation is due in half an hour. About that time the patient in room 13 may be complaining because the steam pipes are making so much noise.

This new superintendent loses no time in calling the engineer, and is perhaps informed by him that it is not his place to look after the laundry, the kitchen, or the operating-room; therefore she must look elsewhere for relief. After a sleepless night or two, with these complaints daily multiplying, she is likely to appeal to some friend, probably, who has had several years' experience in hospital management, and is told that the whole trouble is with the engineer. With much surprise this new superintendent states that John seems to know all about boilers, firing, and, in fact, everything else about a modern heating plant. She feels sure the trouble is with the system and not with the engineer. If the friend with more knowledge and longer experience wishes to enlighten or help her sister superintendent, she will ask her if she has informed herself about how the engineering work of the hospital has been installed, about how it should work; about the pressure of steam to be maintained at the boilers, at the laundry, and for warming the several rooms in the buildings. She will inquire if she knows how much fuel should be burned daily or weekly, on the average; the amount of steam required in all the buildings to keep them at proper temperature; whether the noise of the system is not caused by the improper closing of valves or the blowing of steam through the traps; why the air has become vitiated so that the rooms are unbearable? These are some of the problems that loom up before the new superintendent, and it is not to be wondered at if she begins to feel that her training for institutional work has been somewhat neglected. The many engineering problems of an institution were things she had not even heard about during her training. She, therefore, is wholly at the mercy of the engineer, who often is wholly incompetent. The ever-thoughtful and saving committee had engaged him, placed him in that most responsible position, and then turned him and the plant over to an inexperienced superintendent to manage.

In these days of advanced hospital practice and training it seems essential that the nurse who assumes the responsibility of superintendent of a 50-bed (or larger) hospital should have some knowledge of the duties of an engineer. She should know at least enough so that he cannot impose upon her. She should know something about the proper location of a heating plant, the amount of fuel to be used to properly heat the buildings and furnish steam for other purposes. She should know something about the quality and price of fuel; the wages and hours of an engineer; the general system of heating and ventilating the buildings; the sanitary condition of all plumbing fixtures; the control for giving even temperatures of hot water; the reading of meters, so as to know whether there is a waste of water in the buildings, or careless use of electric current. Much of this information can be best secured by a visit to an adjacent well-organized institution.

If she knows how to handle these problems when she receives her appointment as a superintendent, she will not only save herself many anxious days, but she will find it possible to save a considerable item in the cost of maintenance, a result that will cheer the heart of her trustees at the end of the year.

The following suggestions may prove of value to the inexperienced superintendent, who has been kept particularly in mind during their preparation.

In building a hospital, for the proper construction, location, and equipment of a power-house, the advice of a competent consulting engineer should be obtained.

Location and General Construction.—The ideal power-house is one located apart from the administration or ward buildings. It may be combined with the laundry, and should have, in connection with it, a workshop of ample size for wood working, pipe-fittings, etc. Suitable lockers should be provided with miscellaneous supplies, such as valves, pipe-fittings, and plumbers' supplies. A coal bunker will be required, and should be large enough to store coal for a considerable period, thus making the hospital independent in case of prolonged storms or strikes.

A platform scale of reliable make should be installed, thus enabling the superintendent to be sure that the full weight of coal is received. If soft coal is to be used, the smokestack should be of sufficient height to carry off all smoke; otherwise it will drift into open windows and be a nuisance.

In many small hospitals the boilers are placed in the basement of one of the main hospital buildings, where the delivery of coal is a noisy and dirty nuisance. The removal of ashes from such a location is often difficult, and also a nuisance.

Equipment.—This will, of course, depend upon the size of the hospital and local conditions. It must be remembered that the jacket kettles and steamers in the kitchen, the mangle, dry room, and washing machines of the laundry require, for their satisfactory operation, steam under high pressure—usually from 30 to 60 pounds. In the busy hospital high-pressure steam is more satisfactory for sterilizing than sterilizers equipped with gas.

Electric lighting, if a considerable amount of this is to be done, can usually be done cheaper from a small dynamo located in the engine-room than by purchasing the current. In certain instances very favorable prices may be obtained from public lighting points, so that electric current for power and lights need not be considered in the equipment. It may be advisable to consider having a dynamo for winter use, and connections from outside electric service for summer use in small hospitals, thus saving the salary of an engineer for night duty in the warm months. If this double system is to be installed, care must be taken that the voltage and character of the current produced in the hospital should be identical with those which the lighting company supplies. Reliance should not be placed on expensive automatic appliances in the power-house. At best, they often fail, and tend to make the employees careless and unobserving.

In very small hospitals a low-pressure heating system is all that is required if cooking is done on ranges and the laundry is operated without much machinery.

Employees.—A chief engineer should, if possible, reside in the hospital. In selecting a man for this important position, one who has a taste for mechanics is desirable. The proper man may be expected to attend to ordinary repairs in the power plant, throughout the wards, the sterilizing room, laundry, and also to do the ordinary repair work of beds, plumbing, and furniture. Obviously, such a man can do more if provided with a workshop connected with the boiler and engine-room.

The number and character of additional employees in this department will depend on the size of the plant and the amount of work to be done. It may be possible to provide comfortable quarters for the employees of this department in the power-building. Bath-tub, set bowl, and water-closet should be provided.

Supplies.—Whether anthracite or bituminous coal is to be used will depend on many conditions which cannot properly be discussed here. It is usually economic to buy high-grade fuel. It should always be purchased of reliable dealers, and it is well to have competitive bids for this supply. As stated above, every load of fuel should be weighed when received or before burning. Care in this matter may soon save the cost of installing scales.

Lubricating oils should be purchased in quantities suitable for the requirements.

Other supplies should be of standard makes, and care should be taken to observe that the goods actually specified in ordering are received.

It is suggested that inexperienced superintendents

consult periodically with other large purchasers of similar supplies, to see that prices are not much different. It is a well-known fact that not infrequently supplies for the engineering department are of inferior quality, and exorbitant prices are often paid by the careless or inexperienced buyer.

It is very desirable that the superintendent attend personally to the purchasing rather than to place this important duty in the hands of an employee. It is not meant by this that she should go "shopping" for all small supplies required, but it is meant that all orders should be approved by the superintendent, and, if possible, be ordered through the office in regular form, so that prices may be carefully followed, and a record kept of the transaction.

It is almost impossible to say what supplies should be required in a hospital that has once been equipped, as these will vary very much, indeed, from month to month. In starting up a new plant, the engineer should be provided with a suitable chest of tools to properly care for his plant and look after the general repairs throughout the buildings. These tools cost about $75 to $100. He should also be supplied with the best of fuel, oil, boiler compound, all kinds of packing for engines, pumps, boilers, etc. The writer also considers it economy for a hospital of this size to keep steam-fittings, pipe-plumbing stock, etc., on hand for emergency work—say $100 or $200 worth. This stock should be kept up and inventoried once a year. By keeping these supplies on hand the engineer will soon learn to take pride in keeping his entire system in good repair. It thus proves a good investment. Any competent engineer will, as a rule, soon see the list of stock that is required after he becomes familiar with his plant. Prices cannot be quoted, as they are constantly changing on this class of goods. It is well to get quotations on needed supplies from more than one supply house.

General Suggestions.—The trap spoken of in the second paragraph of this chapter is a steam trap placed on the return side of any system, and is used to prevent the steam from blowing back into the receiver at the pump, and to take care of the water of condensation as rapidly as it may accumulate in the returns, either from radiation or high-pressure apparatus in use. If steam blows through any of these traps, it will not only create a noise in the pipes, but will waste steam, and therefore waste fuel.

The amount of fuel required for any given plant is determined by the grate area in the boilers, and the nurse superintendent should, when possible, obtain this information from the engineer who laid out and figured the system. Then she should see, by keeping a close watch of the engineer's log, that the fuel is kept as near this estimate as possible.

Economy of fuel will be obtained by the engineer firing lightly, and often, also, by keeping grates free from clinkers and ashes. Brains as well as muscle should be used in the boiler-room. A first-class engineer or fireman will study to show economy at the coal pile.

An engineer's log should be kept by him and filed at the office of the superintendent at least once a month. If the plant was turned over to the engineer in good condition, it would soon be observed whether his daily consumption of fuel was increasing over former records, or whether he was making a saving for the institution and obtaining just as good, if not better, results than his predecessor. This is important information to obtain.

More may be learned from these engineers' logs about the proper management of the plant than in any other way the writer knows of. (See Fig. 122.)

The noise in steam pipes is usually caused by the partial closing of radiator valves or the blowing of steam through steam traps to the receiver. When this disturbance occurs, the nurse or attendant should see that all radiator valves are either tightly closed or wide open. If this does not stop the noise, the engineer should be notified and asked to see that his traps are not by-passed, or blowing through to the receiver. When properly handled, no well-installed

ENGINEER'S REPORT

BUILDING _____

WEEK ENDING _____ **19**___

LABOR AND MATERIALS USED

COAL USED, LBS.	SUN.	MON.	TUES.	WED.	THURS.	FRI.	SAT.	TOTAL	
DAY ENGINEER									
NIGHT									
Lbs of Coal at $ per ton									
Cu. ft. Water at $ per 100 cu. ft.									
Pints Oil at $ per pint									
Lbs. Cotton Waste at $ per lb.									
Electric Lamps, 8 c. p., at $ each									
" " 16 c. p., at $ "									
Cu. ft. Gas at $ per 1000 cu. ft.									
Other Supplies									
Average Outside Temp.									
" Inside "									

PERFORMANCE	HOURS	MINS.
Total kilowatt hrs. electricity used for power		
" " " " " " lights		
" hours engines running, No. 1 No. 2		
" " steam on building		
" " live steam on building		
" " " " " laundry		
" " " " " sterilizers		
" lbs. ashes removed		

Fig. 122.

heating system should cause any annoyance when in regular commission. Noise may occur when steam is first turned on the system, but should not continue after the radiators have become warm.

The care of the boiler and engine is a duty that must largely be left to an engineer. He should be questioned, however, at frequent intervals as to whether he is keeping his boilers clean or not, and if his engines are properly adjusted so as to get the greatest efficiency from amount of steam used.

In caring for laundry machinery it is the engineer's duty to carefully inspect all bearings, valves, and adjustments at least once every day that the machinery is in use. He should see that the apparatus is not only in good working order, but he should report to the superintendent any lack on the part of the employees in properly caring for their machines. If the washers and mangle are not kept clean, it often occurs that white goods are spoiled from grease or other discolorations. The engineer should see that the water is not rusty, and that the steam is dry and of sufficient pressure in the mangle and other pieces of apparatus where steam is used.

If these notes should be read by any one contemplating the work of a superintendent and who has not received any instruction along engineering lines, I would recommend that, before taking up such duties, you have a good long discussion of these subjects with some experienced superintendent, or with a competent and reliable heating and ventilating engineer. Go over the items in question not once, but many times, until you feel master of the situation.

IMPORTANT ENGINEERING POINTS FOR THE ENGINEER

See that your plant is complete and in good working condition when you assume charge.

Do not condemn the plant turned over to you by the hospital authorities until you can convince them by your reports that there is something entirely wrong.

Study to get the best and most efficient service out of your plant that is possible, and thereby make yourself a valuable man to the institution.

Acquaint yourself with every valve and piece of machinery around the place so as to be prepared in any emergency to prevent damage or loss.

Make yourself agreeable and helpful to the superintendent and others in charge of the hospital. In other words, be a gentleman at all times and to everybody.

Always see that your boilers and engines are kept in readiness for inspection at any time, as far as it is possible.

Never leave the plant or system in charge of another without explaining to him the condition of the plant, so that he may properly and efficiently handle the same in your absence.

CHAPTER XIII

THE LAUNDRY

By Joseph B. Howland, M.D.

The hospital laundry should not be located in a building used for ward or administration purposes because of the disagreeable odors from soap-tanks and washers and unavoidable noise of the machinery. With relation to the rest of the plant, a central location is desirable, because linen must be collected from and distributed to all parts of the institution at frequent intervals.

A one- or two-story building given up entirely to laundry work or combined with a power-house may be practicable. There should be ample room near the laundry for out-of-door drying and sun bleaching of the wash. If this is not possible on the ground, it may be arranged to use for this purpose the roof of a suitably constructed laundry. It is needless to say that no linen dried within doors can compare in freshness to that which has been exposed to the wind and sun.

Construction.—In this chapter we are only concerned with interior construction. Plastering is undesirable, as it may peel and crack from the excessive moisture. Brick walls painted in light color are satisfactory in every way. Windows should be large and near together. At least one outside door should be made wide enough to admit the largest piece of laundry machinery.

All machinery should be placed well away from the walls to allow thorough cleaning on all sides, and not so crowded on the floor but that ample passage-ways are left. In building, have laundry area sufficient for growth. Good ventilation must be provided for the steam from soap-tanks and washing machines. In a one-story building, sky-lights with ventilators attached will be found satisfactory for this purpose. All laundry work may be done in one large room or several may be utilized. The one advantage of the first plan is that supervision of the whole plant may be more easily accomplished by one person. If separate rooms are preferred, the following may be mentioned: (1) A sorting room for soiled linen; (2) room for soap-tanks, washers,

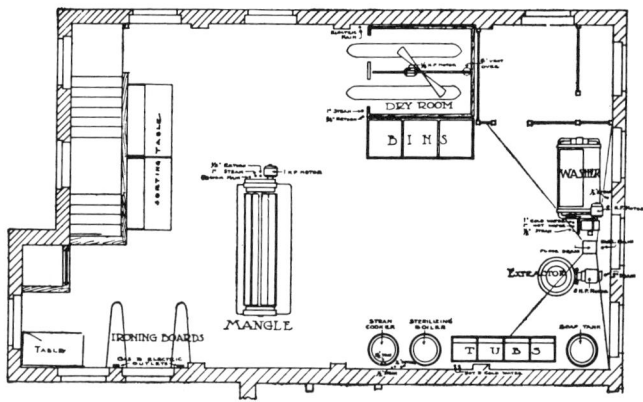

Fig. 123.—Plan of laundry apparatus, Leonard Morse Hospital, Natick Massachusetts.

shakers, extractors, and dry bars; (3) room for mangles, hand irons, and other ironing machinery; and (4) a clean linen room; (5) many advantages will be found in having a sewing room adjacent to the clean linen room.

The sorting room for soiled linen should be accessible from the hospital without the necessity for linen being carried through other parts of the laundry. It should be of ample size, have smooth walls, and a water-proof floor graded to a drain so that it may be thoroughly cleaned.

The washing room should be constructed similarly to the above, and cement floors will be found satisfactory.

THE LAUNDRY

The floors in the ironing, clean linen, and sewing room may be of wood, as it is much more comfortable to stand on continually than those of cement or other inelastic material.

Equipment.—High-pressure steam is necessary if much work is to be done, and if, as is true in many small hospitals, the general heating is done by a low-pressure system, a

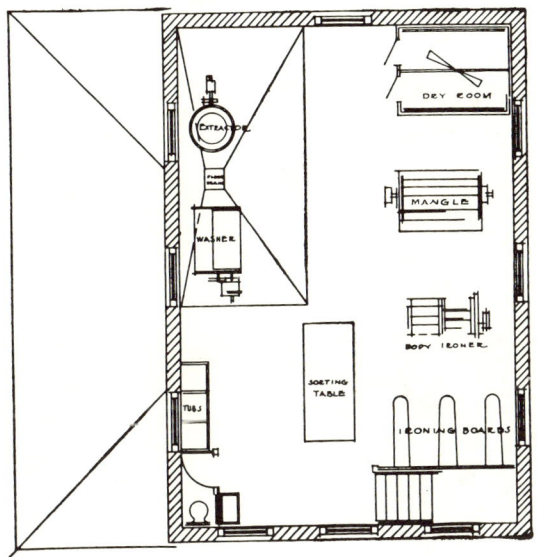

Fig. 124.—Plan of laundry apparatus, Beverly Hospital, Beverly, Massachusetts.

small boiler must be installed for laundry use. Power may be steam or electricity. If the former, a system of shafting must be provided. If electricity is used, one or more motors may be belted to shafting, or a small motor may be attached to each machine. The latter method must be more economic of current, and may be an important item where power is purchased. In many small hospitals it will probably be much cheaper to have a small steam engine. Body ironers and hand irons may be heated by gas or electricity. While the latter is safer, it usually costs more for operating, and electrically heated machinery is expensive to keep in repair. Employees who use gas-heated irons frequently complain of headaches, presumably due to escaping fumes and the heat.

The following equipment may be required for a hospital of from 75 to 100 beds: one wood or metallic

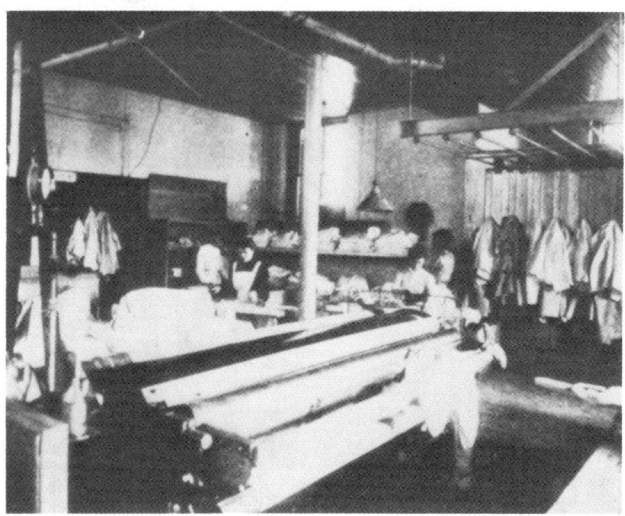

Fig. 125.—Corner of laundry, Hospital for Sick Children, Toronto.

washer, one sterilizing washer, one extractor, one shaker, one or two soap-tanks (one if a soap solution is made from soap chips, two if soft soap is to be manufactured), one mangle, one body ironer, four set tubs, one set of dry bars, four ironing tables, clothes-horses, laundry trucks, etc. A wooden washer will cost less than a metallic one; if properly cared for, will last a long time, and is less hard on clothing.

The sterilizing washer is usually made of iron, with a

brass cylinder, and may be used as a sterilizer, or for ordinary washing, The soap-tank may be made of cast or galvanized iron, and should be equipped with a perforated steam pipe in the bottom for boiling contents. Mangles are made in a great variety of sizes and patterns. The steam chest should be at least 70 inches wide, and 50 to 70 pounds of steam pressure is required for rapid drying. In laundries having few employees it will be desirable to use a mangle to which linen may be fed and removed from the same side. Two persons may do the work instead of four. In selecting a mangle only such should be installed which have devices to protect the operators from having their hands drawn in and burned in feeding. A reversible body ironer, while more expensive than one which revolves in one direction only, is also much better, because the hot roll can go over the same area of goods as many times as necessary without taking the time to pull back the garment or remove pressure to go over the same surface.

Metallic dry rooms are not necessary. Wooden ones lined with sheet metal are less expensive and perfectly safe if properly managed. It is in the dry rooms of hospital laundries that many fires start. The following rules should be observed:

Do not allow lint to collect behind the steam-pipes or on the floor.

Do not allow clothing to remain in dry room longer than necessary, as the heat affects the wearing quality of the goods to a certain extent.

Never leave clothing in the dry room at night.

Do not leave steam turned on at night.

It would be well to install a sprinkler system over the dry bars as a measure of safety, if the above rules were at any time not carried out.

Set tubs may be made of porcelain, enameled iron, soapstone, or wood. Tubs of good quality pine will last a long time if cared for and are the most satisfactory if it is desired to equip with perforated steam pipes for boiling clothes.

Hand-irons.—If electric irons are used, care must be

taken that the current is turned off when not in use, otherwise the iron will become overheated and the connections burned out.

Much thought should be given to the relative location of the laundry equipment. As far as possible machinery should be located in the order in which it will be used, e. g., the washers near the receiving room, the extractors next, then the shaker, mangles, etc. By this method confusion and unnecessary steps will be saved.

Employees.—The number will, of course, vary with the amount of work to be done, but perhaps it may be helpful to have described the system in a successful laundry of a hospital averaging 80 patients. Three women working five and one-half days and one man for two or three days each week should be sufficient to manage well the laundry of a hospital of from 75 to 100 beds. Hours of duty, 7 A. M. to 5.30 P. M., with one hour at noon. The head laundress is responsible for sorting, washing, and entire management of the laundry. She should understand thoroughly the importance of carrying out instructions with regard to infected clothing. The first maid should iron well, and be able to take the place of head laundress when occasion demands it. All three should be good workers.

All household clothing, with exception of table linen, is washed first on Monday morning. The head laundress sorts clothes, attends to the dry room, and assists where most needed. The first and second maid do hand washing in the morning until about nine, when some clothes should be ready for mangling. Washers and extractor should be run by the man, who also looks after the power.

Tuesday morning there will be some drying, folding, and sorting of clothes to do. The first and second maids can prepare starched clothes for ironing, while the head laundress attends to the drying, sorting, etc. Tuesday afternoon the hand ironing begins. The head laundress runs the body ironer, and does the most particular of the hand ironing. By Thursday noon all household clothes should be ironed, sorted, and sent to the proper places. The laundry is closed Thursday afternoon. When adjusting of engine, motors, machines, etc. is attended to, it will be found preferable to close Thursday or some other afternoon than Saturday, for if the latter time is selected, work may not be completed by the end of the week, and a large amount of soiled linen accumulated in the laundry which will be needed before Monday.

Friday is given to washing for wards, after the table linen, which is put to soak Thursday noon, is washed. The laundry should get an extra cleaning Friday evening. Saturday the head laundress can attend to sorting and giving out clothes, while the first and second maids can be sent into the hospital to do work assigned by the housekeeper. On each day of the week, the head laundress should see that any emergency requirements are filled, such as immediate attention to infected or soiled clothing.

Soiled clothes are brought from the wards each day, and the head laundress should see that they are put in proper places, and the empty bags returned to the wards. Two boxes or bins may be provided for unstained clothing, while ventilated metal containers should receive stained and infected clothing in case there may be a little delay in attending to them.

Clothes.—All clothes are sent to the laundry in bags, which have pinned to them the list of clothes signed by persons responsible for them, and the name of the ward or department from which they are sent. Duplicates of these lists are kept. Soiled and infected clothing are put in separate bags marked "rinse house." In the laundry, the head laundress verifies the count, and must see that all clothes are accounted for among discarded linen if not returned to departments from which they come.

Discarded Linen..—All clothes that require mending, or are too worn and torn to be mended, should be kept in baskets after mangling and drying, and on two mornings of the week looked over by the housekeeper, who keeps a list of discarded clothes, which are replaced the first of each month. Care should be taken to provide covers for mangle and ironing boards of new cloth whenever necessary. The housekeeper alone should discard clothes.

Sorting Clothes.—Household clothes are sorted as follows:
1. Collars and cuffs.
2. Handkerchiefs.
3. White dresses, skirts, and aprons.
4. Internes' suits.
5. Table linen.
6. Flannels.
7. Cotton underwear.
8. Flannelettes according to color.
9. Ginghams and prints according to color.
10. Shirts according to color.
11. Towels, pillow-cases, and sheets.
12. Miscellaneous dark clothes.
13. Stockings—(1) cotton; (2) wool.

Collars, cuffs, handkerchiefs, and all small articles should be washed in twine bags and may be put in the washer with white dresses.

Ward clothes are sorted as follows:
1. Sheets, pillow-cases, night-shirts (cotton).
2. Spreads.
3. Cotton wrappers.
4. Flannels according to color.
5. Blankets according to color.
6. Stockings.
7. "Rinse house" linen according to degree and quality of staining.

Washing.—White clothes are rinsed in cold water fifteen minutes, then washed in suds made with warm water and two and one-half gallons soap solution[1] to washer 60 by 32. Turn on the steam, heat water to boiling, and wash one-half hour. Rinse fifteen minutes in hot water, then fifteen minutes in cold water. This completes the washing for bed-clothing and ward clothes and towels. All other

[1] See formula for making soap, p. 293.

white cotton and linen clothes have a blue rinse for fifteen minutes. Dresses, aprons, and clothes requiring starch have a rinse in hot starch, allowing seventeen and one-half gallons starch solution to washer 60 by 32. All clothes are put in the extractor for five to seven minutes. Sheets, pillow-cases, towels, and all pieces suitable for mangling are prepared for the mangle and the remainder of white clothes are dried in dry room. No bleach is used in the laundry.

Blankets.—White and gray blankets are washed entirely in cool water, but never ice-cold. For a washer 60 by 32 use four gallons soft soap and one four-ounce cupful borax. When the suds is prepared, put the blankets in and wash one-half hour. Rinse in two waters of the same temperature that blankets have been washed in, allowing fifteen minutes in each water. Put the blankets through extractor, and when there is no frost in the air, dry out-of-doors. Otherwise, hang on lines in laundry, but never in the dry room.

Infected blankets are soaked in carbolic acid 1 : 20 in set tubs for at least one hour, then washed as ordinary blankets.

Stockings. Wool stockings are washed and dried as blankets, omitting borax in the suds.

Red Blankets and Flannels.—Red blankets and all flannels are sorted according to color and washed by hand. Wash them on a board in suds made with soap solution, one cupful; borax, 1 cupful to three-quarters tub of water. If extra soap is required on soiled parts, use hard soap. Place in the second suds made the same way. If flannels are very soiled, the board should be used again, but generally this second suds is but a rinse. Then rinse in two waters. Have all waters for washing and rinsing flannels of the same temperature, warm, squeeze out excess of water, but do not iron flannels. Dry as blankets. Proper attention to temperature of water and squeezing instead of wringing flannels will produce excellent results.

Colored Prints and Ginghams.—Ginghams, prints,

and cotton stockings are sorted according to color, and washed as blankets. They may be dried in the dry room.

Stained and Infected Linen.—This should be sent from wards in separate bags, the lists marked "rinse." In the sorting room, bags are emptied, and the contents sorted into—(1) Those stained with blood; (2) those stained with vomitus and fecal matter. These are sorted again into—(a) somewhat soiled and (b) very much soiled. They are placed first in set tubs, each division by itself, covered with cold water, and left to soak overnight. In the morning they are washed in the sterilizing washer as follows:

Those not badly soiled—

Washed in successive clear cold waters until the water remains clear. Then soap is added—four gallons of the soap solution to a large washer (diameter, 60 by 32), and steam turned on gradually until five pounds' pressure is reached, which is continued for fifteen minutes, then cold fifteen minutes.

Those badly soiled—

Washed in successive cold waters until water remains clear; then, after adding soap, steam is turned on gradually until five pounds' pressure is reached, and washing is continued one-half hour, followed by hot and cold rinse fifteen minutes each.

Dressing Gauze and Bandages.—These are sent to the sorting room in bags from which they are taken by a sorter wearing rubber gloves. Bandages are separated from gauze, and pins, etc., removed. They are then packed loosely in net bags which are placed in set tubs, and covered with cold water and left to soak overnight. In the morning they are placed in the sterilizing washer, and washed first in clear cold water ten minutes, drained and washed in cold water with three and one-half gallons soap solution and one large cup sal soda for fifteen minutes, drained again, and six gallons soap and two cups sal soda put in, both hot and cold water being turned on. The washer is then sealed, and ten pounds live steam turned on for thirty minutes, followed by hot rinse fifteen minutes, and cold rinse fifteen minutes.

Starch.—Use wheat starch only; other kinds make linen yellow. For collars and cuffs use three-quarters pound starch and one thimbleful paraffin to one gallon water.

For aprons, dresses, etc., three-quarters pound starch and one thimbleful paraffin to one and one-half gallons water.

Dissolve starch in cold water, add hot water and paraffin and boil thoroughly, then add a little bluing.

Always use starch hot, and if too thick, dilute with hot water. Linen requiring starch is starched in washer; after the last rinse, the starch is poured in, and machine revolved seven to eight minutes.

Bluing.—Purchase a reliable make and follow the directions given. If thoroughly dissolved in hot water and a little of this solution is added to rinse water, the clothes will not be unevenly blued or spotted.

No bluing is used for ward linen. Table linen, aprons, dresses, muslin underwear, etc., have a blue rinse in addition to the regular rinses.

Soft Soap.—Twenty-four pounds potash, thirty-six pounds soap grease.

Mix in cauldron and add fifteen gallons water. Simmer for eighteen hours, then add enough water to make one-hundred gallons.

Dyeing.—Red blankets and blanket wrappers which become faded and dingy may be redyed with cardinal dye and in that way kept a good color until worn out.

Method of Dyeing.—Use two packages of "Diamond" dye (cardinal) and two quarts of vinegar in enough water to cover the goods. Use according to directions on package. Rinse thoroughly and dry without wringing.

CHAPTER XIV

THE PURCHASE AND ECONOMIC USE OF SURGICAL SUPPLIES

BY CARLETON R. METCALF, M.D.

It is out of the question for you to learn from rhetoric to purchase surgical supplies economically or to use them wisely. Such knowledge may be gleaned only from practical experience; the best that I can do is to point out some of the pitfalls in the path of economy, and to offer a few suggestions for saving an honest penny.

In your purchasing, go as often as you can to the "man higher up." Deal with the manufacturer, the surgical supply house, or the jobber, rather than with the retail dealer. Make the corner drug-store your court of last resort. With a little time and less energy not a few surgical supplies may be prepared, as we shall see, in the hospital itself.

Many wholesale jobbers publish catalogues, with discounts or monthly bulletins which they are very glad to send; these form a working basis in purchasing, for from them one may gauge the market value of various supplies.

It is a poor plan for a customer to limit purchases in any given line to a single firm. The single firm frequently takes advantage of such devotion. Rather, play one firm against another; if you are buying in considerable quantity, secure quotations from several firms. If the materials are not perishable, ask for quotations for immediate delivery; if the materials are perishable, ask for quota-

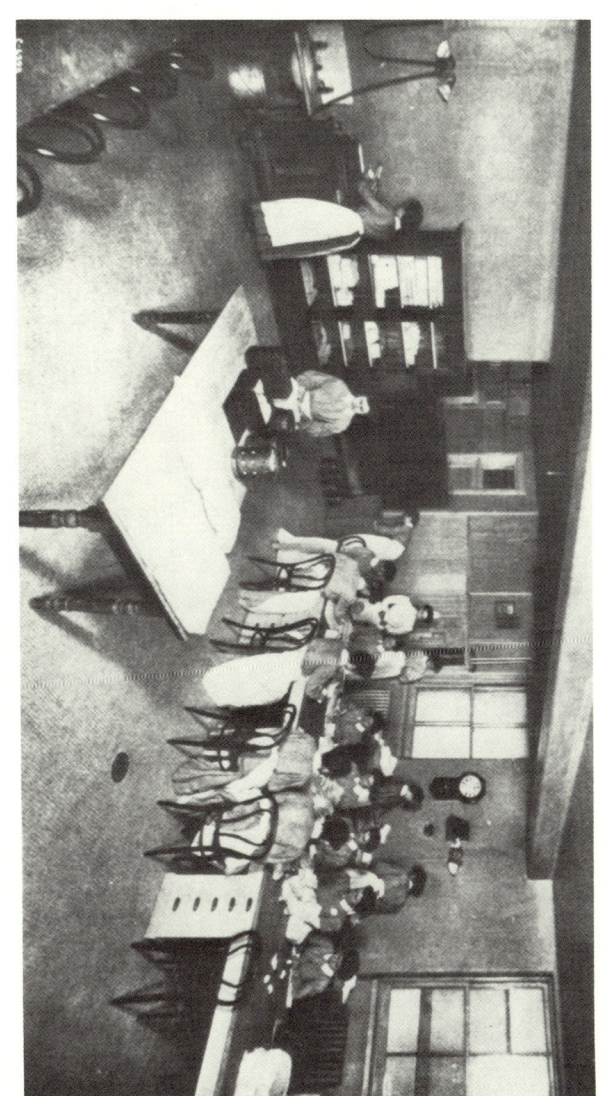

Fig. 126.—Preparing surgical dressings. Presbyterian Hospital, New York.

tions on a given quantity to be delivered piecemeal—so many dozens or so many pounds every month or two.

It is needless to say that the larger your purchase, the lower relatively will be your quotation. It is economic, therefore, to order a sufficient supply for six months or a year, unless the merchandise will deteriorate by prolonged keeping. Buy six months' supply of gauze, but two months' supply of rubber gloves.

If a firm wishes to introduce a new brand of ether or of ice-bags at a suspiciously low price, ask for references; an inquiry at another institution that has tried the questionable goods will resolve your doubts.

I am accustomed to the "return system" in dispensing surgical supplies. All supplies are distributed originally on presentation of a properly signed requisition from a central storeroom. When any article becomes unserviceable, it is returned with a second requisition. A leaking ice-bag or a broken instrument comes back, either to be replaced or repaired. In the repair of supplies a "junk-box" is highly desirable. The box contains odds and ends of all sorts,—portions of instruments, an atomizer stem, a syringe bulb,—all saved from some previous catastrophe and now useful in supplying some defect in a utensil.

Let me take up seriatim the more important surgical supplies and make a few concrete suggestions about their purchase and use. I have divided supplies roughly into eight classes:

1. Dressing materials.
2. Rubber goods.
3. Suture material.
4. Glassware.
5. Surgical instruments.
6. Anesthetics.
7. Drugs.
8. Miscellaneous.

1. **Dressing Materials.**—*Gauze*, which is subject to fluctuations in price, should be purchased in quantity

when the market is low. We are accustomed to secure samples and quotations from several mills and to buy about 100,000 yards at one time, which is delivered in lots at stated intervals. Bolts are ordinarily 100 yards long and one yard wide; the bolt is folded once lengthwise, so that the apparent width is one-half yard.

The different grades, four or five in all, are identified by the number of strands or threads to the square inch. For bandages, a close mesh (40 by 52 strands to the square inch) is desirable; for sponges, secure a medium mesh (14 by 20 strands to the square inch), because a close mesh prevents adequate drainage. Gauze should be cleanly bleached.

Gauze bandages should be bought by the pound. Ask for "seconds." First quality bandages are sterilized and neatly wrapped in paper—theoretic advantages for which a purchaser pays two-fold. "Seconds" are not ravelled on the edge and vary slightly in width and in length from standard; yet they are quite as serviceable as their more esthetic brethren. It is evident that bandages which are removed without the aid of scissors may be washed, rewound, and used again.

Cotton.—The price of absorbent cotton varies directly with the length of the fiber. A cheap absorbent cotton has a short fiber or is not thoroughly freed of oil. For plugging test-tubes a long-fiber cotton is essential. For other surgical purposes a short-fiber cotton answers every purpose, although, in pads, it tends to "lump." Test the presence of oil by dropping a bit of the cotton in water; if oil-free, it will fill and sink immediately. An oily absorbent cotton is dear at any price.

Cotton sheeting is used for sheets, pillow-cases, and nightshirts. Old sheeting may be utilized for compresses, swathes, slings, and for cleaning rags. The only disadvantage of a cotton swathe is that safety-pins go through it with difficulty.

Cotton wadding comes in pieces a yard square. Each piece should be torn into strips six inches wide. Three such strips sewed end to end and tightly rolled form a suitable cotton roller for dressings.

Iodoform Gauze.—All surgical supply-houses market it in glass jars—1, 5, or 10 yards to the jar. Strength, 5 or 10 per cent. Keep it in a tight jar and in a cool, dark place. Avoid a supply that will last longer than six months, because iodoform is volatile.

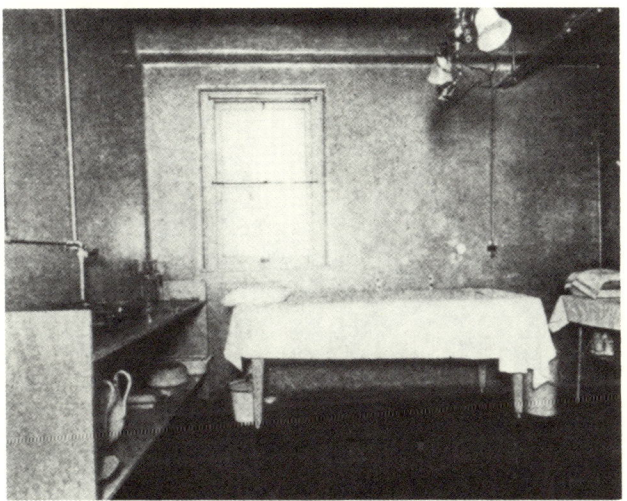

Fig. 127.—Dressing-room, Minnequa Hospital, Pueblo, Colorado.

Poultice paper or "parchment paper" may be had from any paper dealer in rolls twelve inches wide. It is used to cover wet dressings or to protect splints. *Oiled muslin* has the same uses, but its expense disqualifies it.

Suspensory bandages are made from cotton, linen, silk, silk and linen, and in five sizes. It is desirable to carry in stock the three smallest sizes made from cotton.

Adhesive Plaster.—Zinc oxid plaster is non-irritating and therefore desirable if the plaster is to come in contact with skin; with this exception plain plaster is the choice.

Adhesive plaster is made by nearly all surgical supply houses. Send to several houses for samples and for quotations on a year's supply to be delivered in monthly lots.

A good plaster adapts itself to all needs. Some is too adhesive—it takes off the skin. Some is not adhesive

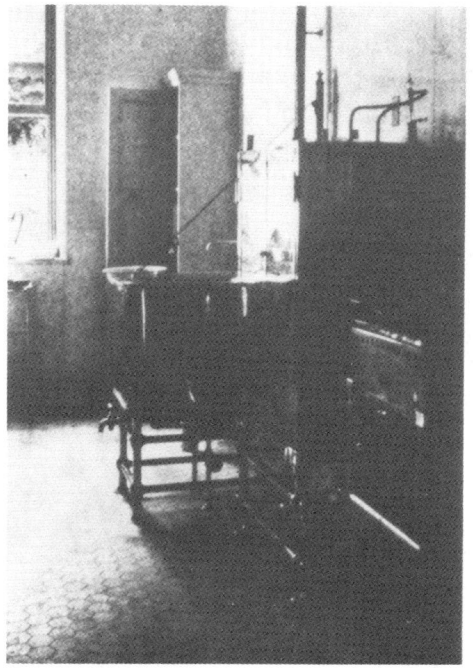

Fig. 128.—Half view of sterilizing room, Royal Victoria Hospital, Montreal, Canada.

enough. Some will stick to a wooden splint, but will not stick to skin. Some has starch added in place of zinc oxid—hence the need of samples.

Buy your plaster in 5-yard rolls, 12 inches wide. For general use tear a roll, with cheese-cloth still adherent, into strips $\frac{1}{2}$, 1, and 2 inches in width. Cut pieces of broom-handle to match these widths, and roll the plaster on the wood, removing the cheese-cloth as you wind.

Plaster Bandages.—If you use these only occasionally, buy a good plaster from a reliable dental supply-house or, better, from a statuary manufacturer. Be sure that the plaster is fresh, and keep it in air-tight containers.

Buy a medium-grade crinolin from a wholesale dry-goods firm. Unsized crinolin is desirable; if sizing is present, wash the crinolin. The preparation of plaster bandages requires a shallow box about three feet long and one and one-half feet wide, with sides two inches high. A supply of plaster is put in the box at one side. A crinolin strip is pulled across the bottom and buttered with a very thin layer of plaster. As it reaches the further edge the excess of plaster should be scraped off or shaken out and the strip should be rolled. An acceptable bandage needs sufficient plaster to fill the interstices and a little more. Two people can do better work than one. The first worker rolls the bandage; the assistant feeds the strip across the board and scrapes the plaster over the strip from the supply at the side.

Don't buy plaster bandages already prepared. Make their preparation a home industry and save money.

2. **Rubber Goods.**—Rubber is expensive. On this account, it is wise to pay a fairly good price for rubber goods and to buy from a reliable manufacturer. The man who quotes a very low price on rubber goods is putting mighty little rubber in them. Old rubber brings sixteen cents a pound at the present time; don't throw any away. Rubber vulcanizes, thereby growing brittle. Therefore, it is wise to carry in stock a supply that will be exhausted in two or three months. Rubber keeps best in a cool place. Any form of grease causes it to rot.

Rubber gloves are made in four weights, and with fingers of three lengths: long, medium, and cadet. A light-weight glove tears easily and is therefore not economic. Steam-cured are more durable than acid-cured gloves. Punctured gloves may be renewed by patching with thin rubber dam, not with a piece of an old glove. **Repair them thus:**

Put the glove on the hand and wash the site of puncture with benzin. Smear with rubber cement (pure rubber dissolved in benzin or chloroform) an area as large as a finger-nail. Treat the patch in the same way. In about twenty minutes, when the cement becomes sticky, press the patch over the puncture, being careful not to move the patch after it has been put in place. Several brands of rubber cement may be had in the market.

After use, gloves must be thoroughly washed with soapy water, rinsed, and dried in the air.

Sterilize gloves in boiling water. Steam sterilization is injurious. If the surgeon wishes dry gloves, powder the interior, tie the open ends of each pair with a piece of $\frac{1}{16}$ inch rubber tubing, put on like a tourniquet, and boil. This procedure sterilizes the exterior of the gloves but does not kill bacteria on the inside.

Pebble-gloves won't slip, but are expensive. Household gloves (very heavy) are suitable for handling dirty dressing material or typhoid stools and for rubbing in ointment. Obstetric gloves have cuffs extending to the elbow; they are useful in autopsy work.

Finger-cots are made of rolled tissue, with or without reinforced tips. One may be put on during an operation if a glove-finger is punctured. Their use in making rectal examinations is obvious.

Hot-water Bags.—Here again the purchaser gets what he pays for and no more. Bags come in three varieties: pure gum, rubber composition, and cloth inserted. A cloth-inserted bag, *i. e.*, a bag with a cloth body, coated on either side with rubber, is economic and will last from eleven to eighteen months. Mark on a bag with indestructible ink the date on which it goes into service, in order to test its wearing qualities.

Instruct nurses not to fill the bags full. A full bag is heavy, and is liable to burst, with disastrous results for an unconscious patient.

Punctures may be mended with a piece of an old bag, following the technic used for gloves. But punctures are rare if the bags, instead of being pinned in cloth, are placed in a woolen bag fitted with draw-strings. It is economy to keep a liberal supply of such covers.

Some dealers will guarantee a bag against wear and tear for a given number of months. See if your dealer will do so.

Ice-bags come in the three varieties just mentioned, save that spinal ice-bags are not commonly made with cloth insertion. An ice-bag with a brass collar is expensive but economic. An aluminum collar is readily bent, whereupon the cap fits imperfectly and the bag leaks. Avoid aluminum. Don't change the cap on an ice-bag, for the slight variations in size cause leakage. If a bag leaks, it may be due to this; it may be due to a bent collar or to a puncture; it may be that a new washer is needed; or, finally, it may be merely condensation on the outside, and hence an error of observation.

Cigarette drainage tubing may be purchased ready for use; more economically, it may be made by cutting suitable strips of light-weight rubber dam and affixing the long edges with rubber cement.

Rubber dam is used also, you remember, for patching gloves. On very foul dressings it sometimes pays for itself in that it protects a splint and the nearby clothing. For other purposes its place may usually be taken by rubber tissue, and as dam costs much and disintegrates quickly, it should be largely eliminated from hospital impedimenta.

Rubber tissue is made in two grades: (*a*) plain tissue and (*b*) silk tissue. Plain tissue costs about $1.00 a pound. Silk tissue costs nearly twice as much, but it does not rot, has no grain, is less brittle, is stronger, and, being lighter, has a larger area per pound. Buy "silk tissue" every time.

Rubber tissue should never be boiled or even placed in hot water. Prepare it for use in this way:

Wash with soap and water. Rinse in cold water,

Keep in a solution of 1:1000 biniodid of mercury. The ingredients of the mercury solution are:

```
Mercuric iodid............................ 1 gram
Potassium iodid...  ....................... 1  "
Distilled water to ........................ 1 liter.
```

Mercuric iodid is soluble in a solution of potassium iodid. Therefore mix the salts thoroughly, add a small amount of water, and, after solution occurs, add the remaining water.

Rubber tubing may be had in many sizes and in three colors—white, red, and black. White tubing is stiff and brittle. Red tubing is fairly pliable. Black tubing is preferable to either. For surgical drainage, buy an absolutely pure gum. An impure gum contains too much sulphur to be safe. Cheaper grades of tubing may be used for other purposes, *e. g.*, for bladder drainage, but care must be used that the two qualities are not mixed. Tubing cut for drainage may be kept in boric-acid solution.

Stomach-tubes become hard and stiff very quickly. Don't carry them in stock. They may be had in various sizes, and with open ends and sides or with closed ends.

Both stomach and rectal tubes form an exception to our rule to buy from a wholesale dealer. It is more economic to have only one or two of each on hand.

Catheters.—Soft-rubber catheters are sold at all prices from $14 to $38 a gross. This variation depends on the quality of rubber and on the presence or absence of an import duty. Surgeons have a choice of stilet or solid ends.

A pure gum catheter is so pliable that it cannot overcome the least resistance of an irritated urethra; nor will it retain its rotundity if used for constant drainage. It will last for a long time, but is relatively expensive.

It is better then to buy a cheap catheter—one that costs, say, from $14 to $18 a gross. But inasmuch as such a catheter gets brittle with age and fails to return to its original shape after stretching, one should procure a supply sufficient for not over three or four months. Manufacturers are always ready to send samples of catheters. Let me repeat that rubber goods are injured by any form of grease. Immediately after use catheters should be thoroughly washed with soap and water and dried.

Bulb syringes have a much longer lease of life if they are properly cared for. Many enemata contain some form of grease which rots the rubber and clogs the valves. If a syringe refuses to work, take it apart and clean the valves. If the tubing wears out, a new piece may be applied. The bulb itself is the only part not amenable to repair. Metal valves are better than hard-rubber ones. A "continuous flow" syringe (Parker, Stearns and Co., New York City) has much merit. Bulb syringes, ready for use, should be kept in sterile boric-acid solution.

Air-cushions are made round or horse-shoe shaped, and of three colors—white, red, and slate. They are equipped with a valve. Most cushions have a fiber interlining, along which air readily travels.

When punctured, then, the actual site of injury may be at some distance from the apparent site. Repair is often a hopeless task.

It is our practice merely to loan air-cushions to the various wards. They are so fragile that they are kept at the store-room except when they are actually in use.

Pessaries are of many varieties—"doughnut," hard-rubber, solid rubber, etc. The soft-rubber "doughnut" is perishable; the hard rubber, enduring. A hard-rubber pessary may be modified in form if it is boiled until pliable, molded, and quickly plunged into cold water.

Atomizers come in all sizes. The rubber arms sometimes become distorted, but may be straightened by boiling and molding, after the method suggested for pessaries. Atomizers need frequent repair from the "junk-box."

3. **Suture Material.**—*Catgut* is made in many sizes, and both chromicized and plain. Before adopting any one of the many brands on the market, it is wise to test the tensile strength and the sterility of samples.

The sterile tubes in which the gut is sold should not be

boiled. Wash them and keep them in glass jars containing a 1:1000 solution of corrosive sublimate. Catgut on spools and remnants from operations are usually unsterile; avoid their employment scrupulously.

Kangaroo tendon is analogous to catgut.

Silkworm gut is of various sizes, and either white or black. The highest grade includes only strands which are smooth and regular. The cheaper grades have some irregularity that forms a point of lowered resistance, at which the gut is apt to break. Such gut is suitable for minor lesions where short lengths are commonly used, but is debarred from major surgery.

Two sizes—fine and extra heavy—form an adequate stock in trade.

Horsehair is sold in skeins similar to those of silkworm gut. It should be boiled and kept, ready for use, in corrosive sublimate.

Silk is prepared in sizes running from 1 to 20, either braided or twisted, and black or white. Braided silk has three strands. Surgeons commonly use the sizes between 5 and 19. If much silk is required, buy in pound lots on one-half or one ounce spools.

An assortment of spools may be steam sterilized and kept in sterile jars in the operating room; or the various sizes may be threaded into needles, run through strips of cotton cloth, sterilized, and kept in sterile jars until required.

4. **Glassware.**—*Clinical thermometers* should be aged before being standardized. As time goes on, a green thermometer varies from its original standard. Ask the manufacturer to give a guarantee to replace all thermometers which change from the standard advertised at the time of sale. Do not buy cases with the thermometers; cases are useless luxuries. A serviceable article may be had from $30 a gross upward; six months' supply should be purchased at one time.

Bath thermometers vary in price with length. They are made in three sizes—6, 8, and 12 inches. The two larger sizes are preferable. Either a spirit or a mercury column may be ordered. The mercury column is more accurate and, therefore, preferable. A bath thermometer should register as high as 140° F.

Inexpensive thermometers, which are deficient in age, register inaccurately.

Glass syringes are needed for washing out wounds and sinuses and for male urethral douches. A "male" (snub-nosed) syringe with a cotton packing is cheap and serviceable. Sizes range from 00 to 6.

Medicine-droppers have nozzles of varying size. If they are used for measuring in minims, specify accurately adjusted tips.

Irrigation tips are merely thick medicine-droppers. Do not throw them away when they become dirty; clean and resterilize them.

The most convenient *drinking tube* is bent at an angle of 120 degrees with arms of equal length—3 inches. These, like irrigation tips, may be cleaned by boiling, either in water or in 10 per cent. nitric acid.

Blood counters may be had from any surgical supply-house. The pipets must be thoroughly cleaned immediately after use, first with water, then alcohol, and finally with ether. Of counting slides, the Türck is most highly esteemed. The slides should be washed only in sterile water. Alcohol dissolves the cement of the counting chamber. Prices are subject to little or no variation.

Slides and *cover-glasses* should be purchased directly from a microscope dealer. Slides are of different thicknesses, either white or blue-white, with edges rough or ground.

Cover-glasses, either square or round, come in two sizes: ¾ inch and ⅞ inch. They are graded by thickness. Most laboratory workers prefer a fairly thin, ⅞ inch, square cover-glass. It is economic to buy a good quality of both these wares.

Slides and covers may be used several times. Discarded

slides should be collected periodically and boiled for four hours in a porcelain dish in the following solution:

```
Nitric acid................................ 1 pint
Water..................................... 1 gallon.
```

Rinse in water. Stand on edge to drain. If the slides and covers are not perfectly clean, repeat the process. Do not attempt to scrape off the adhesive balsam. Such a procedure does little but scratch the glass and make it unfit for further use.

Flasks may be secured from a "druggists' sundry" house in sizes from a half-pint to a half-gallon. Quart flasks are suitable containers for salt solution. The glass should be well annealed. Do not allow glass to come in contact with hot metal—*e. g.*, in steam sterilization; insert an intervening pad of cloth or felt. In ordering glassware, have the shipper agree to replace all breakage above 5 per cent. which occurs during transit.

5. **Instruments.**—All surgical instrument manufacturers provide a comprehensive stock. Some of them specialize. Buy only the best quality of steel. With jointed instruments—snaps and scissors, for example—insist on a screw lock. A slip joint may choose as the psychologic moment for slipping, the critical period of an operation; or, if not, the halves surely become separated when the instruments are being washed. Dried blood engenders rust. Clean dirty instruments with scouring soap and rinse them without delay. A tooth-brush is a valuable asset in cleaning. If the vagaries of each surgeon are consulted, instruments in infinite variety must be on hand. Ask your staff to agree on a limited number of styles.

Corrosive sublimate will spoil the best of steel. If a surgeon deems it unnecessary to boil knives or other instruments, they may be sterilized in a 5 per cent. solution of carbolic acid.

Save portions of broken instruments. It is sometimes possible to make a new pair of scissors or a new snap from the odds and ends.

Needles.—Buy in quantity lots from a large surgical supply-house. The jobber need be patronized only for a small lot of a special needle.

Hypodermic Needles.—The ordinary length is ¾ inch. We prefer a ⅞-inch needle, 23 gauge. A needle of this size will neither bend nor penetrate too far, and the extra ⅛ inch allows for sharpening. For antitoxin, buy a needle of 20 or 21 gauge, 1½ or 2 inches long. Here again the wise

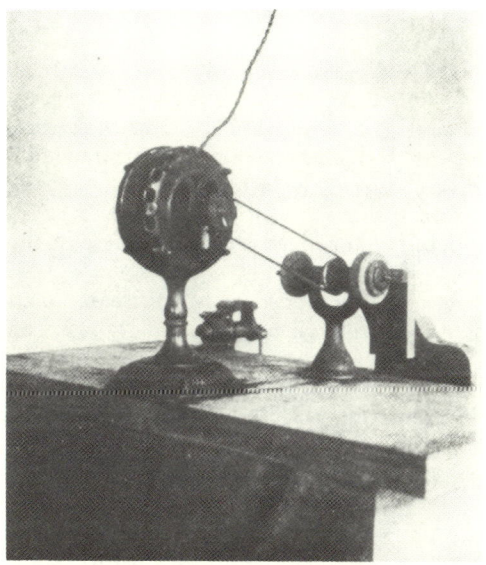

Fig. 129.—Machine for sharpening operating-room scissors, etc. Made at Presbyterian Hospital, Chicago.

man eliminates the jobber; he buys directly from a manufacturer.

Old hypodermic needles should not be thrown away. When 30 or 40 have accumulated, send them to an instrument repairer to be cleaned out and sharpened.

The most serviceable *hypodermic syringe* is of metal with a metal plunger. If a plunger becomes worn and fits loosely, it may be nickel-plated to increase its diameter.

Glass hypodermic syringes break easily, and the asbestos packing, commonly employed, soon shrinks. The parts of a glass syringe are not interchangeable. For these reasons glass syringes are not economic. For antitoxin we like a solid metal syringe of 12 c.c. capacity.

Clean and oil a syringe occasionally, and don't forget to run a wire completely through the needle after it has been in use. For all syringes, extra wires, washers, and needles may be had.

A *knife-edge* demands careful nursing. Rust spoils it. A prolonged bath (more than three minutes) in carbolic acid or in boiling water is detrimental. A clever instrument repairer grinds off very little when he sharpens a knife; he can transform an old amputation knife into a breast-knife, or, from the latter, make a serviceable scalpel for the ward. For ward dressings, instruments are adequate which have outlived their usefulness in the operating-room.

One side of a *needle-holder* always wears down. Your instrument repairer will give it a new lease of life by affixing a plate of brass or copper. Brass is preferable. He can file new teeth for a worn pair of *toothed forceps*. A supply of brass ribbon *retractors* will enable one to eliminate some of the fanciful retractors that flood the market. Double-headed retractors comprise two sizes at the price of one.

A poor *razor* is unworthy of notice. Its steel is soft, improperly annealed, and its edge is sure to turn. Buy a blade of good quality, $\frac{3}{4}$ or $\frac{7}{8}$ of an inch wide—the extra width allows for repeated honing. Never boil a razor.

Platinum *cautery-tips* require an absolutely pure benzin of a low boiling-point. Ordinary benzin spoils a tip.

6. Anesthetics.—Buy the same *ether* that some other hospital has found satisfactory. Buy it from a reliable chemical house, and buy ether prepared "for anesthesia." Cans containing either $\frac{1}{4}$ or $\frac{1}{2}$ pound are serviceable, and the contents keep indefinitely until the cap is broken.

After the cap is broken the liquid, exposed to the air, becomes "stale" and inefficient in a day or two. For this reason ether must never be bought in bulk.

Chloroform should read: "Purified for anesthesia." Packages containing either two or four ounces are appropriate in size. This anesthetic keeps indefinitely, even with a broken package. If it is poured into a bottle, seal the bottle with a cork rather than a glass stopper.

Nitrous oxid comes in cylinders containing 100 gallons each. The gas keeps indefinitely.

Oxygen is marketed in both large and small cylinders. In a small cylinder, the gas is under great pressure. For hospitals, it is better to employ a large cylinder containing 100 gallons. See to it that the product is absolutely pure; the presence of nitrogen lessens its efficiency. Oxygen is viable for one year. Gas remaining in a partly used cylinder does not deteriorate.

For inhalation, have the gas flow through a wash-bottle affixed to the side of the tank. The water in the bottle does not wash or purify the oxygen, but permits one to see just how fast the gas is escaping. At the distal end, the proverbial funnel is an extravagance. Less gas is required if a hard-rubber tip is inserted in mouth or nostril.

Ethyl chlorid should be guaranteed to comply with the Pharmacopœia. A supply for three months may be safely bought in glass tubes of 60 grams each. Ethyl chlorid is also put up in metal tubes of 30 and 100 grams. Your dealer will give a rebate on the latter tubes when returned empty.

The price of *cocain* fluctuates with the supply of coca leaves. It is wise to secure quotations from two or three chemical houses, and to buy a lot of from 5 to 25 ounces when the market-price is low.

Cocain is soluble in distilled water or in ½ per cent. carbolic solution. The addition of carbolic acid prevents contamination, but this drug should, of course, be absent from solutions intended for eyes.

It is well to place bottles in the wards containing a 4

per cent. solution, which may be readily diluted to a greater or lesser degree for each individual case.

7. **Drugs.**—A small hospital should submit to several jobbers a list of all drugs and chemicals, with a request for quotations. The order may then be split among several bidders or given in toto to one. The jobber will usually pay expressage if you ask him to do so.

Corrosive Sublimate.—The ordinary tablets are convenient, but expensive. If the salt is used regularly, it is much cheaper to procure it in bulk.

Buy from 1 to 25 pounds, specifying "small crystals." To make a saturated stock solution, mix:

Corrosive sublimate	1 pound
Sodium chlorid	2 pounds
Water to	2 gallons.

From the above stock solution, a 1 : 1000 solution is thus made:

Stock solution	10 drams
Water to	5 pints.

The 1 : 1000 solution should be poured into distinctive 5-pint bottles and kept, ready for use, in the wards.

Corrosive sublimate solution should be colored. A red dye has the following formula:

Anilin-red or fuchsin	5 grains
Alcohol	1 ounce
Water to	5 pints.

Three drams of the dye thus made will color a 5-pint bottle of corrosive solution.

A blue color may be imparted by adding 1 to 3 minims of saturated aqueous methylene-blue to each 5-pint bottle of solution.

Carbolic acid is supplied in tin drums holding from 10 to 100 pounds each. Eighty pounds is not too much to buy at one time.

Puncture the top of the can. Add $\frac{1}{20}$ part of water or glycerin to its contents. Melt the acid in a hot-water bath—not over a fire, for the *fumes of carbolic acid are inflammable.* Siphon the melted acid into glass containers, using care that it does not spill on one's hands. (Alcohol externally is the antidote.) Dilute with *warm* water to an appropriate strength, or rather weakness—usually 5 per cent.—and place in distinctive 5-pint bottles. Add an anilin dye. Globules of carbolic acid tend to sink to the bottom; be sure that the acid is thoroughly in solution.

It is impossible, with water, to make a carbolic acid solution stronger than 5 per cent. If a stronger solution is necessary, glycerin must be used as a solvent.

Carbolic acid sometimes turns brown with age. Its quality is not thereby impaired.

Formaldehyd is a 40 per cent. solution of a gas in water. If used extensively, formaldehyd should be bought in original kegs of 125 pounds each. Ordinarily, it is had in smaller lots from a pound upward. The drug keeps well in a cool place, but should not be allowed to freeze.

It may be used (2 per cent.) as a disinfectant for hoppers, stools, etc., and in 10 per cent. strength for preserving pathologic specimens.

In combination with *permanganate of potash*, formaldehyd forms a cheap and adequate fumigant. I am familiar with the following method of fumigating a room that has contained a patient with a contagious disease:

Arrange, or disarrange, the bed-clothes, mattress, and all other articles in such a way that the fumigant may have free access. Obliterate with cotton cracks and crevices about doors and windows. Place in the middle of the floor a large galvanized iron can. We use a receptacle one foot in diameter and 30 inches high; a metal ash-barrel is a respectable substitute.

Deposit in the can 400 grams of permanganate of potash; pour over this a mixture of—

```
Formaldehyd............................ 1 liter
Water.................................. 1  "
```

and beat a hasty retreat.

The amount of gas generated by these quantities will fumigate 1000 cubic feet. In buying permanganate specify "small crystals."

Hydrogen peroxid has 3 per cent. by weight, and 10 per cent. by volume, of available oxygen. It should be bought in carboys or demijohns containing about 5 gallons, and should comply with the Pharmacopœia. The liquid keeps well in a cool place.

Chlorinate of soda may be had in carboys holding 10 or 12 gallons. A 1:10 dilution may be kept in the wards in 5-pint bottles.

For *boric-acid solution* buy crystals, which are soluble in the ratio of 1 part to 25 of water. Dissolve in warm water and filter through cotton. For ointment use boric-acid powder rather than crystals.

A boric eye-wash demands U. S. P. acid. When not so guaranteed, the acid is slightly contaminated with sulphates, arsenic, and other irritants.

Vaselin may be put up conveniently at home in collapsible tubes. The latter cost 40 cents a dozen. The vaselin, bought in bulk, should be melted and poured in at the bottom of the tubes, which may then be closed and sterilized by boiling.

Ointments are much more economic if purchased in large quantity. Ointment containing lard, however, becomes rancid.

Liquid petrolatum is either colorless or colored. The yellow variety derives its color from impurities, but if one specifies U. S. P., he may secure a fairly good product at a reasonable price, that answers all purposes. Colorless petrolatum is expensive.

Liquid petrolatum is used to lubricate and to suspend iodoform or bismuth. It is a serviceable polish for soapstone sinks.

Glycerin is used for enemata, for dressings, and as a lubricant in cystoscopy. It pays to buy a good quality drug in any quantity up to 50 pounds. Cheap glycerin may be adulterated with glucose syrup; yellow glycerin contains organic impurities.

Green soap may well be bought by the barrel. Any soap manufacturer will quote a price on a soap conforming with the U. S. P. test, although he'll substitute cottonseed for linseed oil.

Glycerin soap is a mixture of:

> Green soap...................... 1 part (by weight)
> Glycerin......................... 2 parts.

Heat the mixture over a flame until it dissolves. Do not boil. Stir occasionally.

Glycerin soap is used as a lubricant in rectal or vaginal examinations and for scrubbing the hands before operations.

Soap solution consists of:

> Green soap............................... 1 pound
> Hot water to............................. 1 gallon.

It is both better and cheaper than cake soap for scrubbing a patient before operation.

Flaxseed keeps best in tin, whereby the escape of oil is prevented. For poultices the meal is used.

Castor oil.—Use only the best grade. Its keeping qualities permit the purchase of large quantities at one time.

Lime-water may be made at home and kept in a 10-gallon keg, prepared especially for the puprose in this way:

Slake a small piece of lime in a bucket or pan. Add water to form a thick cream. With an old brush coat the inside of the keg, and when the first coat is thoroughly dry, add a second coat. (Unless coated in this manner, a keg will leak and will discolor its contents.)

The preparation of a keg of lime-water requires:

> Water.................................... 10 gallons
> Unslaked lime............................ 15 ounces.

Place the lime in a large pan. Add water gradually until it slakes or becomes pulverized. Then add 3 gallons of water and stir thoroughly. Allow two hours for the mixture to settle. Decant the water and throw it away. Add 3 gallons more of water to the precipitate and stir. When the lime has settled a second time, decant, and add the precipitate to 10 gallons of water in the keg. Mix thoroughly. When the lime in the keg has settled, the water is ready to use. Lime is soluble in 760 parts of water. Washing it in this way eliminates soluble alkalis and their carbonates. The keg should be equipped with a tightly fitting cover.

Carron oil consists of lime-water and linseed oil in equal parts. Olive oil is usually substituted for linseed, but mixes less readily. Linseed oil may be had of the jobber in any quantity from a gallon upward.

Ringer's solution has the following formula:

```
Sodium chlorid................ 18¾ ounces (Troy)
Potassium chlorid.............  105 grains
Fused calcium chlorid.........  154½ grains
Distilled water to............  5 pints.
```

To make normal Ringer's solution add 2 ounces of the above stock solution to 5 pints of distilled water.

Calcium chlorid is used also to absorb moisture in instrument cases. Place the lumps in a glass dish in the case; renew at the end of a few weeks, when the salt liquefies. On account of its hygroscopic properties a stock of calcium chlorid should be kept in a dry place and in tight containers.

Commercial *talcum powder* is suitable for gloves which are to be dry sterilized. Purified talcum is a luxury. Buy in 25- or 50-pound lots.

A good *bathing solution* may be made of:

```
Powdered boric acid...................... 40 grams
Alcohol,
Water ..........................of each 500 c.c.
```

A small amount of the powder may fail to dissolve. Allow it to settle and decant.

PURCHASE, ECONOMIC USE OF SURGICAL SUPPLIES **315**

Liquors should be procured, not from a jobber, but from a liquor dealer. A straight liquor gives full medicinal effect and has the advantage of being less palatable than a blend.

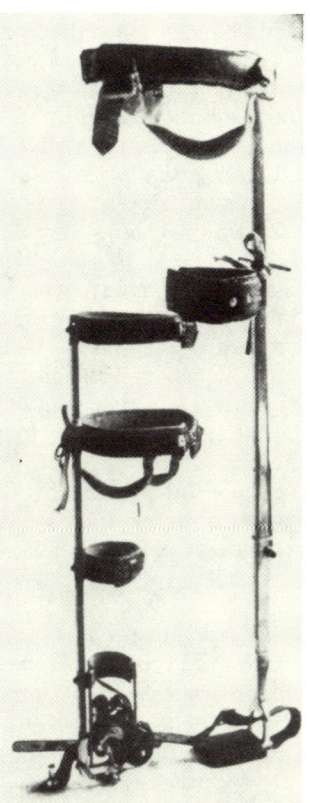

Fig. 130.—Brace made in workshop. Hospital for Sick Children, Toronto.

Whisky should be at least four years old and should contain 44 to 55 per cent. of alcohol by volume. Brandy should be of good quality: a cheap brandy is nauseating.

Sherry is used chiefly in egg-nogs. It should be "dry." For cooking, use a "sweet" sherry. California sherries are quite as satisfactory as the more expensive brands.

7. **Miscellaneous.**—*Splints.*—The internal angular variety can be made by any tinsmith from a drawing or a sample. Price, 50 cents each downward.

Ham splints are carried in five sizes by surgical supply-houses. Coaptation splints may be had from the same source; or they may be made by gluing Canton flannel to splint wood and scoring the latter at half-inch intervals with a sharp knife. Splint wood may be had of any lumber dealer. Ask for white wood, 36 by $2\frac{1}{2}$ inches, and $\frac{3}{16}$ inch thick.

Crutches are made from many woods. A rosewood crutch is ornamental, but one equally serviceable may be had in birch, cut regardless of grain. Birch crutches cost from \$3 to \$3.50 per dozen. The joints should be held with copper rivets; iron rivets rust and weaken the joints. "Sticks"—rough T-shaped supports—form a cheap substitute for crutches.

Crutch-tips are either—(a) rubber or (b) fiber—inserted. The latter cost a little more, but are more economic. It is safe to buy tips in gross lots.

For applying collodion or iodin use a *camel's-hair brush*, size 8.

Nitrate of silver sticks do not need a fancy wooden handle. Cut off the point of a quill tooth-pick, insert the silver nitrate into the quill, and bind the junction with a bit of adhesive plaster. When the stick is not in use, embed it in a small glass bottle filled with whole flaxseed.

Orange-wood Sticks.—Buy the "large" stick, 5 inches long, and sharpen it. Avoid pointed and bladed sticks which have been whittled down to half their original size.

Tongue depressors may be purchased most reasonably at a seed store, where they are made for tagging plants.

Card-board for ether cones should be 6 by 18 inches, and cut across the grain, so that it will not break when folded.

CHAPTER XV

THE HOSPITAL DRUG ROOM

By John E. Groff

It has been said that there is no such thing as an economic woman; that all women are either extravagant or niggardly. Allowing this to be more apparent than real, the saying may be applied to hospitals. If the attempt is made to satisfy the multifarious demands of all the attending and resident doctors, the resulting expenditure appears extravagant to those who pay the bills. On the other hand, if the management provides strictly according to the amount of money on hand, always with a working balance in the bank, it appears to the doctors to be stingy. There are two general plans upon which hospital dispensaries are conducted. One always appears penurious, and it is difficult to prevent the other from appearing extravagant. One plan equips the dispensary with ready made preparations of all kinds. All fluidextracts, tinctures, ointments, syrups, tablets, pills, solutions, chemicals, everything but the most simple things, such as lime-water and simple syrup, are purchased, and practically no manufacturing is done on the premises. Under this plan the medicines in stock correspond closely to the requirements of a more or less extensive formulary, to which the hospital doctors must confine themselves in prescribing. As will be shown further on, this is not an economic method, speaking of the cost of the medicines alone. It is cheaper in that it restricts the quantity used and permits of the employment of a man or woman of little knowledge or experience at a low salary.

The other plan calls for a first-class operative pharmacy—one equipped with the utensils and apparatus, together with the drugs necessary for the manufacture of as many of the Galenic preparations as can be made more cheaply than they can be purchased. This plan calls for a man or woman of experience as well as knowledge, and a consequent higher salary. When this plan is followed, there are usually no restrictions placed on the doctors as to the medicines they shall prescribe. Therefore, more medicine is used, and it would seem as though more money should be spent, but this is not necessarily so. Before entering into the respective merits of these two plans, it will, perhaps, be best to consider the location, etc., of the dispensary. In many cases the basement appears to be the best place. It is a quiet place, and the least liable to disturbance from visitors, both of hospital employees and the public. But whether in the basement or on a floor above ground, it should be centrally situated, easy of approach to those having business there, well lighted by day-light, and capable of perfect ventilation. There should be several rooms, three at least. The dispensary proper, where all the medicines are prepared for the wards, should have wall space sufficient for shelving to hold all the dispensing bottles, one row deep, so that there never will be any bottles in the rear. There are firms all over the country who make a business of fitting up business places of all kinds. If they are given the dimensions of a room with a statement of the purpose for which it is to be used, they will design the fixtures, and their great and varied experience enables them to give perfect satisfaction. The room itself is best if small. The larger it is, the more traveling there is to do. A table in the middle of the floor at which the occupants can work on four sides at once is better than a wall table for rapid work. There should always be a counter with a gate, to hold the ward baskets while being filled, and to keep out those having no business there.

The laboratory should be connected directly with the

dispensary, and constructed after the manner laid down in the recognized works on practical pharmacy. It should be equipped for all kinds of manufacturing purposes, as well as chemical and microscopic work in testing and identifying chemicals and drugs. Adjoining the laboratory there should be a storeroom for glassware and sundries. The storeroom bins ought to be inclosed. This allows of the storage glassware being washed as soon as received and preserved in a clean condition. The stock of drugs may be kept in the laboratory, in the glass and sundry storerooms, or in a separate room if there is one.

Conducted after the manner of either of the plans mentioned, the matters of greatest importance are the prices paid for supplies; the determination of the quantities to be purchased; the prevention of waste, and the guarding against the accumulation of dead stock. There are some drugs and chemicals which are with us to stay and which are used in large quantities. Such drugs as ether, cocain, cascara, cinchona, gentian, carbolic acid, glycerin, corrosive sublimate, potassium iodid, phenacetin, sulfonal, ammonia, formaldehyd, and others are used in large quantities every year. Whenever it is possible to make an estimate of a year's supply, it is a good plan to do so, and, after obtaining quotations from various reliable manufacturers and dealers, to make a contract with the lowest bidder. If the ebb and flow of the market is watched through the journals and price-lists, a great saving can be effected by placing an order during a low-priced period. If the saving amounts to more than the interest on the money tied up, that must be regarded as an economic deal. The same rule, of course, holds good with regard to tablets or any supplies used in large quantities. A considerable saving over jobbers' prices may be effected if, when ordering large quantities from the manufacturers, there can be included with the order such items as are used only in small quantities. In securing quotations from all parts of the country, it is generally considered wise to give the business men of the home city an opportunity, and if their prices are right, to give them the preference. Indeed, this preference is shown by some institutions even though the price is not the lowest, if the difference is only slightly in excess. It helps to create a good feeling and sometimes brings contributions.

It must be remembered that the above-mentioned plans are for large hospitals, of which there are comparatively few. The smaller hospitals, which far outnumber the others, seldom have the funds to support an apothecary, nor do they need an extensive pharmacy. For such institutions the plan best adapted to their needs is to select the best apothecary in the neighborhood and engage him to buy and prepare for the institution such articles as they find themselves in need of. As far as manufacturing those preparations involving the use of alcohol is concerned, there can be no question as to its economy. Hospitals, as a rule, buy their alcohol tax free, and this means a very great advantage in manufacturing such preparations as are used.

The determination of the quantities to be bought is closely related to the accumulation of dead stock. Changes occur in the practice of medicine, as in everything else, and drugs that were largely used in other days are of no use now, while many of those in use now will be dropped in the future. Fortunately, such changes happen mostly in connection with drugs used in small quantities, and the loss on each drug is small; but on the accumulation of years it is considerable. Dead stock will accumulate, and all one can do is to make it small by anticipating the changes as closely as possible. To this end, of course, the head of this department should consult the superintendent.

While in most hospitals the bookkeeping is done by a corps of bookkeepers in the office, there is usually some of it done in the dispensary. There is the matter of discounts of 1 or 2 per cent. allowed for cash in ten days, and which it is perhaps needless to point out amounts to a tidy sum in a year. A book for entering the goods received, with the consignee's name and the date, is of occasional assistance in tracing lost packages or settling disputes over bills. All bills should be promptly checked up as to quantities and prices on receipt of goods and handed into the office. The habit of tabulating all the goods in stock in the storeroom is an efficient check against overstocking and a great aid in keeping track of articles seldom used, while a card index of prices, with quantities purchased and dates of purchase, is also of great value. Under the head of dispensary bookkeeping we include the care of prescriptions. All prescriptions should be preserved. The manner of their preservation rests with the people in authority. They may be kept on file, pasted in a book made for this purpose, or copied in a specially ruled book. Either way, they should be numbered and ready for reference at all times.

Hospital work is peculiar, inasmuch as there are times when the work must be done with a rush and other times when there is nothing to do. To accomplish the work promptly while the rush is on, assistance is necessary, and to keep that assistance busy after the rush is over is one of our problems. Much, but not all, of this time is used up in getting ready to meet the requirements of the rush hours. The remaining time may be filled in according to individual ideas. One man or boy during these hours can fill a day's supply of siphon soda and ginger-ale. The cost of the apparatus for filling and of the ingredients for making is small, and if a considerable amount of these beverages are used, a proportionately large saving may thus be effected.

Experience teaches that small quantities frequently given will be better taken care of and more economically used than large quantities. An order from the superintendent breeds consideration before asking and care after receiving. On the part of the druggist and his help, care in handling will save much loss by breakage. Help should be made to understand its cost. It is an excellent idea to keep account of it, with its cost, charged against the name of the person concerned. In a business of any kind a boy incurs the disapproval of his employers by reckless handling and waste of material, and if he fails to mend his fault, he loses his job. The same should hold good in a hospital dispensary. As a rule, it does not, and yet breakage and spilling of material in handling it, make deep inroads on a hospital's funds.

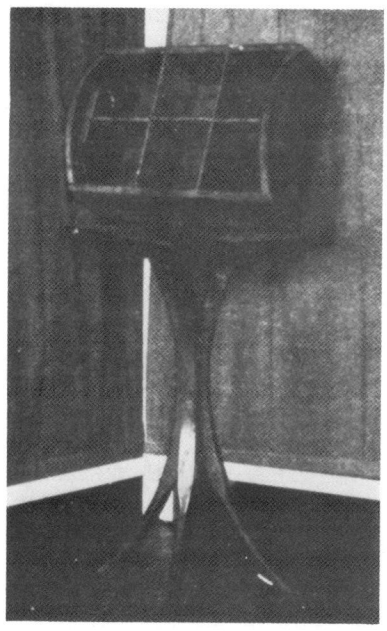

Fig. 131.—Wooden basket for carrying drugs and solutions. The large compartments will hold a gallon bottle. Rhode Island Hospital, Providence, R. I.

The hours of a hospital apothecary vary with the notions of those in authority. With all the ward medicine-closets well filled with medicines, the accident and operating-rooms well furnished, with a surplus of supplies, with the key of the dispensary in the hands of the night matron in case anything should be needed in the night, it is assumed

THE HOSPITAL DRUG ROOM 323

that if the dispensary is opened at 7 A. M. and closed at 6 P. M., all requirements will be met. The medicine baskets should be at the door of the dispensary at 7 o'clock and all stray bottles should be brought in by 9 o'clock. If this is done, the apothecary will, as a rule, be able to have them all back in the wards at 10 o'clock. Sometimes the

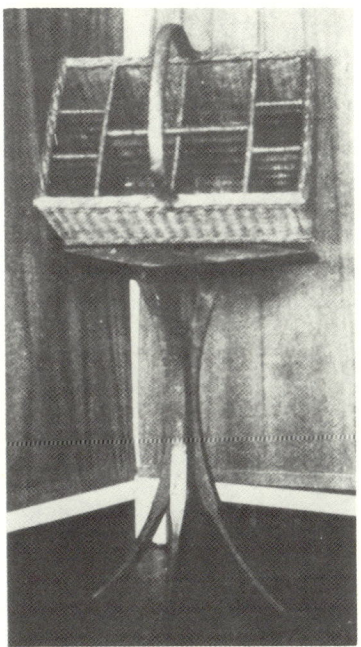

Fig. 132.—Wicker basket for carrying bottles. Rhode Island Hospital, Providence, R. I.

apothecary delivers them, sometimes the ward orderlies come after them. Prescriptions, accident room, and operating-room orders must be taken and attended to promptly, as they arrive at all hours of the day. Nothing should be delivered without an order from the head nurse. In case of expensive preparations and liquors of all kinds, an order from the superintendent of nurses or house officer, countersigned by the superintendent, should be required, and this should be a hard-and-fast rule.

The apothecary in a hospital should be a college of pharmacy graduate, a man or woman of experience, and

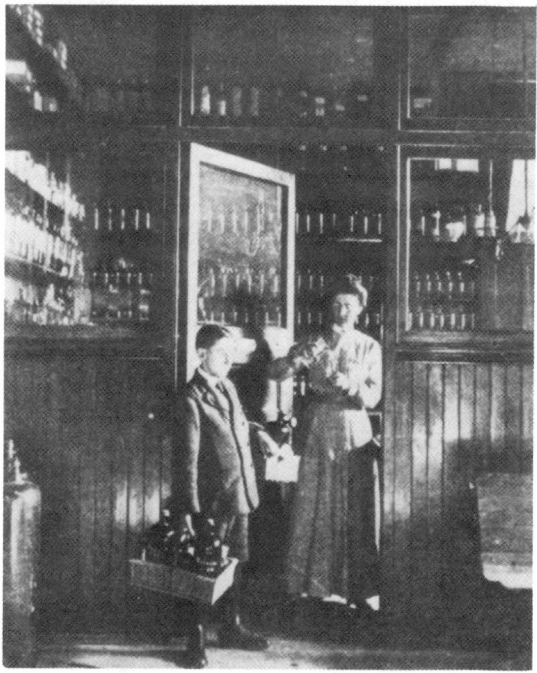

Fig. 133.—Morning orders for the dispensary. Hospital for Sick Children, Toronto.

disposed to keep abreast of the progress being made in the field of work. Sufficient salary should be paid to secure and hold such a person. If assistance is needed to render prompt service at all times, it should be provided, and if further assistance is needed to keep the dispensary spotlessly clean, that, too, should be given. The matter of making the dispensary self-supporting or of making it a paying investment rests with the hospital authorities. Medicines may be given away. A nominal price of ten cents, or a price nearly approaching that of the retail druggist, may be charged. Every hospital knows its own running expense and must decide for itself whether or not the dispensary should be made a source of income.

The question of making a short term of service in the dispensary a part of the nurse's training is a difficult one. In a small hospital, where there is plenty of time for the pharmacist to devote to such work, he might, if it could be arranged, impart much useful knowledge to the nurse. The latter could not, in the time allowed, gain very much more than a greater familiarity with the general appearance of drugs and mixtures of various kinds. Much would depend on the knowledge and attitude of the apothecary. Some have the instinct of training and teaching; most of them have neither. A plan like the following in any case would be most feasible:

Let one nurse enter the dispensary for one month's service there. Let her be instructed in the art of measuring and weighing accurately and allowed to take part in all the operations connected with receiving, properly caring for, and compounding drugs and chemicals. At the end of two weeks another nurse should enter and begin work under the first one, both, of course, being under the direct supervision of the apothecary, while at the same time aiding each other. By such an arrangement the benefit to the nurse would be greater, because two nurses, each with the same end in view, would be learning together, while if there were but one, she would get the apothecary's view only. The really essential parts regarding materia medica are learned from the text-books upon that subject in the classroom. But the kind of knowledge which one gains by working among drugs and talking about them might be acquired in the dispensary. It cannot very well be classified, because it is dependent upon daily occurrences. Such service requires constant vigilance. Accuracy first, rapidity second; care in reading prescriptions; care in noting the doses ordered; care in correcting incompatibilities and immiscibilities; care in taking the right bottle from the shelf, and accuracy in measuring and weighing; silence while compounding and writing labels—are some of the important lessons that may be learned under the apothecary's direction. The work cannot be well done if talking is permitted, but after the work is finished, a review of it would be beneficial, and make the nurse better acquainted with the medicines she handles, and with the necessity of constant watchfulness against mistakes.

It is impossible to give a satisfactory minimum list of drugs, such as should be included in the first stock of a hospital. In these days of rapid transit and telephone communication, it is easy to supply deficiencies with little delay. There are, however, some drugs in constant use, and they should always be on hand from the beginning. The following list includes the more important ones:

Acetanilid	4 ounces.
Acetic acid	1 pound.
Boric acid	25 pounds.
Carbolic acid	25 "
Hydriodic acid syrup	1 quart.
Chloroform	
Hydrochloric acid	1 pound.
Nitric acid	1 "
Phosphoric acid	1 "
Sulphuric acid	1 "
Tannic acid	1 "
Benzoinated lard	1 "
Lanolin	1 "
Ether	
Ethyl chlorid (in tubes)	
Alcohol	
Ammonium chlorid	½ pound
Ammonium carbonate	½ "
Amyl nitrite pearls	1 box.
Starch	5 pounds.
Ammonia water	
Distilled water	
Silver nitrate (crystals)	1 ounce.
Silver nitrate (stick)	1 "
Atropin sulphate	1 dram.
Bismuth subnitrate	½ pound.

THE HOSPITAL DRUG ROOM

Caffein citrate	1 ounce.
Camphor	1 pound.
Capsicum (pulverized)	½ "
White wax	1 "
Cantharides cerate	½ "
Chloral	½ "
Cocain hydrochlorid	1 ounce.
Codein phosphate	1 "
Collodion, flexible	1 pound.
Digitalis leaves (Allen's)	1 dram.
Elixir three phosphates	1 quart.
Elixir compound orange	1 "
Adhesive plaster	
Fluidextract buchu	1 pound
Fluidextract cascara	1 "
Fluidextract ergot	1 "
Fluidextract hydrastis	1 "
Extract malt	1 quart.
Iron and quinin citrate	½ pound.
Iron and strychnin citrate	½ "
Glycerin	1 "
Corrosive sublimate	1 "
Calomel	¼ "
Mercury	¼ "
Iodin	¼ "
Iodoform	1 "
Liniment, ammonia	1 quart.
Liniment, chloroform	1 "
Liniment, soap	1 "
Liniment, camphor	1 "
Basham's mixture	1 "
Formaldehyd	1 "
Fowler's solution	1 "
Calcined magnesia (heavy)	1 pound.
Magnesium sulphate	10 pounds.
Brown mixture	1 quart.
Morphin sulphate	1 dram.
Oil of wintergreen	1 pound.
Cotton-seed oil	1 gallon.
Cod-liver oil	1 "
Linseed oil (raw)	1 "
Castor oil	1 "
Spirits turpentine	1 quart.
Pepsin	¼ pound.
Vaselin	5 pounds.
Compound cathartic pills	
Lead acetate	1 pound.
Cream of tartar	5 pounds.
Potassium bromid	1 pound.
Potassium chlorate	1 "
Potassium iodid	1 "
Potassium permanganate	1 "

Dover's powder	¼ pound
Quinin sulphate	1 ounce.
Mustard	1 pound.
Sodium bicarbonate	5 pounds.
Borax (powdered)	5 "
Sodium bromid	1 pound.
Sodium salicylate	1 "
Spirits of nitre	1 "
Spirits of anise	1 pint.
Spirits of camphor	1 "
Spirits of chloroform	1 "
Whisky	
Brandy	
Sherry	
Spirits of peppermint	1 pint.
Strychnin sulphate	1 dram.
Sulphur precipitated	1 pound.
Syrup iodid iron	1 pint.
Syrup ipecac	1 "
Syrup sarsaparilla compound	1 "
Syrup squill	1 "
Syrup senna	1 "
Aconite tincture	
Tincture belladonna leaf	1 pint.
Tincture benzoin, comp	1 "
Tincture capsicum	1 "
Tincture cardamom comp	1 "
Tincture cinchona comp	1 "
Tincture digitalis	1 "
Tincture iron chlorid	1 "
Tincture gentian comp	1 "
Tincture hyoscyamus	1 "
Tincture iodin	1 "
Tincture lavender comp	1 "
Tincture myrrh	1 "
Tincture nux vomica	1 "
Tincture opium	1 "
Tincture opium, deodorized	1 "
Tincture opium, camphorated	1 "
Tincture rhubarb	1 "
Tincture strophanthus	1 "
Tincture valerian	1 "
Tincture ginger	1 "
Mercurial ointment, 50 per cent	1 pound.
Nitrate of mercury ointment	¼ "
Zinc oxid ointment	1 "
Zinc sulphate	1 "
Zinc stearate	1 "

The hospital, be it large or small, should, in all respects, be a pattern in its line to the community in which it exists.

It is a school in all its departments. **Therefore, the pharmacy should be first class in everything it undertakes.** Its appointments should be ample for doing the work required. All the preparations made should be made according to the accepted standards. **The purity of all** chemicals should be proved by the apothecary, and the apothecary, as has been stated elsewhere, should be the best obtainable. The assistants should be encouraged to attend a college of pharmacy; time should be given them to do so, and they should receive careful training from the apothecary. It is clear enough that a hospital dispensary must be managed with the same care and business acumen required to make any business successful. **Profit is not** usually considered, but saving by watching the market and buying at the right time and at the lowest figure, and constant study of the needs in order to distribute supplies plentifully but not extravagantly, are the main factors in the problem.

CHAPTER XVI

THE TRAINING-SCHOOL AND ITS MANAGEMENT

By Charlotte A. Aikens

In training-school work we are slowly changing from the old order to the new. The old haphazard methods of the past are gradually being abandoned, and surer, saner methods, based on sound pedagogic principles are being adopted. Under all such conditions more or less anxiety, uncertainty, and confusion of thought are inevitable. Periods of transition are apt to be characterized by difficult problems as well as great opportunities. Patience combined with perseverance are virtues necessary to be cultivated by all who have the practical good of hospitals and training-schools at heart. "Let your moderation be known unto all men" is a motto well worth adopting by hospital and training-school workers at the present time. It is well to remember at the outset that the hospital school differs from every other educational institution in that it carries by night and by day tremendous responsibilities which cannot be set aside. Its problems must be worked out with those responsibilities always in view. Therefore it is wise and necessary to make haste slowly in making changes if we would avoid the necessity of having to retrace steps which should never have been taken in hospital schools.

Within the last few years many conflicting opinions regarding training-school policies and development have been advanced. Here and there are found people who unhesitatingly and sweepingly condemn the whole present training-school system. One ambitious speaker is quoted as publicly stating that there is not a training-school in the whole United States worthy educationally of the name. The criticism seems largely to be based on the fact that nurses are doing very little laboratory and research work. This is an extreme view. At the opposite extreme are found hospital people, not a few, who apparently regard system and methods in the training-school as of very little importance. The main thing is to get the nursing done. What the nurse learns while doing it is given little thought or attention. Others wish to see the training-school entirely separated from the hospital, and developed as a separate institution or organization, with the nursing service of the hospital provided for by graduate nurses, the pupils being only assigned such duties as seem to the teachers absolutely necessary to give opportunity for acquiring the required skill—much greater attention being given to the theoretic part of the nursing course. Between these extremes of thought all grades and shades of opinion and policies exist, though doubtless more uniformity in what is taught is found than ever before.

What the future holds in the way of development along these lines no one can predict, but for the present at least we must deal with conditions as they are—not as we might wish they were. The greatest possibilities of improvement seem to rest in closely observing present methods and general conditions, and studying how, without adopting revolutionary measures, we may bring all training-schools up to that fair degree of efficiency now reached by many of the schools. The claims of the sick cannot be set aside. Neither should the claims of pupil nurses to the best training our facilities afford be ignored. A system which has produced as many thousand capable women as are found in the ranks of trained nurses to-day cannot be wholly defective. Some leveling up is undoubtedly needed—possibly also some leveling down at some points and in some schools. There is no reason whatever to be discouraged regarding the progress which has been made in American nursing affairs in the last forty years. In the past quarter of a century experiments of many kinds have been tried in hospital schools. Many of these have been found wanting. Others have stood the test of time and practical utility. Through these latter, much improvement has been effected; the good results have been published and become the common property of all concerned in this work. It remains for the workers of to-day to reduce to system and continue to publish the results of the best methods, so that newer schools and future students of training-school management may study the methods of this age and profit thereby.

Some one has said of a noted educator that this man sitting on one end of a log with a student on the other end was the nucleus of a university—so well informed was he, and so highly developed were his teaching faculties. It is coming to be clearly recognized in the training-school field that the woman at the head of the school, to a very great degree, determines its standards, and means either the making or the undoing of the school. Given an intelligent woman full of enthusiasm for the fullest development of her nurses, with a determination to adopt the best nursing and training methods as far as possible, to make the most of the teaching opportunities that are present in her special corner of the field—given these, and intelligent pupils willing and anxious to please, and ambitious to excel, and a good school is possible under otherwise discouraging conditions. Such a woman is worth more and means more to a school than elaborate buildings, hundreds of occupied beds, finely appointed laboratories, or splendid class-rooms, valuable as all these aids are. Without a superintendent of this kind a school is poor, indeed, however well equipped it may be along other lines. The constant daily teaching and practicing of correct methods at the bedside, in the operating-room, and in all departments where nurses are employed, is the chief object of the training-school, and however elaborate the teaching of theory may be, it can never compensate for a lack of attention to this point.

Before assuming charge of a hospital or hospital school,

the superintendent should have had experience in an executive position in a hospital—preferably other than the one in which she trained; for, however thorough and up-to-date one school may be, or may think itself to be, no one school can claim to have the best methods in every particular. There is no school, no hospital, which has not yet something to learn from others. When it comes to careful, thorough personal care of individual patients, many of the small schools could teach sadly needed lessons to larger schools; while many of the latter could teach to some smaller schools much-needed lessons regarding disciplinary methods and internal organization, as well as exactness in surgical technic and advanced methods in other departments. All large schools are not good schools, nor all small ones inferior.

The demands on hospital and training-school superintendents increase every year. Hospital problems become more intricate, and the nurse who has nothing but her nurse training as an equipment for hospital work is more and more hesitating to undertake such work. And rightly does she hesitate. It is generally believed that normal training for such work—a possibility of securing in some well-organized teaching hospital special training in how to teach, how to manage a department or a training-school, how to organize nurses and direct their efforts, is one of the lines on which great developments may be expected in the near future. A beginning has already been made in this direction, and the results are so satisfactory that it is confidently hoped increased provision for the training along rational, practical lines of hospital superintendents and training-school principals, will be made. The American Hospital Association, if it fulfils its highest mission to the hospitals of America, must needs give closer attention to providing efficient superintendents, trained according to the best known methods; for of all plans for promoting efficiency and economy in hospitals and training-schools, no method promises so much as that of providing trained, efficient superintendents who will know when they begin service with hospitals as executives something definite regarding the best methods to be used in the different departments for whose good management they are responsible.

While it is true that in training-school work we are in a transition stage, finding the need of constant adjustment to meet changing conditions, it is also true that some few principles of hospital organization are, or seem to be, quite firmly fixed. However desirable it might have been to have had the training-school for nurses develop as a separate institution or organization, in more than ninety-nine cases out of a hundred, the school came into existence as a part of the hospital, to meet a definite need in that institution and community, and has developed as a department of the institution. In a large measure the existence of the hospital is quite as dependent on the training-school as the latter is upon the hospital, and both must stand or fall together. Any attempt to separate that which custom has wisely or unwisely allowed to grow together, and which the experience of many thousands of physicians, hospital trustees, superintendents, and nurses shows to have large benefits to mankind to its credit, is fairly certain to end in failure. There are practical problems involved, of vast moment, when the demand is made that "training-schools must be freed from bondage to hospital needs." The divorce of the two may come in the future, but there are many who believe that a divorce of this kind would be just as deplorable as divorces usually are. For the present, at least, however important the average school may be, it is not the whole institution. However strong and flourishing it may be, it is not a separate organization. It is a department—a part of the whole—and its development must never be allowed to divert the main institution from the real purpose for which it was founded.

In every well-organized institution there is one head—one person whose duty it is to coördinate the different factors concerned in the institution, and so organize the different departments, that the objects for which the whole institution was founded may be realized to the fullest extent. This person may be called the superintendent, or general manager, or some other name, but he (or she) is the official representative of the board of managers, the real head, the chief executive of the institution.

In the smaller hospitals the superintendent is usually a woman and a trained nurse. As a rule, she is expected also to assume the duties of superintendent of the training-school. This rule is sometimes observed in hospitals of 100 beds or more where the superintendent is a trained nurse. She may, in fact must, have one or more assistants, termed first and second assistant, according to rank and responsibility. The first assistant acts as general supervising nurse, but the accepting and dismissing of pupils, arranging of the course of study, appointment of teachers, etc., are held to be a part of the duties of the superintendent of the whole institution. This plan has much to commend it. It works well and is highly approved by experienced nurse superintendents who have tried it for years. It centers the authority and main responsibility for the personnel and work of the nursing corps in one woman, and is generally productive of harmony and strength in an institution.

There is gradually developing a conviction that one superintendent is enough for any institution, and that the title "superintendent of nurses" or of nursing should be dropped, and the title "supervising nurse" or "principal of the training-school" substituted.

Where the superintendent of the hospital is a man, the arrangement referred to would be less satisfactory, and is rarely, if ever, attempted. He, under authority from the governing board, appoints the principal of the training-school, her assistants and head nurses, and assists in organizing the school. If the board wishes to retain the appointing power in these matters, it is customary and right that the superintendent should nominate the candidates for these various offices. He also with the consent of the board terminates the appointments when such cease to be satisfactory.

The rules relating to the training-school department may be formulated and arranged by the principal, but always subject to the approval of the superintendent, and in the last resort to the board of managers, who are held responsible for good government by the public or by those who maintain the institution. The details of the daily work, the general discipline of the pupils, and the personal care of patients, will, of course, become a part of the principal's responsibilities or duties, but always subject to the executive head of the institution. The head of an institution (male or female) must be the head of it. If there is any one in the institution who is bigger or better fitted to assume the responsibilities of the chief executive, he (or she) should unquestionably be promoted to that place. The superintendent must be the final arbitrator when difficulties arise. His oversight is, of course, general. He sustains exactly the same relation to the training-school as to all other departments. He may not have specific or technical knowledge of the details of the various departments, but he should have general knowledge or be working diligently to acquire it, and his suggestions regarding any department should be respectfully received and carefully considered.

Not long since a training-school principal rather severely criticized a leading medical superintendent for what she termed "petty meddling." It developed that he had called the attention of the head of the training-school department to the condition of some of the beds in the institution, and asked her to see that greater care was taken regarding this matter. She resented his suggestion, and complained to some of her associates about his meddling in her province. Unfortunately, this attitude is by no means rare. It seemed to the writer that the principal in question had a very faulty conception of the superintendent's position, and of her own. There is no department of the hospital which it is not the superintendent's duty to be interested in—none regarding which he is not entirely in his province in making suggestions regarding

THE TRAINING-SCHOOL AND ITS MANAGEMENT

its management. The wise superintendent will interfere as little as possible regarding daily details, but he is certainly neglecting his duty if he fails to interfere, or make suggestions when the reputation of the institution for neatness and cleanliness or the comfort of the patients is concerned.

Training-school Supervisors.—The essentials of a training-school are, first of all, pupils to train, second, a principal for the school, and third, patients and facilities for nursing. However, experience has taught that it is not enough to accept pupils, teach them in regular classes, and appoint them to different wards to gain their experience. Some one must work with them constantly, must supervise them and see that they practise the methods taught. Lack of supervision means waste—of time, energy, and supplies, as a general rule. It means also slipshod work, and is bad for the hospital as well as for the nurse. For this reason, even in small hospitals, the superintendent should have an assistant or a head nurse who can follow the details of the daily nursing, as no one woman can who has to meet the public, attend to the office work, do the purchasing, and oversee the whole institution. In larger hospitals each large ward should have a head nurse. The practice of appointing senior pupil nurses to executive positions seems a necessity in many institutions, and as the construction and character of hospitals vary greatly, no fixed rule can be made which would hold good in all institutions. The plan of some buildings is such that small corridors with accommodations for a half-dozen patients or thereabouts, makes it a practical impossibility for a graduate head nurse to be appointed to each department of this kind. The result is that often either a junior pupil nurse must be left there entirely, or for the most part, without supervision of the details of the work, to meet doctors on their rounds, get orders, provide for supplies, etc., or a senior pupil nurse must be detailed as charge nurse. Where a sufficient number of patients grouped together are found, a permanent graduate head nurse is very desirable. For efficient institutional work, either as head nurse or superintendent, experience is necessary to the best results. The custom of letting senior pupils assume the responsibility of head nurses, with the necessity of periodic changes in order to do justice to the nurse, robs the hospital of the accumulated experience it greatly needs in its different departments. Knowledge of hospital values, of the cost of the various supplies in common use, and the amounts necessary, of the best methods of preventing waste, and a hundred other kinds of knowledge necessary to efficient supervision does not come quickly or by accident, and it is the exceptional senior pupil nurse who has enough of it to do the best by the institution.

A graduate night supervisor who will take the superintendent's place at night should also be added to the working force in every hospital as soon as possible. When a nurse superintendent tries to be on duty night and day, seven days in the week, as many of them do, she is simply paving the way to premature health bankruptcy. No factory would expect to keep open at night without an efficient night foreman. No business firm would expect the day foreman or manager to be ready for duty night and day. Then why should philanthropic institutions demand double duty from superintendents? The reason is chiefly that such institutions start small. There is not enough work at first to warrant a night supervisor, and the superintendent, anxious to economize and to keep things running smoothly, cheerfully responds to the occasional calls that come. But, unfortunately, when the number of patients doubles and trebles, and the night calls mean every-night calls, and sometimes three or four calls in a night, no change in policy or methods is made. The superintendent hesitates to complain. The board does not know how real and pressing the night duty of the superintendent is—does not know conditions as they really are—and the bad practice is continued until the superintendent is no longer equal to the burden. She goes away for a long period of enforced idleness, tries to recruit her shattered health, and some one else takes her place and makes the selfsame blunder. No woman can long do justice to an institution or keep at her maximum of efficiency who is unjust to herself in the matter of sleep and recreation. Unbroken rest is as much the right and necessity of a nurse superintendent as of a hospital trustee. A few years of constant broken rest is about all the average woman can stand. Hundreds of splendid women within the last twenty-five years of American hospital work have attempted to carry this double burden. They have drawn on their reserve nerve capital until it was exhausted, and have been obliged to prematurely retire from work for which they were eminently well fitted, and leave the field to beginners. The experience of the past quarter of a century ought to teach some useful lessons regarding this matter to boards of managers as well as to overambitious nurse superintendents.

The Training-school Committee.—Not all hospitals have a training school committee, and the idea of such a committee is both strongly approved and disapproved by experienced hospital executives. Many feel that with a capable superintendent and training-school principal, a committee is unnecessary. They think they are better without it. There is much to be said on both sides. As a general rule, a good committee which had a proper respect for the superintendent or principal and did not attempt to interfere in details of daily routine—a committee which had a fair and wise conception of its functions and limitations, should prove helpful in the ordinary hospital. In the smaller hospital, where the superintendent is alone in her daily responsibility, a committee should be a source of strength. Whether they always are is a question. Experience has shown that a training-school committee has very often proved as a broken reed on which to lean when difficulties arise. Undoubtedly, also, much confusion has resulted from some committees who objected to giving the superintendent or principal authority to act in certain matters, and refused to act themselves or delayed action or shirked responsibilities or disagreeable tasks. Many times when the superintendent's judgment regarding a pupil, for instance—judgment based on firsthand observation and close daily contact—should have been accepted without question, the committee has insisted on keeping the pupil when the superintendent recommended that, in the interest of the good reputation of the school and hospital, she be dropped. Such a condition is disastrous to any institution, and the frequent changing of superintendents in many institutions can often be traced to unwise interference in matters which should either have been left entirely to the superintendent to work out, or in which the committee did not respect her judgment. Capable men and women will not long be content to remain where they are constantly hampered by petty rules and small-minded committees, and the policy may easily prove the undoing or handicap of an institution which otherwise had every chance for a high degree of practical success. There is a decided possibility of *overmanaging*, and many committees have shown a zeal that was not according to knowledge—a zeal that was unnecessary.

In any case the personnel of such a committee should be carefully weighed and the scope of its functions clearly defined. The principal of the school and the superintendent of the hospital should unquestionably have a place on the committee. The other members of the committee should represent both the trustees or managers and the medical staff. A committee of five or six, consisting of one or two representatives from the managing board, one from the medical staff, and the superintendent and principal, is as large a committee as is desirable in any hospital. The representatives from the managing board should be selected from those persons of a judicial temperament—never from the impulsive, meddlesome class, which unfortunately, for various reasons, are occasionally found on voluntary managing boards of hospitals.

It is the newer institutions which are most liable to blunder in this respect. Time will usually reveal the usefulness or uselessness or mischievousness of all such members—and, given a capable, tactful president of the governing board, useless and mischievous members of committees can usually, in due time, be shorn of their power to do harm. Patience is a prime necessity in working out many such problems, and the principal or superintendent who is discouraged or hampered or worried over the well-meant efforts of certain members of such committees may perhaps derive a crumb of comfort from the reflection that "there are others"—that faithful service is not always overlooked, even when it seems to be, and that many superintendents have been able to achieve a fair measure of success in spite of such difficulties. Time works many changes in hospital policies. Experience is one of the best of all teachers in this respect, as well as in many others.

In general, it will be found best to have the committee decide only on questions of broad general policy, and leave the details to the officials appointed to take care of them. The superintendent and principal will together decide on the course of study, the general order in which the different branches are to be taken up, and the lecturers or teachers it seems desirable to appoint. They may or may not bring their recommendations before the committee for revision or confirmation. The superintendent will usually make the preliminary arrangements with the different lecturers and teachers for the year, leaving final details and dates to be worked out by the principal.

When new equipment of an expensive nature is desired for the school, the committee as a whole should be consulted. In many cases the members from the managing board appointed to the school committee have undertaken to secure new reference books for the library, have furnished magazines and other reading matter for the school, secured donations of anatomic charts and other teaching helps, studied how to increase the comfort and pleasure of the nurses, and in a variety of different ways have contributed much that was very valuable to the daily life and upbuilding of the school. The principal can do much to arouse enthusiasm and direct activity along these lines by making her needs and desires known. If a thing is worth having it is worth asking for, and a common fault with many otherwise capable principals is that they are altogether too modest in their requests, too easily satisfied with school conditions. There is no reason except inertia, or timidity, in many cases, for the training-school being as poorly equipped with teaching helps as it often is. Medical men expect to be supplied with instruments and conveniences for work and demand them. Why not hospital teachers also? A good blackboard is quite as much of a necessity in a school for nurses as in any other school, yet even this inexpensive help to teaching is often conspicuous by its absence from the class-room. Books are tools; so are charts and blackboards and specimens—tools for teaching and study—and no school is too poor to start to secure a good working equipment, which can be added to yearly.

The Pupils.—The preliminary correspondence with pupils, their selection and admission on probation, naturally, is a part of the principal's work. The committee or the superintendent having decided the size of the staff necessary and the number to be admitted to fill vacancies, the subsequent details should be left to the principal. With or without the superintendent's approval in each case, as may be determined by the individual school, she notifies the candidate of her acceptance on probation, and fixes the date for the probation to begin. During the probation term she observes each candidate as carefully as possible, weeds out the undesirable ones, and at the end of the trial period recommends their acceptance or rejection in each case. The superintendent or in some cases the entire committee approves the recommendations, and the probationer is accepted as a pupil of the school.

The probation period should be of sufficient length to determine the candidate's fitness for nursing. Beginning some years ago with a trial term of one month, the period

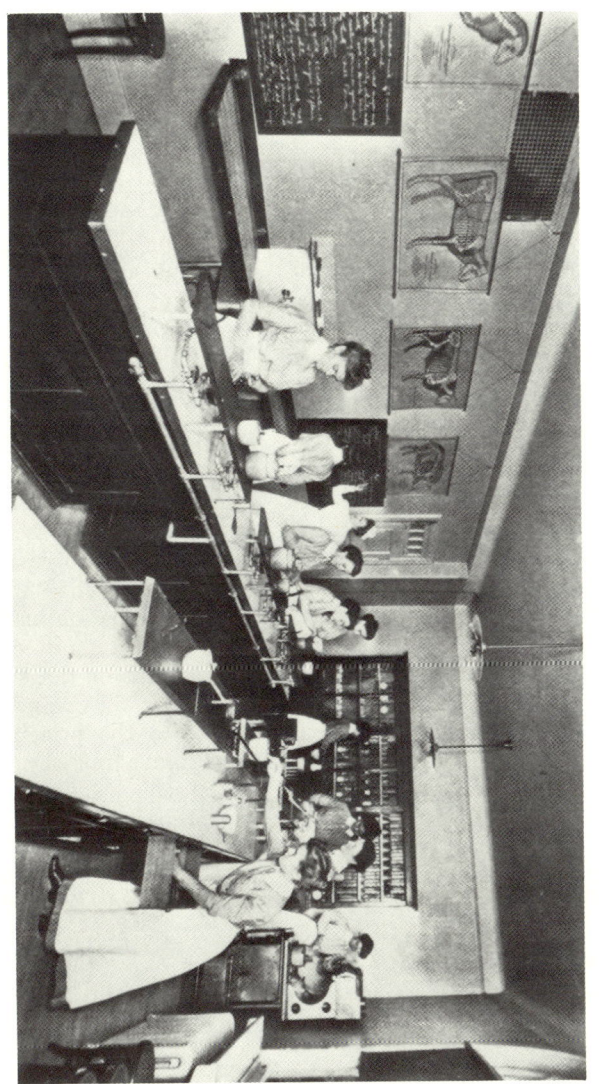

Fig. 134.—A class in dietetics. Presbyterian Hospital, New York.

has been gradually lengthened to two or three, and in some schools to six months. Three months seems a fair trial period, but many experienced superintendents lean to the six months' term, believing that it is better to have a longer term of trial than to dismiss a pupil after once having been accepted, as often is required to be done. In the case of the average candidates three months' trial will usually determine their fitness or unfitness, but it is undoubtedly true that every school which has had a half-dozen years of experience has had many nurses whose virtues or defects have shown much more clearly in the second or third three months than the first. It is much easier and better to terminate a pupil's relation with the school during probation than to accept her, give her reason to look forward to successful graduation, and then later on discover her unreliability or unfitness generally, and dismiss her with her course half finished. Where the case is doubtful, an extension of the trial period is desirable.

This period gives the candidate an opportunity to judge of the quality of the training she is likely to receive and of the general conditions under which she will have to work and study during training. The probation term is as fair for one party as for the other, and a dissatisfied probationer who withdraws is by no means to be condemned. Once the probation term is ended, and both parties to the contract accept the conditions, only an offense or circumstance of a serious nature should form ground for withdrawal or dismissal. However carefully a principal may select pupils, she will find as the training period progresses that she has accepted some "undesirables." Since the beginning of history, round pegs have occasionally gotten into square holes. Misplaced lives, misplaced talents, misplaced energies, human souls busy with some one else's work, are among the sorrowful spectacles of life which are all too often seen. They are not peculiar to the nursing profession. Every profession has its share of them. People who might have achieved success in some other walk in life somehow get into the wrong place, and according to ordinary human measurements of success, they fail. Why allow such to graduate? Why not peremptorily reject them if, at any time during training, undesirable qualities manifest themselves in pupil nurses, or if they do not come up to a certain standard of work and study or theoretic attainments? There are many questions bound up in the answers to these problems. Toleration with human infirmities is one of the prime essentials to success in hospital work, or probably in any work, for perfection is not found anywhere this side the sky. It is just possible that some people's ideals may be wrong, and that a closer knowledge of individual cases would show that there were possibilities of a fair measure of success, even when lives apparently have become misplaced. The conditions regarding the supply of probationers tend to make superintendents and everybody concerned more tolerant, for sickness does not tend to grow much less, judging by the admissions to hospitals. Many nurses drift out of the work after a few years, and there are many who believe that whether or not a young woman practises nursing, she is the better for the education which can be obtained in the ordinary hospital. There are a great many sides from which this question should be viewed.

In former years, dismissal was a very common form of discipline, and many a promising nurse was unjustly and harshly dealt with. We are beginning to give more consideration, and rightly, to the future of the pupil and the rights of the individual. Suspension for a few days or weeks will often teach a lesson that can be taught in no other way, and lessons taught in this way have a salutary effect on the whole school. Every principal should have power to temporarily suspend any pupil pending further investigation, or to give time for consideration, or for violation of known rules or neglect of duty. But after a candidate has been accepted as a pupil of the school, the termination of her connection with the school should never be made without due consideration of all the facts and conditions in the case. The sanction of the superintendent or the training-school committee, or, lacking such consulting authorities, of the president of the board, should be asked for before final rejection is accomplished. Quite serious results have occurred in connection with church hospitals by the dismissal of some nurse whose relatives were prominent in a local or often a distant church. The dismissal may have been very necessary for the discipline and welfare of the school. It may have been entirely just, but the girl herself did not think so. Her story as told at home, fifty or a hundred miles from the scene of action, may have badly twisted and colored, or suppressed important facts, but it was believed. Bequests to institutions have many times been canceled, annual contributors have stopped their contributions, and in various ways the results of such dismissal have been far-reaching.

Serious results to the hospital, of course, do not always occur, but a dismissal is always a serious matter to the nurse concerned. While many training-school superintendents or principals may question the need of consulting members of the board regarding such matters, there is a legal aspect of the case which should not be overlooked. The board of managers can be held legally responsible in case of accidents or injuries due to pupil nurses' neglect or mistakes. While the board members may not have first-hand knowledge regarding each pupil nurse, they should, in a general way, have their authority and responsibility recognized. It is a safeguard to the executive officer as well as to pupils. Every principal should endeavor to observe the distinction between indiscretion and more serious offenses, and, as far as possible, give the candidate the benefit of the doubt. In every case the offender is worthy of a fair hearing before two or more representatives from the board if she desires it. The rights of the lowest and most unimportant employee are respected in a well-governed institution.

Monthly Allowances.—Should pupil nurses be paid an allowance while in training is a matter which has come up frequently for discussion in recent years. It is a question which each individual school must largely settle for itself. Telephone companies find it absolutely necessary to pay young women from the very beginning to learn to manage the telephone board. The public demands continuous service. It demands efficient service, and to get these, the companies must offer inducements to young women to enter, or at least make it possible for them to do so if they are fitted. S milar conditions are found in hospitals. Well-established schools which have a reputation for excellent work and a large number of graduates, and which are otherwise advantageously situated, may—and numbers of them do—find it possible to secure an ample supply of candidates without giving an allowance. Such schools usually furnish board, room, laundry, tuition, general school supplies, and uniforms. A few schools supply shoes, but the custom is not general. Some schools have the uniforms made, and it seems fair that they should, as it is well known that the cost of making is often in excess of the cost of material. Anyway, material is not a uniform until it is made in uniform style, and where no allowance is paid, it should be arranged to have the making of the uniforms attended to by the institution without cost to the pupil who is giving her services.

Newer schools, most of the smaller schools, and many of the large schools, still provide a monthly allowance sufficient to cover the ordinary expenses of the average girl in training. The experience which several well-established schools have had in trying to make the change which would abolish the allowance shows very clearly that under present conditions, it is perilous to the nursing side of the hospital to try to adopt such a policy. Some schools, after a six months' experiment in trying to fill vacancies in the corps after cutting off the allowance, finding the nursing force of the hospital greatly weakened, and the practical care of the sick sadly suffering in quality, have returned to the allowance method, sadder and wiser because of the experiment. The testimony of hundreds of superintendents goes to show that they are able to secure a greater number of applicants by offering an allowance, and are, therefore, able to provide a better quality of nursing, and turn out, on the whole, a better grade of nurse, than would be possible without it. Many believe that practically all schools will ultimately return to the allowance system. In any case it is the exceptional new school which will find it possible to secure or to maintain a sufficient nursing force without the allowance.

Hours of Duty.—This is another important question of policy on which varying opinions are held. Theoretically all will agree that an eight-hour day is very desirable, not only for nurses, but for workers in general. However, things which are best theoretically, often prove to be worst practically. Experience and inquiry from the superintendents of a large number of institutions confirm the writer's convictions that at present the eight-hour day is not feasible or desirable for the average hospital, large or small. A recent report in a foreign journal shows that after a fair trial of the eight-hour system in government hospitals, and after due investigation of conditions, the graduate nurses' association, which at first had highly recommended it, passed a resolution or recommendation that it be abolished. A few American schools have devised a system which is called the eight-hour system, but its superiority over the old system is disputed. Where the eight-hour day means the loss of the customary weekly afternoon off duty, and the half day or extra time off on Sunday, with the daily eight hours possibly broken into fragments, the advantage of the system is surely open to question.

A nine-hour day for day nurses can be accomplished in most institutions with two relays of nurses with and often without the addition of a few relief nurses, to the regular staff. The pupils are allowed one hour for meals, and two hours out of the wards each day—making nine hours of actual nursing. This plan includes the weekly afternoon off duty, and a half day or extra hours on Sunday, and seems as fair an arrangement as can be arrived at for the majority of hospitals under present conditions.

Every superintendent will bear willing testimony to the cheerful response of nurses when extra pressure of work makes it impossible for pupils to get the hours off duty which they need and are supposed to get. On the other hand, a great many hospitals generously grant nurses now and then extra days off duty for various reasons, or overlook or cancel the time, or part of it, lost by illness, which time, as a rule, is expected to be made up. But it is better to be just than generous, and no system can be entirely just which does not keep accurate daily account of the hours of extra duty given by the pupils, and which does not make just as accurate plans to grant this off-duty time as an extra as soon as possible. In the trades, if a workman is obliged to work overtime, he is usually paid either double for the extra hours, or a considerable advance is made in payment for his willingness to oblige the company by serving after regular hours. In hospital work we have been so absorbed in caring for the sick that we often forget to be truly just to those on whom we depend for the actual labor involved in serious cases or emergencies. To announce in a prospectus, or to candidates, that the hospital is working under the nine-hour system, or that nine hours constitutes a full working day, and then habitually or even frequently keep nurses on duty for twelve or thirteen hours with no effort or plan to make up this week the extra time given by the nurse last week, is not strictly honest or business-like, even if custom has for years sanctioned this method. The world moves, and our conceptions of justice should move also. Our conception of training has broadened. Extra burdens in the line of study are demanded of nurses, and the old system under which a nurse was obliged to stay, or allowed to stay, hours after the regular time off duty, with no account of the hours of service thus rendered, should be abandoned as soon as possible. This plan is carried out in some of the best hospitals, head nurses being obliged to render to the principal's office each day an account of the extra hours of duty required, the name of the nurse who gave the extra service, and the reason for it.

Head nurses differ widely in their ability to plan for the pupils, and manage so that they will get the stipulated time off each day. Nurses are often detained unnecessarily when a little forethought, a little better management, would have prevented it. Once a system is established in a hospital by which head nurses are called to account for their management of the pupil's recreation and duty hours, it becomes a stimulus to head nurses to make better plans; it means more to pupil nurses than many realize. It involves a principle of justice which hospitals cannot afford to ignore much longer. It is an advance step which should be taken in every school.

Thus far no satisfactory plan has been devised of making the hours of night duty less than twelve, but since the terms of night duty are relatively short,—a month to six weeks being the rule,—the nurse who is physically fitted for nursing at all, should have no difficulty in fulfilling this necessary requirement. If she is not equal to twelve hours of night duty as a pupil nurse, she is hardly fitted either for private nursing or institutional work after graduation, and should seek some other line of work. Some schools plan for a half night off each week. A large number of schools have a plan of granting a day or two off duty after each night term is completed, and whenever this is possible to arrange, it should be done.

The Nurses' Home.—From the time a hospital building is first planned the nurses' home should be kept well in the foreground in calculations, since nurses constitute a large part of the machinery by which the human repair shop is to carry on its beneficent work. It may seem to some unnecessary to emphasize this point, but experience and observation have clearly shown that architects and managers—new boards particularly—are very liable to forget the nurses altogether in their plans. The writer knows of a hospital built in the twentieth century, costing over $200,000, in which not even a nurses' dining-room could be found in the plans, or in the building, or anywhere on the grounds. When the managers were asked where they expected to house the nurses, they frankly said they had forgotten to make any provision for them at all, but they would "put them somewhere." But there were no less than five operating-rooms in the building with elaborate plans for fitting up and equipping them. This is not an isolated case at all. Hospitals galore have made

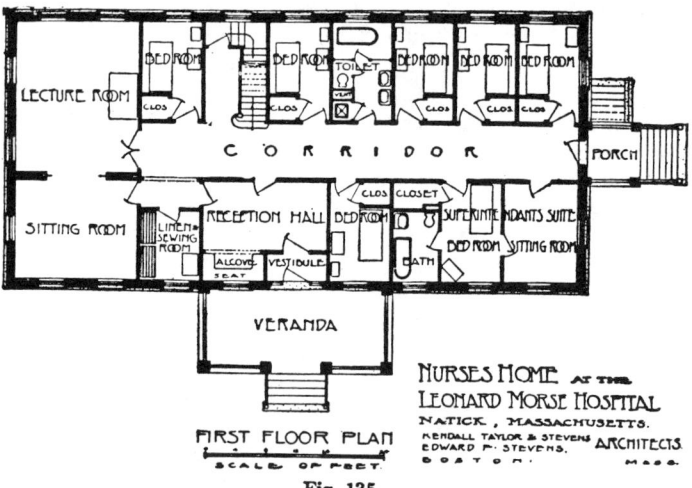

Fig. 135.

a similar blunder in the beginning; in fact, it is a rather unusual thing to see a hospital building and a nurses' home building planned at the same time, and progressing together. Addition after addition is often made to hospitals, making a much larger nursing force necessary, while the capacity of the nurses' home remains the same as when the hospital was small. This results in overcrowding, which is detrimental to all concerned. The past ten or fifteen years have seen much progress in this direction. New splendid training-school buildings have been built all over

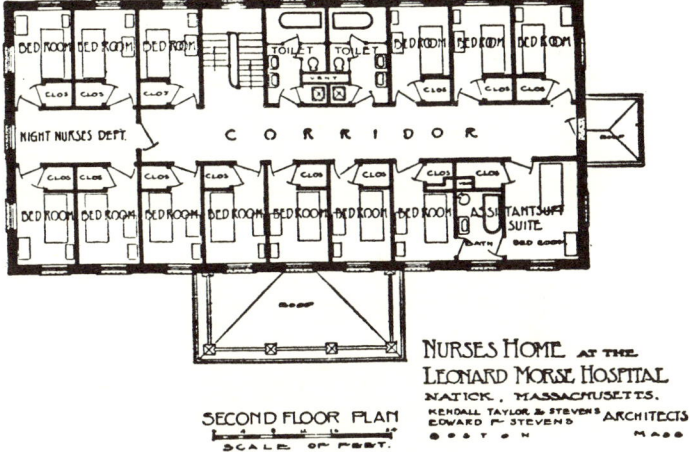

Fig. 136.

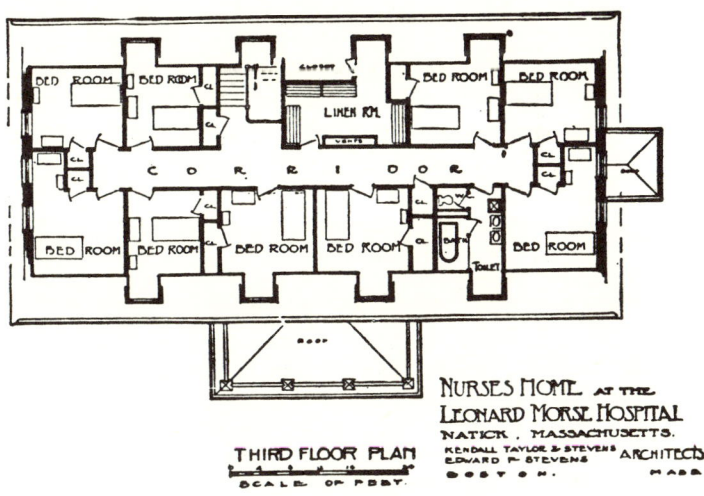

Fig. 137.

the country. Business men have long since found that it pays to look to the employees' welfare—that better service is given by workers who are well treated and cared for in the matter of holidays, working hours, and living conditions generally. And the same rule holds good in hospital work. Better service, with more heart in it, may be expected from nurses who realize that the hospital trustees are doing all in their power to render their life in the hospital comfortable and pleasant.

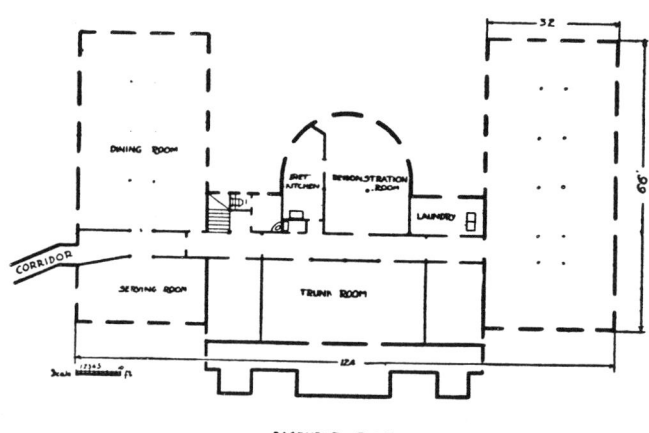

Fig. 138.—Nurses' home, Rochester Homeopathic Hospital.

Nurses are surrounded during their working hours by extremely depressing influences, and for this reason it is desirable to house them in a building separate from the main hospital building, where they can make merry and give vent to their emotions without disturbing the sick. The building need not be elaborate, but it should be comfortable, and as homelike as it is possible to make an institutional building. Fortunately, one need not travel far in any direction in the United States or Canada before finding splendid illustrations of what a nurses' home should be. The cost may range all the way from $4000 or $5000

THE TRAINING-SCHOOL AND ITS MANAGEMENT 353

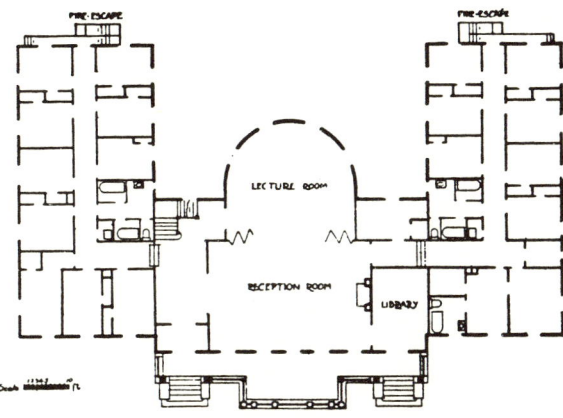

FIRST FLOOR PLAN
Fig. 139 — Nurses' home, Rochester Homeopathic Hospital.

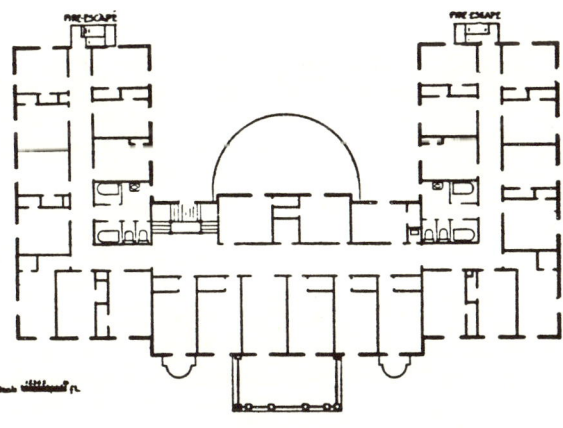

2ND FLOOR PLAN
Fig. 140 — Nurses' home, Rochester Homeopathic Hospital.

to $130,000, buildings being readily found at these extremes of figures, which seem well adapted for their purpose. When planning a new building, it is extremely desirable to arrange for each nurse to have a separate room of her own. Even though it must be very small, there is much comfort in having a few feet of space which the weary nurse may call her own. This plan is a very great convenience also n that it makes unnecessary separate rooms for night nurses, though when space permits, it is better to have the quarters for night nurses entirely shut off from the main building. When two nurses occupy the same room, one being on day and the other on night duty, neither one gets much comfort, undisturbed, in her own room.

The Maria Louise Robertson Home for Nurses connected with the Hospital for Sick Children, Toronto, is regarded as probably the most luxurious type of nurses' home in America. It owes its existence to the generosity of one man who apparently believes that nothing is too good for nurses who spend their strength in service to the sick and helpless. Probably the most complete nurses' library to be found anywhere is there. Besides spacious parlors on different floors, a general reception room, music room, writing room, lecture room, etc., this building has a well-equipped gymnasium, a swimming pool, and a special diet-kitchen for the instruction of the nurses, with facilities for individual cookery provided as in the regular domestic science schools.

The nurses' home, known as Kay House, in connection with the Polyclinic Hospital, Philadelphia, is one of the newer buildings of its kind, and is a good type of a comfortable, homelike training-school building at a moderate price. The plans were drawn by the lady superintendent, with the assistance of the secretary of the board of trustees and the builder. No architect was employed. After some years of experience with this building and with a wide knowledge of other similar homes, one who knows much about it states that for practical comfort she would not exchange it for any other building she knows of. Others who have lived and worked in the same building have made similar commendatory statements. The building itself cost $36,596.42, and the furnishing and equipment, $3,557.90. There are four stories and a roof-garden, forty-seven single rooms, with three suites of

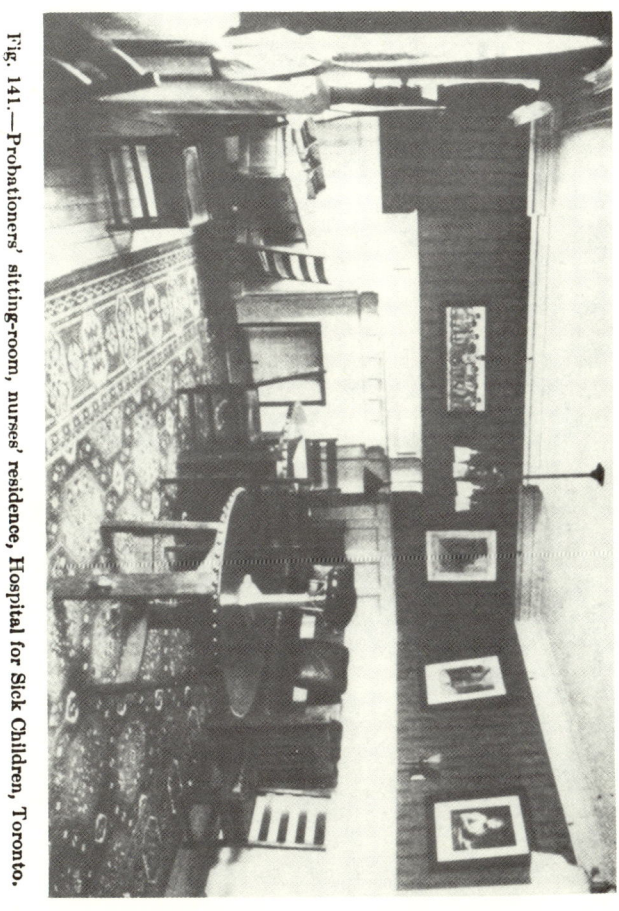

Fig. 141.—Probationers' sitting-room, nurses' residence, Hospital for Sick Children, Toronto.

rooms, consisting of bed-room, bath-room, and sitting-room, for the officers of the school. Of the forty-seven rooms mentioned, six are large rooms with two windows, which could, if necessary, be used for two nurses. Every detail seems to have been carefully considered, with the thought

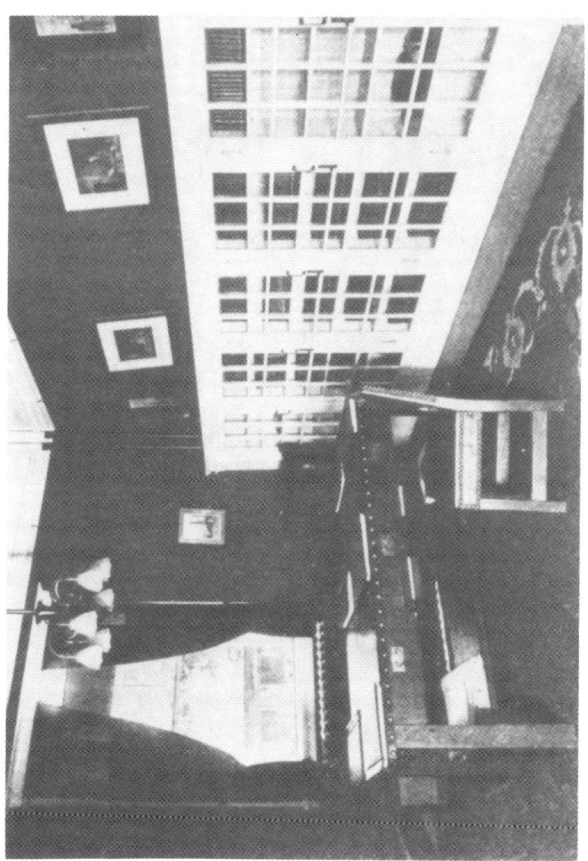

Fig. 142.—A corner of the reading-room, nurses' residence, Hospital for Sick Children, Toronto.

of having the home and furnishing as simple and effective as possible. The book-cases in the library were built into the building when it was constructed. Every nurse has a single room, each room having a closet, making wardrobes unnecessary. Each room is provided, as a minimum,

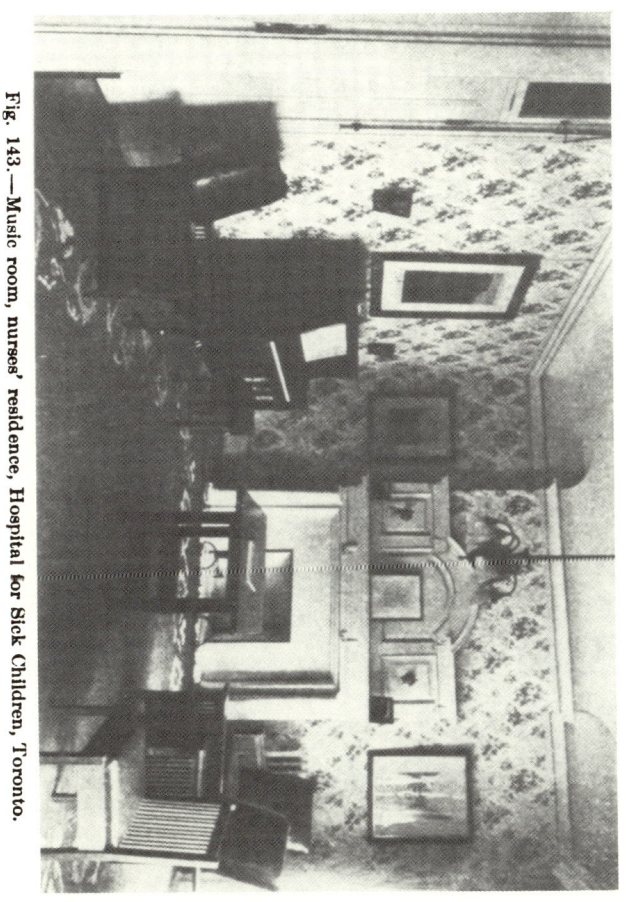

Fig. 143.—Music room, nurses' residence, Hospital for Sick Children, Toronto.

with writing table with drawer, book-shelves, bureau and mirror, rocking-chair and straight chair, and bedstead. On each floor there is a tea pantry, with gas stove and hot and cold water. Besides these, there are the usual sitting-rooms, class-room, dining-room, and library.

The Nurses' Home of Grace Hospital, Detroit, is another example of comfort, convenience, and simplicity. It was constructed in 1900, and provides accommodation for sixty nurses and ten orderlies. It is a four-story, hard-brick structure of colonial architecture, costing $25,000. To build the same building now would require a much

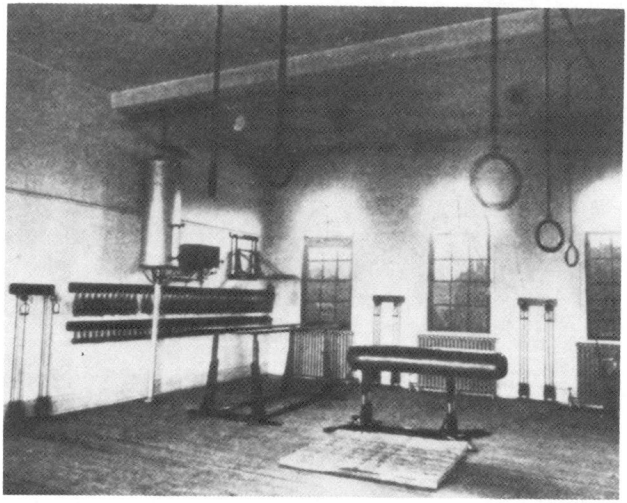

Fig. 144.—Gymnasium, nurses' residence, Hospital for Sick Children, Toronto.

larger outlay. It has accommodations for the principal, her assistant, several head nurses, and the maids necessary for the care of the home, in addition to the number specified. All the bed-rooms are for one or two beds. The first floor is entirely devoted to the library, reception room, music room, large reception hall, and quarters for the principal and her assistants. The rooms on this floor are so arranged that they can be thrown together for parties, receptions, or amusement purposes. The lecture room is in the basement, which is a furnished half-basement. In the basement there are also a small kitchen and two dining-rooms en suite for the purpose of serving lunches at receptions, etc. There is an outfit of spray baths, and two scrub-up rooms with bath, toilet, etc., for the use of nurses who have been exposed to contagious diseases, a large trunk-room, and other conveniences.

At the Rhode Island Hospital, Providence, may be seen some excellent features well worth considering in

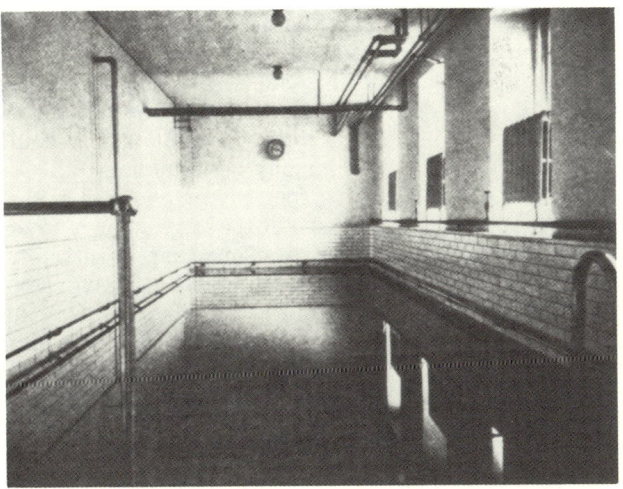

Fig. 145.—The swimming pool, nurses' residence, Hospital for Sick Children, Toronto.

planning a nurses' home. The large addition to the George Ide Chase Home for nurses recently completed at that institution contains 95 separate sleeping-rooms for nurses, each room being of an average size of ten by eleven feet, with a clothes closet adjoining. On each floor are toilet rooms, and on the several floors are placed a library, sewing-rooms, sitting-rooms, etc. In the basement a special laundry has been built for the nurses who may wish to do certain parts of their own personal laundry work. Leading off the main hallway on the ground floor is a one-story building given up to class-room and recreation purposes. This space, 56 by 32 feet, can be divided into five class-rooms by sliding vertical partitions, or can be thrown into one room for lectures and amusement purposes. A small stage with a dressing-room on either side makes it an ideal place for purposes of amusement and entertainment.

In the nurses' home of the Natick Hospital, Mass., the superintendent and her assistant are each provided with a suite of two rooms each and bath. The lecture room adjoins the nurses' sitting-room, making a large room for special purposes when needed. Single rooms are arranged for, with large closet for each nurse. A small laundry is provided for the use of the nurses, a point which should not be overlooked in plans for any new building.

A feature which might be specially emphasized is that the bath-room or lavatory should be large enough to accommodate a number of nurses at one time in the morning. This is in the end a real economy, since it saves labor and the expense of providing washstands and china for each separate room. An equipment of a dozen or more wash-basins or lavatories with running water is none too many for a school of twenty to forty nurses. The bath-tubs may wisely be in a separate room, or at least separated by partitions from the main lavatory.

In the nurses' home at the Evanston (Illinois) Hospital there is a bath-room between each two rooms, so that each nurse has a room connected with a bath.

A vacuum cleaning system has been installed in many of the recently built homes for nurses, a modern convenience well worth considering when finances admit.

A point at which many otherwise well-planned nurses' homes are deficient is in the matter of provision for head nurses. The question of securing and retaining suitable head nurses for the different departments of an active growing institution is in many cases a real problem. One reason for this is that in numbers of institutions the position carries with it so little in the way of material comforts for the head nurses or supervisors of departments, so little in the way of salary, and so little prospect of advancement in knowledge, that it proves unattractive to capable workers. It is used by nurses in many cases to tide over a period until something else is found. An inquiry into conditions will show that the accommodations provided for head nurses are often no better than those provided for the probationers, the salary is about half what it ought to be, and no provision is made for special training or study along any line. So long as this condition continues, the head nurse question will continue to be a problem. It is therefore well in planning a building to keep in mind the needs of these workers who are so important in the daily routine of the hospital.

When the training-school building or nurses' home is separate from the hospital, as all agree it should be, it means that two distinct households must be planned for and supervised. The principal cannot be in the hospital and in the nurses' home at the same time. If no one is in the latter place in authority, difficulties are likely to periodically occur. In England the 'home sister" presides over the nurses' home. In America, various arrangements more or less satisfactory are made regarding the matter. When the school is large enough, the ideal arrangement is to place a graduate nurse in charge, make her responsible for the supervision of the cleaning, etc., the general condition of the home, for much of the theoretic instruction of probationers, the care of nurses with minor illnesses, the distribution of letters, etc., the charge of the linen and uniforms, and the variety of other details which otherwise the principal would be obliged to see to. Her work can be arranged so that she relieves the principal in her office occasionally and assists in numerous other ways as occasions arise.

When a school has finally decided to carry several paid instructors on its staff, it has been found advantageous to combine the duties of matron of the nurses' home and instructor of probationers. Where an untrained woman has acted as matron of the home, it will be found to require but little increase in expenditure to secure a nurse graduate who can assume the supervisory duties in the home, and those of teacher also, and it is a step toward systematic practical teaching which means better nursing for patients and better training for nurses.

Rules and Regulations.—However much one may dislike to take up the subject of rules and regulations and restrictions, the fact remains that where a number of individuals are congregated and closely associated in daily life, rules and regulations are necessary if any degree of order and general comfort is to exist. Some one has said that "rules are recorded experience." As a general thing, rules should be and are the outgrowth of conditions. All rules should be plainly stated to each new pupil by the proper official—never left to be handed down from class to class, never allowed to become obsolete. If necessary, rules should be enforced; if unnecessary, they should be abolished. All nurses will not need all rules to restrain them. Some nurses in every school will.

Rules for nurses are important considerations in the comfort and general welfare not only of nurses, but of the entire institution. They need at least annual consideration on the part of officials, so that suitable changes may be made as needed.

The list of rules appended is in use in several hospitals, and is the result of the combined wisdom of experienced hospital and training-school superintendents. If any rule seems unduly severe, the reader may be absolutely sure that "there's a reason."

House Rules.—The hour for rising for day nurses is ......A. M. The roll will be called by the night supervisor at....... Nurses failing to answer to their names will forfeit their time off duty for the day. Rooms and beds must be thoroughly aired each morning, and rooms kept in condition for inspection at all times. Day nurses must be in their rooms by 10 P. M., and light in sleeping apartments extinguished by 10 P. M. Visiting in each other's rooms after 9.45 P. M. is forbidden.

Night nurses are required to remain in bed from 9 A. M. to 4 P. M., during which hours quietness must be observed in the entire nurses' department. The piano may not be used during those hours without special permission.

When off duty, nurses are not allowed to visit in any part of the hospital proper. Negligée attire must not be worn in the reception room, dining-room, hospital, or grounds.

Lights must be extinguished when the room is left even for a short time. Soiled linen of any kind must not be left in the bath-rooms, except where receptacle is provided. Personal belongings or dishes must not be left in bath-rooms.

Bath-tubs must be cleaned immediately after use, and slops must not be emptied in them. Baths must not be taken after 9.45 P. M.

Personal laundry must be marked as required and must be deposited in bags in the places appointed before ....A. M. on .... Twenty-four pieces are allowed every nurse each week, not including handkerchiefs. Only plainly made underclothing, plain shirtwaists and hospital uniforms will be received. White skirts are not permitted to be worn when on duty.

Nurses are not allowed to entertain friends while on duty. No visitors shall be invited to visit any part of the hospital without permission. Discharged nurses may not be received as callers in the hospital without permission from the superintendent.

Gentlemen callers may be received from 7.30 to 9.30 P. M. on Wednesday and Sunday evenings in the parlors of the nurses' home. Appointments may not be made with patients or ex-patients without permission from the superintendent or principal. All intercourse with the staff, internes or employees connected with the hospital must be strictly professional. At no time shall nurses supply internes with meals without permission from the principal, nor shall appointments be made with internes to meet outside or to go from the hospital. Violations of this rule will be considered sufficient cause for suspension or discharge.

Unless in cases of extreme emergency, nurses will not be called to talk with friends over the telephone while on duty. Messages will be delivered from the office. When off duty, nurses may use the telephone for a limited time on permission from the person in charge of the office.

Dishes and food must not be carried from the dining-room, kitchen, or store-room to nurses' rooms.

Nurses are cautioned not to leave money or valuable jewelry in their rooms. Valuables or sums of money should be deposited in the safe.

Visitors may not be invited to meals nor to spend a night on the premises without permission from the principal.

The appropriation by any nurse or employee of any article of food or drink belonging to a patient or provided by the hospital for the use of patients will be deemed an offense justifying the dismissal of the person found guilty of this offense.

The affairs and conditions of all patients are to be considered strictly private. The discussion of patients or their affairs or matters concerning the hospital or the doctors outside the hospital is forbidden.

Nurses who require medical advice or treatment must report promptly to the principal. Doctors' offices must not be visited without permission from the principal. Drugs, except those specified, may not be procured or prescribed without her knowledge.

Nurses who have been excused from duty because of illness must report to the principal before going on duty again.

Nurses are cautioned to observe all possible precautions to avoid damage to, or interference with, plumbing.

Nurses are required to register their names in the office when they leave the hospital and also the hour when they expect to return. This rule does not apply to short walks in the immediate vicinity of the hospital. Some exercise in the open air is obligatory on every nurse daily. At least one-half hour should be so spent.

Nurses must not appear in public places nor go on board street-cars when dressed in their uniforms or parts of uniforms. Street clothing should be worn when on the street except in the immediate vicinity of the hospital.

Nurses will be excused from class or lecture only when illness or duty requires their absence. Social engagements must not be made nor invitations accepted that will interfere with studies or classes.

The making of new articles of personal wearing apparel or sewing, beyond the ordinary mending, is not allowed during the months when lectures and classes are held. Needed additions to the personal wardrobe should be made while on vacations.

The vacation period is given for rest and recreation. Nurses are not allowed to nurse during vacations. In cases of serious illness of relatives special arrangements may be made.

General Ward Regulations.—No patient must ever be left without a nurse in charge. Nurses may not leave the department to which they have been assigned for even a few minutes without permission from the head nurse of that department. When on duty, nurses must wear the full uniform, including shoes with rubber heels. Rings, flowers, or unnecessary jewelry must not be worn when on duty.

Nurses who are in charge of wards are expected to see that visitors comply with the hospital regulations relating to visitors. It is the nurse's duty to notify the visitor when visiting hours have expired. Violations of rules must be reported to the head nurse.

Nurses are required to confine their conversation with each other while on duty to necessary professional matters, and to use all possible efforts to keep the hospital free from unnecessary noise. Loud talking or visiting with each other while on duty is not permitted. Talking in corridors is to be avoided as far as possible.

Nurses are not allowed to visit in any wards or rooms except those to which they have been assigned, without permission from the head nurse. All possible care and economy in the use of hospital appliances and supplies must be observed. Breakages or accidents must be immediately reported to the head nurse or principal. Broken or worn-out articles must not be destroyed. They should be taken by the head nurse to the principal and exchanged for new ones.

Nurses are strictly forbidden to give any medicine without a written order. Except in serious emergency, nurses are not expected to carry out verbal orders regarding treatment.

Nurses are required to notify the head nurse, or if necessary the principal, when it is found impossible to carry out orders.

All supplies needed for the night must be procured by day nurses before going off duty.

All lights not actually necessary must be extinguished by 9 P. M. Extravagance in the use of light at night will be reported to the superintendent. Borrowing supplies is prohibited.

Screens must be used to avoid exposure of any patient.

Upon entrance of an officer, physician, or stranger, the nurse in charge of the room or ward shall rise and give the visitors prompt attention.

When a patient is discharged, the nurse who has had charge of him during the hours immediately preceding his discharge is expected to take his discharge card, signed, and go with the patient to the office.

No legal papers shall be executed or signed by nurses for patients without the knowledge of the superintendent. Nurses shall preserve as strictly private any affairs relating to patients which shall come to their knowledge in the course of their duty.

A list of the clothing and effects of each patient on his

admission must be made in the clothing book or record provided for that purpose, together with the number of the locker to which the effects have been sent. The entry must be signed by the nurse on duty.

Nurses are strictly forbidden to use the printed blanks of the hospital for any other purpose than that for which they were designed.

All entries on bedside records must be made promptly at the time the event recorded takes place.

When a nurse expects to be engaged in such manner that she cannot attend to her bells or calls promptly, arrangements must be made for a temporary substitute. Failure to answer signals or calls promptly may be considered sufficient cause for suspension.

Hot-water bottles must not be filled with water at a higher degree than 115° F. All such bottles must be carefully protected, and must never be left with unconscious patients without special permission.

Nurses are especially enjoined to use all possible precautions in handling medicines and to leave no drug within reach of any patient. Medicines must be taken in the presence of the nurse. As far as possible strongly poisonous drugs should be kept separate from other drugs.

A nurse who is found sleeping while on duty shall be suspended for not less than two days. For a second offense, she shall be suspended for a week and reported to the executive committee, with the facts in the case. Such committee may recommend discharge, or another trial may be given.

For violation of rules of a serious nature, the matter shall be reported to the superintendent, who will confer with the executive committee regarding it. If, after investigation, the executive committee so recommends, the nurse shall be suspended or dismissed. Minor violations will be dealt with by the principal. Unavoidable violations of known rules shall be promptly reported to the principal, with the reason therefor.

The Instructors.—In the early days of training-schools the instructors were necessarily doctors who selected out of the wide field of medicine such knowledge

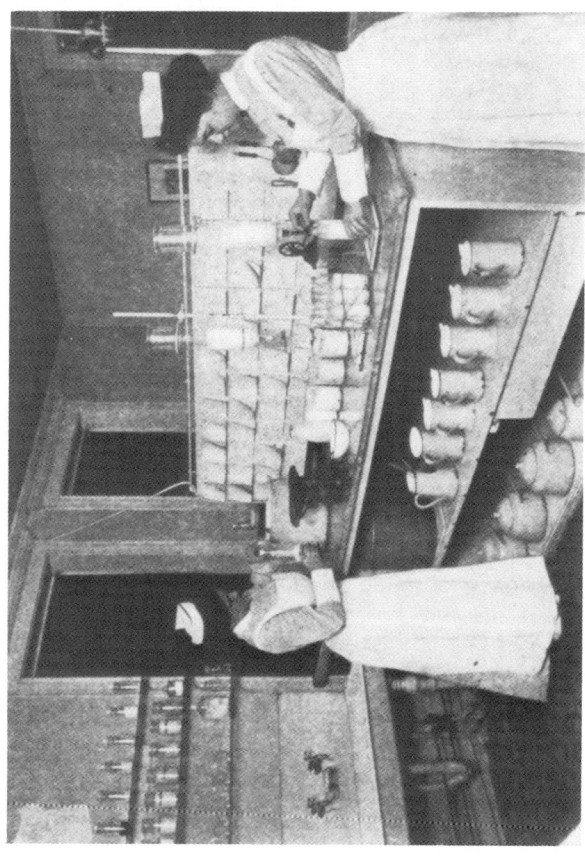

Fig. 146.—Milk laboratory, Wesley Hospital, Chicago.

as they felt should be imparted to nurses, and delivered it in lecture form. Each man had his own individual ideas about the knowledge which was worth while for nurses, and naturally each man who had a specialty, emphasized its importance. The nurses were expected to take notes on the lectures or pick up as much as they could in any way they could. The announcement of the school often contained the names of brilliant well-known medical men as included in the faculty, and the number of instructors under this plan frequently reached astonishing proportions. This was the old way. Experience, however, has shown that the multiplying of instructors beyond a certain point has proved a source of weakness to the school, and a positive handicap to good, enduring results. The best schools have abandoned this promiscuous haphazard method and are limiting the medical instructors who are really depended on to teach the required theory, to three or at most four, outside of the resident corps, who occasionally are detailed to hold regular classes. Instead of a class being taught by a half-dozen or more different men, one or two are appointed to carry the studies through the year and are paid a sum ranging from $2.50 to $5.00 for each class period. This is especially desirable in the first half of the course. The cost is a trifling part in the total of the year's expense of the average hospital; the instructors take more interest in the work, and the school acquires a degree of control over the instruction impossible under the old volunteer system. Instead of depending on pupils taking notes from which to study, text-books covering all the important subjects taught are provided by the school, or the pupil, if paid an allowance, is required to possess her own text-books covering all branches taught. This change in methods is taking place gradually but surely, and it marks a long step in advance in every school which adopts the new method.

The practical and theoretic instruction given during the probation period is an exceedingly important part of the training. When possible, it is wise to make one nurse responsible for the teaching of correct practical methods during that period. In many of the larger schools a graduate nurse devotes herself solely to the probationers and is termed the "instructor of probationers."

The value and importance, both to patient and nurse, of giving a short course of preliminary practical instruction to every nurse before giving a nurse any actual nursing responsibility need no discussion. The plans for this course will vary according to facilities and conditions, but every school can plan for at least a fortnight or a month to be spent in preliminary training before the probationer is made responsible for actual bedside work. This does not

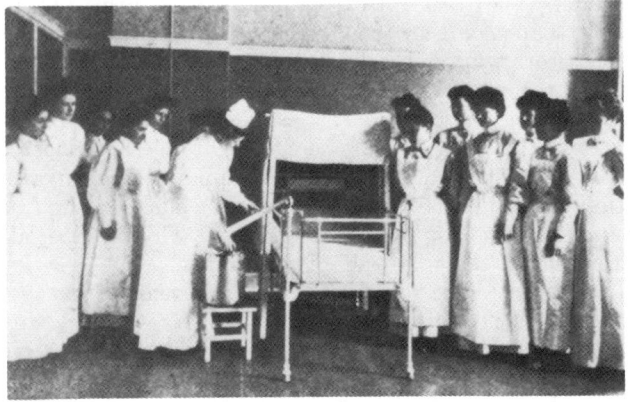

Fig. 147.—A class in the demonstration room, nurses' residence, Hospital for Sick Children, Toronto.

mean that she may not be admitted to the wards for demonstration of bedside methods or to assist in minor duties, but it does mean that she shall be taught how to do properly the ordinary nursing duties before she is detailed to perform them for a patient.

Occasionally one sees a statement published that instructors of nurses should be nurses exclusively, and another giving the opposite view, that "the instruction of nurses should be intrusted entirely to physicians." Neither of these methods seems the ideal. So long as

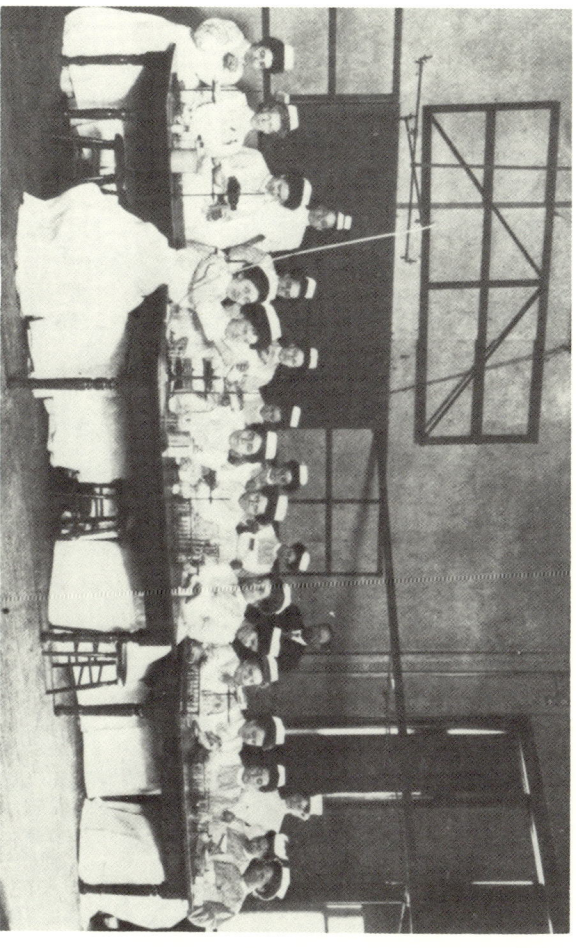

Fig. 148.—A class in the laboratory. Wesley Hospital, Chicago, Illinois.

they have to serve under the direction of physicians, the nurses should receive instruction from physicians regarding many points. At the same time, experience has shown that many physicians who admire thoroughness and appreciate the best results of training have but very vague ideas as to the detailed measures needed to produce in the nurse the results they admire. There is much which goes in the makeup of the well-trained nurse for which nurses must be responsible, and both nurses and physicians should be numbered among the instructors.

The Course of Study.—For the first time in the history of training schools on the American continent it is possible to approach this subject feeling that an authoritative answer that is more than an individual opinion can be given to the question, "What should nurses be taught?" Believing that uniformity regarding essential points in the training of nurses was both desirable and possible, the American Hospital Association, representing the hospitals of the United States and Canada, appointed a committee to study the whole training-school question and bring in recommendations, with a view to standardizing the training in the two countries represented. The report of the committee, which was unanimously adopted by the Association, will be found in the appendix. There is no hospital capable of managing a training-school, which cannot give one of the courses recommended, and hospital authorities generally are hereby urged to give the recommendations of the committee serious consideration, and join in the general movement toward greater uniformity and thoroughness in training.

General Matters.—The vexed question as to whether a two- or three-year course should constitute a training has been much discussed. The recommendations of the committee appointed by the American Hospital Association suggest two years, and three months of probation extra, as a minimum. Whatever term is decided on, proper grading of classes and instruction is necessary for thorough work. In a small school it is next to, if not wholly, impossible to carry three separate classes through and do justice to them. Enthusiasm dies when a class dwindles to two or three. Doctors object to spending their instructive efforts on two or three, so it happens that in many schools the foundation principles of teaching are thrown aside. Probationers are sent in to study and receive lectures side by side with nurses in their third year, and thorough work in any year becomes impossible under such conditions. The foundation work of the first year is by far the most important, and practical methods cannot be too thoroughly taught. Two classes are all that can be successfully carried through in the average small school, and a term of two years and three or six months seems fair to pupil and hospital.

The skipping of classes sometimes for weeks at a time during the school year, a custom which in the days of our ignorance of training-school methods was winked at, is one which should be speedily abandoned in every school which pretends to offer thorough training. Various excuses are made in defense of this habit when it exists. Among these are—"We were so busy"; "There were so many nurses on special duty"; "Dr. Blank seems to get a call somewhere else every class night," etc. Back of all these excuses is the real fact that the superintendent does not care very much whether the nurses have their class periods regularly or not. If he did (or she did), he would manage so that none of these time-honored excuses would be accepted as a reason more than once. If Dr. Blank is so busy that he cannot attend to the duties he accepted, then the superintendent should see that some substitute is provided, or that Dr. Blank is relieved altogether of class work. If there are not enough nurses to do the duties that need to be done during the class hours, so that the nurses can go to their proper classes, then the staff should be increased. Emergencies will arise which may require the postponement of a class, but these should be the exception. When there is a man or woman in charge of an institution who has a proper conception of what a training-school should be and should do, there will be few class periods missed in any school during the school year. This is a matter which boards of managers or training-school committees may very properly inquire into each month. There is some danger of overdoing the matter of class periods, and unduly exalting theoretic instruction, but there is much more danger of minimizing its importance, and many schools in all parts of the country need to be called to repent of their shortcomings in this matter.

The matter of records of training-school graduates is another point which should not be overlooked. It should be possible, however many changes of principals or superintendents may have taken place, to obtain, by writing to any institution, the main facts regarding any graduate of the school. A suggestive form for this record will be found appended.

Another question which has excited considerable debate is whether pupils who have begun training in one school and for some reason have left the school shall be admitted into other schools. When nursing material was plentiful, many, probably most, schools adopted as a fixed policy that no pupil who had had even a few weeks' training or experience in any other school should be considered as a candidate. This policy is still adhered to quite generally, but the rule has found more exceptions in recent years than ever before. It is a two- or three-sided question, and at the present time it seems desirable, if this rule is made, to make it of some more flexible material than cast-iron. To generally relax in the enforcement of such a ruling would create a disastrous condition of affairs both for hospitals and nurses, yet undoubtedly there are many cases where such a rule may be stretched without disadvantage, and often with great good, to both pupil and hospital. Several cases have come to the writer's attention recently where the pupil nurses were doing faithful work; they were desirable nurses who had a wholesome ambition to secure a complete well-

374 HOSPITAL MANAGEMENT

HOSPITAL OF THE GOOD SHEPHERD—SCHOOL FOR NURSES,
SYRACUSE, N. Y.

STUDENT'S HISTORY CARD.

Date

Name
Address
Birth place   Age on admission
Religious belief
Character
Education
Name and address of nearest relative or friend

Acceptability to private patients
  "   " ward patients
  "   " doctors
  "   " student nurses
Quality of work—Medical
  Surgical   Obstetrical
  Children
Executive ability
Illness, No. of days   —nature
  Time
  Time made up
Absence, No. of days   —cause
  Time made up
Special discipline—cause
  Character
Expulsion—time ·   cause
Vacation—1st year   2nd year   3rd year
Final rating—practical   theoretical
Graduation   No. of pin
Time completed
State examination
  Registration   No. of certificate
  Joined Alumnae Association

Fig. 149.—Student's history card. On the reverse side of same card is printed the record for instructions and work (Fig. 150).

THE TRAINING SCHOOL AND ITS MANAGEMENT 375

Fig. 150.—Record of instruction and work. This is printed on the reverse of card containing matter shown in Fig. 149.

rounded training, but the pernicious habit of skipping classes, often for weeks at a time, had prevailed in the hospital in which they began their course, until they despaired of getting the theoretic training they felt they should have, that had been promised, and that other nurses were receiving. It is not the business of pupil nurses to effect changes in the policy or methods of the school they have entered, but when they are being defrauded of the training they should receive, when classes are irregular or entirely dropped for weeks or months during the school year, it seems hardly just to such nurses that a cast-iron rule should be erected as a bar to keep them from securing admittance to any other school. A dissatisfied pupil nurse is not always to be condemned. If all hospital and training-school superintendents were perfect, living up to the best they knew in training-school matters and dealing justly and fairly with pupil nurses, blanket rules in this matter would be in order. But since they are not all just, not all perfect, while adopting the general rule of exclusion of candidates who have had previous experience or training, it seems desirable that it be made a somewhat flexible rule which will allow of consideration of individual cases when vacancies exist in the school. In all such cases the courtesy of a note of inquiry to the school which the pupil had previously been connected with should be observed. This is not only a matter of courtesy, but a safeguard to the institution to which the nurse desires admission.

A custom which has prevailed to a considerable extent in recent years, and which is well worthy of consideration, is the matter of awarding prizes annually—a certain number to each class. These prizes are often offered by staff physicians, trustees, occasionally by the superintendent personally, sometimes by the graduates of the school. These prizes are awarded for a variety of reasons, among which are neatness in the care of the nurse's room, neatness in wards, practical nursing, general proficiency in theoretic work, surgical technic, quietness in daily routine, for the best essay on a certain subject assigned, etc. The general effect in such schools as have had experience has been such as to justify a continuance of the practice of prize-giving after the experimental period has passed. It is quite probable that if prizes were more generally given, some difficulties along other lines would be lessened. If more prizes were given for general good deportment and observance of institutional rules, there might be less need to consider methods of enforcing rules and management of discipline.

CHAPTER XVII

THE OUT-PATIENT DEPARTMENT

By Louis H. Burlingham, M. D.

The out-patient department[1] has three duties:
1. Toward the patient.
2. Toward medical teaching.
3. Toward society.

1. The chief sphere of an O. P. D. is to care for the ambulatory sick poor of the following classes:

(a) Those whose illness or injury is not sufficiently severe to require treatment in bed, as compensated cardiac cases, minor injuries, and skin and throat diseases.

(b) Those who come to an O. P. D. for further treatment after discharge from the hospital wards.

Another function is to serve as a place from which patients who are still ambulatory, but should be in bed, or who require treatment which the O. P. D. cannot furnish, may be recommended to the hospital wards.

2. The O. P. D. affords an opportunity to members of the medical profession to acquire experience and do research work through the large numbers and the wide variety of cases which are presented there, and for teaching medical students, profitably and practically, by direct personal contact with the patients and the various conditions which may be found.

3. The O. P. D. serves society by aiding struggling individuals over a period of greater or less stress because of

[1] Throughout this chapter the abbreviation O. P. D. will be used instead of the words out-patient department, dispensary, or polyclinic.

THE OUT-PATIENT DEPARTMENT

sickness or injury, and enabling them to return as soon as possible to occupations profitable to themselves and society. And more recently, through social service departments, which see to it that the course of treatment advised by the physicians or surgeon is carried out, and which in various ways improve home, hygienic, and moral conditions, it becomes a prominent factor in the chief end of medicine, prevention.

Because of the wide differences in the requirements as to the number of patients to be accommodated, as to the size of the building, and also in the amount of money available for construction and maintenance, only general principles can be laid down as to the construction and conduct of an O. P. D.

Location.—The O. P. D. should be easily accessible for the patients. It should be connected with a hospital to provide beds for patients needing them, to provide for easy transportation for patients from the O. P. D. to the hospital in emergencies, to facilitate consultations between the hospital and O. P. D. staff in regard to difficult or obscure hospital or O. P. D. cases, and to permit the use of the hospital laboratories when needed. This connection with the main hospital will diminish the expense of running the O. P. D., through the use of the hospital power plant and laundry, by obtaining supplies through the hospital store, through utilizing the regular hospital employees in making repairs, and by providing for the feeding and housing of the O. P. D. employees.

However, an O. P. D. should always be located in a thickly settled district, and if the hospital is not so located, it may be wise to have the O. P. D. separate from the hospital to attain this end. Patients can be transported from the O. P. D. to the main hospital in ambulances when necessary; the laundry can be taken care of at the hospital, and the regular employees of the hospital can be utilized in repairing and similar work.

A quiet location is necessary if good work is to be done in physical diagnosis.

An abundance of light is greatly to be desired, both for diagnosis and treatment, where close inspection is necessary, but it is not so absolutely required for the welfare of the patients as it would be in the ward buildings, as the stay of each patient in the O. P. D. is so brief.

The Building.—There seems to be no objection to the use of the many-storied building as compared with an O. P. D. of one story only, and it has the following advantages: the cost of construction is thereby diminished, the problems of heating, ventilation, and plumbing are simplified, for similar departments with similar requirements in equipment may be superposed, the cost of up-keep and administration is diminished, the distances to be traversed are less, thus aiding economy in administration, and the comfort and convenience of the patients and staff. The disadvantage of superimposed stories is obviated by the use of an elevator for those unable to climb stairs easily. This form of building renders more easy the problem of keeping the sexes separate, for on one floor may be located the rooms for male medical, male surgical, and genitourinary departments, and on another the rooms for female medical, female surgical, and children's diseases.

The building should preferably be of fire-proof or semi-fire-proof material, though this is not so important as in the hospital ward construction, for in the event of fire, few, if any, of the individuals in the building would be entirely helpless. Interior ornamentation should be avoided, for this, with the construction advised, makes the attainment of scrupulous cleanliness more easily possible. The windows, especially in the examining and operating-rooms, should be large, to admit all the light possible, and so arranged as to admit of easy and frequent cleaning; they should be screened in summer.

Heating may be by the direct or indirect methods.

Ventilation should be carefully looked out for, for though patients remain in the O. P. D. but a short time, still they are usually present in large numbers during the hours when the clinic is in session, and many of them have yet much to learn in regard to personal cleanliness. The Plenum system has been found satisfactory.

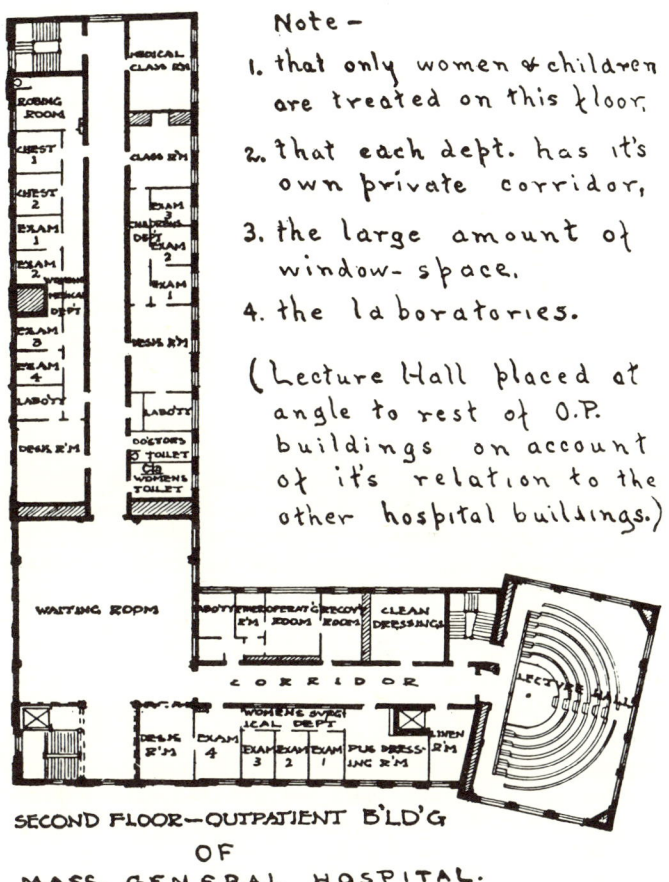

Note —
1. that only women & children are treated on this floor.
2. that each dept. has it's own private corridor.
3. the large amount of window-space.
4. the laboratories.

(Lecture Hall placed at angle to rest of O.P. buildings on account of it's relation to the other hospital buildings.)

SECOND FLOOR—OUTPATIENT B'LD'G
OF
MASS. GENERAL HOSPITAL.
Fig. 151.

The plumbing should be open, and pipes, sinks, hoppers, and radiators, if used, should be placed at such a distance from the walls and corners that cleaning may be done behind them with ease.

There should preferably be but one door for the entrance and exit of patients, for convenience in admitting them, that they may be better controlled, and that a patient may not leave by one door while his friends are waiting for him at another exit. This door should be at the ground level, because of the number of patients who have some impediment in walking and who can ascend or descend stairs with difficulty; and, for the same reason, in a building of several stories for out-patients, there should be at least one elevator; by locating this near the entrance, such patients can be easily taken to the proper floors.

There should be a general waiting-room near the entrance, where those who have come to the O. P. D. for the first time may await registration, and where the friends of patients may remain until the patient returns from the clinic to which he has been sent. It is wise to have a common waiting-room for each group of related departments, as male medical, male surgical, and genito-urinary. In connection with the general waiting-room there should be one or more rooms or booths where the admitting physician may examine such cases as he considers necessary, and where contagious cases can be detained until they can be transported to a contagious hospital.

Arrangements should be made in each department so that a patient, by means of a corridor within the department, may be taken from one room to another or go from dressing-room to examining-room without leaving that department.

Every O. P. D. should have one or more laboratories in which examinations of smears, urine, sputa, stools, etc., can be made.

The Patients.—To avoid "dispensary abuse" only the following classes of patients should be admitted to the privileges of an O. P. D.:

1. The "poverty stricken."
2. Those whose wages or incomes are never more than

enough to meet the regular expenses of living, and frequently not enough to do that, and who are never able to save anything for a time when misfortune overtakes them.

3. Those who have a small sum saved up, but who, through old age, the chronic nature of their illness, or the number of those dependent on them are not able to make any further savings, and whose small stock of savings alone keeps them from absolute poverty.

4. Those who have been treated in the hospital and are unable to pay a private physician, or require more skilful care than the average practitioner can give, or cases possessing especial scientific interest.

5. Those who in ordinary circumstances could pay a private physician, but through loss of position or illness cannot do so at the time when they apply for treatment; for such patients and those in the second and third classes under (4) a special form of admission ticket may be provided, which shall be good for a limited period only, but which may be renewed in suitable cases.

As a general rule, any patient who has employed a physician should bring a letter from him, recommending the patient to the O. P. D. for treatment.

Among those who should not be treated in an O. P. D. are the following:

1. Those who are able to pay a physician his fee, even if small. Such individuals should be referred back to their family physician, or, if none has been employed, they may be given the cards of members of the O. P. D. staff, if they (the applicants) desire them.

2. Those who have been treated by a physician and bring no letter of recommendation—they should be referred back to him.

3. Those who have been treated at some other reputable dispensary—they should be referred back to it.

4. Those who come for confirmation of a physician's diagnosis or are referred by a physician for consultation to avoid a consultant's fee.

The following questions should be asked of every person on his first visit to the O. P. D.:

1. What is your illness?
2. Have you consulted a physician or visited a dispensary?
3. Do you not feel that you can pay a doctor's fee?
4. What is your total income?
5. How many are dependent on you?
6. Have you ever visited this O. P. D. for treatment? (This question to avoid duplicating records.) The above questions may be varied and added to according to the necessities in each case.

It goes without saying that no patient should be refused treatment if his condition is so urgent that he will receive serious injury thereby.

Administration.—The superintendent of the hospital should also be the superintendent of the O. P. D., but the major part of the actual work can be delegated to an assistant superintendent. The assistant superintendent in charge of the O. P. D. has general charge, and is responsible for the discipline of that department, including the O. P. D. visiting staff, externes, student assistants, and the employees whom he hires. He orders supplies and interviews all persons who apply for treatment for the first time, using the questions under "The Patients," or modifications of them, and decides each case on its merits.

Important questions, as of policy or making radical changes, are decided by the superintendent of the hospital.

The hospital training-school furnishes the nurses which may be necessary to aid in the administrative work, chaperoning, making supplies, and assisting the O. P. D. physicians and surgeons.

The O. P. D. Staff.—The physicians elected to the staff of an O. P. D. should be the members of the local profession who have shown the most ability and aptitude for work of that sort. When vacancies in the hospital staff occur, the men who have best demonstrated their worth in the O. P. D. may be elected to fill them. It would seem wise to have the heads of the various departments in the hospital at the head of the corresponding departments in the O. P. D.

The staff of attending physicians and surgeons, with their assistants, should always be large enough so that every patient may have a careful history taken, a careful examination made, and a course of treatment carefully mapped out and explained to him. Hasty work should never be permitted in an O. P. D., as it is an injustice to the patients, the visiting staff, and the institution.

Punctuality on the part of the visiting staff should be insisted upon.

Records.—For keeping records the separate leaf system seems the best, because of its greater flexibility through the addition of extra sheets as needed, because it allows a separate leaf for each department, when a patient is referred from one department to another, and because of the ease with which a particular record can be obtained when wanted. It also allows of easy expansion of the records in the record room by the addition of filing cases when needed. Two indices only are needed—one of names and one of diseases.

If, after an interview, the assistant superintendent in charge of the O. P. D. considers a patient worthy of treatment, he is sent to a member of the record-room force, who gives him a card made of durable material, with the name of the hospital and the hours when the patient may come to the clinic printed on it. On this the department to which he is assigned is stamped, and his name written, and he is told to preserve this card carefully. At the same time, in the proper place, on the first sheet of his history, the name, age, residence, birthplace, and social condition are written, and the department stamped to correspond with that on the patient's card. The same number is stamped on both the history and the patient's card. In recording the name of a patient, the full name should be used in every instance, thus: John Henry Smith, not John H. Smith, or John Smith. The history is sent to the proper department, and the patient pays his fee, and is given a pass, which directs and admits him to the proper department. On his next and all subsequent visits, the patient presents his card at the door, the number is taken and sent to the record room, that the history may be sent to his department, pays his fee, and is then given his pass to the department stamped on his card. If his card is lost, the patient is referred to the record room, where his number and department are looked up and a new card is issued to him. If it is necessary to transfer a patient from one department to another, this fact is stamped in the body of his history, and the department to which he is transferred is written after it. The old department is crossed off on both history and patient's card, the new department stamped on them, and the patient and history are taken to this department by a messenger. On his next visit the patient will go directly to the new department, as that is the department which will be evident on both the patient's card and history. At the close of the clinic the records are returned to the record room by the externe or person in charge of each department.

It should be an inflexible rule that no patient is ever to have his history in his possession; he should not be allowed an opportunity to read it, and also to avoid the possibility of its destruction or loss.

By the use of the method outlined a history is very rarely lost.

The messengers, during the hours of the clinic, direct patients to the proper departments, carry histories, and act as errand-boys, and during the remainder of the day are employed in the cleaning.

Fees.—It seems a wise provision to charge nominal fees, as in this way the self-respect of many poor patients is preserved, and a portion of the expense of maintaining the O. P. D. may be met.

The following scale of charges seems just:

Admission	10 cents.
X-ray (plates or treatment)	25 cents.
Hydrotherapeutic treatment	25 cents.
Massage	25 cents.
Ether	$1.00 or $2.00.

Medicine, surgical and orthopedic apparatus may be supplied at prices slightly above actual cost. Any of the above except the charges for apparatus can be remitted (by the executive in charge) in worthy cases, and the apparatus can usually be obtained through charitably inclined individuals, or societies when necessary, thus avoiding any hardship to patients.

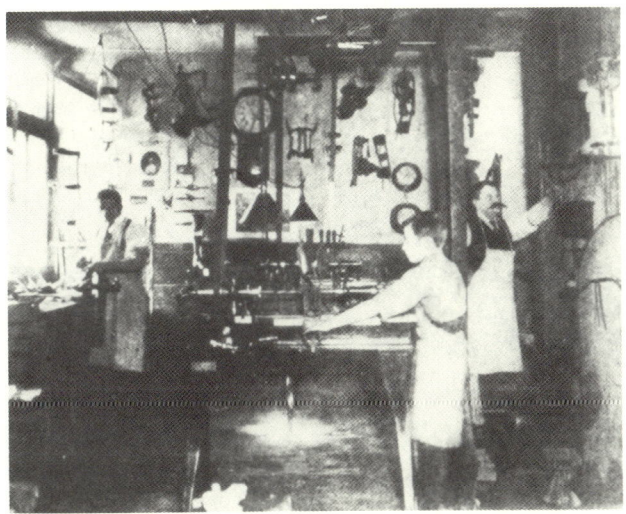

Fig. 152.—Orthopedic workshop, Hospital for Sick Children, Toronto.

Departments.—In addition to the regular departments, as male and female medical, male and female surgical, genito-urinary, children's, nerve, throat, skin, orthopedic, eye and ear, there should be *x*-ray (where may also be installed apparatus for electric and light treatments), and hydrotherapeutic departments, unless these departments in the hospital are available. Arrangements should be made so that massage can be given manually, and if funds and space permit, active and passive movements by the use of machines.

Social Service Department.—Whenever funds are forthcoming, and a sufficient amount of interest is displayed by the O. P. D. staff, a social service department should be established. To this department may be referred all patients whose disease or general condition seems to require aid, either material, mental, or moral. Through this department the physicians and surgeons in charge are brought into closer contact with the patient and his life conditions, thus aiding in diagnosis and treatment, and giving assurance that the treatment prescribed will be carried out. The social service department is thus an aid both to patient and physician. It also assists the executive department in that through its closer contact with patients and their home condition unworthy patients may be detected and excluded.

PARTIAL LIST OF REFERENCES

"Remarks on the Function of an Out-patient Department," Dr. William Osler, British Medical Journal, 1908, p. 1470.

"Hospital, Medical Science, and Public Health," an address by Sir Clifford Albutt at the opening of the Medical Department of the Victoria University, October 1, 1908.

"The Out-patient Department at the Massachusetts General Hospital," Dr. F. A. Washburn, National Hospital Record, April 15, 1909.

"Dispensary Ideals, with a Plan for Dispensary Reform, Based upon the Adoption of the Principles of Restricted Numbers," Dr. S. S. Goldwater, American Journal of Medical Science, September, 1907.

Massachusetts General Hospital Reports, 1880, pp. 33–38.

"The Development of the Work and the Restriction of the Abuse of the Out-patient Department," Dr. J. M. Peters, National Hospital Record, February 15, 1909.

"The Abuse of Medical Charity," Dr. G. W. Gay, Boston Medical and Surgical Journal, March 16, 1905, with discussion by Drs. Derby, Elliott, Worcester, Cobb, Munro, Washburn, Cushing, Crowell, and Cook.

"Hospital and Dispensaries," copied from Medical Times in National Hospital Record, June, 1905.

"The Abuse of the Privileges of the Free Dispensaries and Hospitals," Dr. Clyde Pence in National Hospital Record, February, 1906.

"Medical Charities," Dr. J. J. Nutt in Charities, copied in National Hospital Record, September, 1905.

"Uses and Abuses of Dispensaries: Opinions of the Medical Profession," by Franklin B. Kirkbride, in Proceedings of the Fifth

Annual Conference of the Association of Hospital Superintendents, 1903.

"The Abuse of Medical Charity and a Remedy," Dr. M. O. Magid in American Medicine, January, 1909.

"The Dispensary Abuse Again," copied from Lancet-Clinic in International Hospital Record, January 15, 1910.

"Coöperation in Dispensary Work, as Exemplified by the Association of Tuberculosis Clinics of New York City," Dr. J. A. Miller, International Hospital Record, March, 1909.

"Suggestions for the Reorganization of Hospital Out-patient Departments, with Special Reference to the Improvement of Treatment," Dr. R. C. Cabot, Maryland Medical Journal, March, 1907.

"Why Should Hospitals Neglect the Cases of Chronic Curable Disease in Out-patients?" Dr. R. C. Cabot, St. Paul Medical Journal, March, 1908.

"Dispensary Abuse," Proceedings of the Fourth Annual Conference of the Association of Hospital Superintendents, pp. 119–139, 1902.

SOCIAL SERVICE

"Social Service and the Art of Healing," Dr. R. C. Cabot, Moffat, Yard and Co., 1909.

First, Second, and Third Annual Reports of the Social Service Department of the Massachusetts General Hospital.

First Report of Social Service Work at the Massachusetts Charitable Eye and Ear Infirmary.

"A Glimpse of Social Service in the Hospital," Convalescent Relief Work at the Bellevue Hospital, New York, 1908.

"The Social Service Department of a General Hospital," Dr. C. P. Emerson, National Hospital Record, March, 1909.

"Social Service Work in a Hospital," Helen M. Glenn, International Hospital Record, January 15, 1910.

"Some Unexpected Implications of the Intentions to be Thorough in Medical Work," Dr. R. C. Cabot, copied from Charities and the Commons in National Hospital Record, February, 1906.

"Social Service and the Abuse of Free Work Done by Hospitals," editorial comment, National Hospital Record, February 15, 1909.

"Social Service Work for Graduate Nurses," Ida M. Cannon, The Courant, 1909.

"Visiting Nursing Plus Social Service in Framingham, Massachusetts," International Hospital Record, January 15, 1910.

"The Social Function of the Hospital," Sidney Goldstein, National Hospital Record, July, 1907.

CHAPTER XVIII

THE HOSPITAL LABORATORY

By F. T. Fulton, M.D.

It has been only about a decade since the problem of furnishing adequate laboratory facilities for the ordinary hospital has been really seriously considered. Previously, any sort of a room or closet in the garret or basement, in which a few simpler tests in urinalysis could be carried out was considered sufficient, but every year the need of a well-equipped and well-directed laboratory is more imperative, and year after year the work which is necessarily done in a laboratory has a closer relationship to the welfare of the hospital patient.

In any laboratory there may be two general lines of work—one which is wholly practical and concerned with the diagnosis and treatment of cases within the institution, and the other wholly scientific, concerned only with the questions of research or with the study of pathologic conditions which are met with in the daily hospital routine.

As a matter of fact, it is rare that these two lines of work are entirely separated, and in every laboratory connected with a modern hospital they should be closely interwoven. That which is practical should be of the first importance, and in the regular routine this includes the examinations of surgical specimens, of bacteriologic cultures, the performing of autopsies, making blood examinations, Widal tests, sputum examinations, preparation of vaccines, urinalysis, etc.

THE HOSPITAL LABORATORY 391

The number of rooms necessary and the equipment will depend, of course, upon the size of the institution.

That for a small hospital need be comparatively inexpensive. The best accommodations can be afforded by an entirely separate building close to the main hospital, in which there should be a small autopsy room, with an adjoining room for immediate bacteriologic and microscopic work in connection with the autopsy. There should be a main laboratory room equipped with a first-class in-

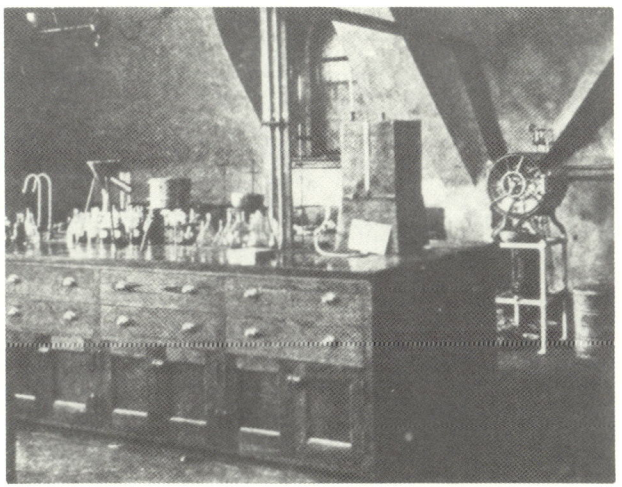

Fig. 153.—Pathologic laboratory, Rhode Island Hospital, Providence.

cubator for bacteria; sterilizer for preparing culture-media; microtomes for cutting sections; a sufficient number of microscopes, and the numerous smaller articles which are necessary for carrying on the work in the laboratory. Besides the main laboratory room, it is desirable to have two or three smaller rooms which may be used for special lines of work, and a room for urinalysis, of sufficient size to accommodate all the apparatus necessary for the simple urine examinations and some of the more complicated tests. A room in which the smaller animals may be kept, such as guinea-pigs, rabbits, etc., is essential. All these rooms should be outside rooms, well lighted, the light being suitable for the use of microscopes. A northern exposure is the best, but windows to the east and west are satisfactory. The main laboratory room, which should be 20 by 30 feet or more, should be provided with desks about the sides, especially along the windows, for the use of mi-

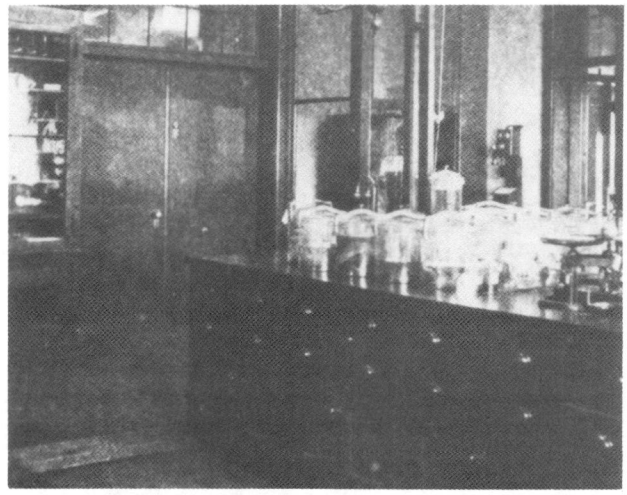

Fig. 154.—Another view of pathologic laboratory, Rhode Island Hospital, Providence.

croscopes. In the central part of the room permanent tables may be built, one or two containing drawers and cupboards beneath. These afford considerable table space, and at the same time add greatly to the drawer and cupboard room which is so essential. In this room there should be an inclosed, ventilated hood in which the sterilizing or operations requiring considerable heat could be carried on.

If it is not possible to have these rooms in a separate

building, arrangements can sometimes be made for them in some part of the hospital building proper. If it is possible to have them in the vicinity of the operating-room, it will be, many times, a great inconvenience.

But the problem of furnishing adequate laboratory facilities for the smaller hospital is, perhaps, not so serious as that of obtaining a properly qualified man to carry on or direct this department. If a hospital is closely connected with a medical school, or if it is situated geographically near a medical school, the matter is always simplified, for under such circumstances there is usually some well-qualified man of the younger generation who is glad to avail himself of the opportunity to have even a small laboratory under his own direction, while he is at the same time engaged in teaching in the medical school or in conducting some research investigations. Such a man can generally be obtained at a nominal salary, or if the hospital is very small, it is possible that the services of some such individual may be obtained without remuneration. The majority of small hospitals, however, are situated away from medical centers or teaching institutions, and unless they are endowed so that they can pay a fair salary, it is impossible to secure a man well trained in pathologic work who is willing to devote his whole time to the laboratory interests. And even when the institution is financially able to pay such an individual, the opportunities which are offered in a small isolated institution are such that no one whose ultimate ambition is advancement in pathologic work is willing to separate himself from the larger institutions, where pathologic material is so much more abundant. Indeed, we must look for a different solution of the question, for, after all, the smaller hospital, and the laboratory which it needs or which it can maintain, is not a very satisfactory place for carrying on research. On the other hand, there are more and more of the younger generation who are coming to see the value of a certain amount of laboratory training as a qualification for a general medical practice or for the practice of more strictly internal medicine, or of surgery. Such men are usually willing to devote from one to several years of their time entirely to laboratory work for the training and experience which it gives to them. After one or two years of time spent in a well-equipped laboratory under the direction of a skilful pathologist, such a young man is well qualified to undertake the direction himself of a laboratory of a small hospital. The question is to make such a place attractive enough so that the institution may be able to obtain a man who has been trained in this way. As stated above, it can be taken for granted that no man who wishes to devote his life to pathology will accept such a position, and the candidates must necessarily be obtained from among those men who are taking a pathologic training for the sake of its bearing on clinical medicine or surgery.

In hospitals where advancement to positions of responsibility on the staff are made largely by virtue of seniority in service, the time which a man may have spent in laboratory or pathologic work should be taken on a par with that which he may have spent in performing the duties of some clinical appointment.

A directorship of a laboratory of a small hospital can be made most attractive to any ambitious medical man who has had a fair experience in pathologic work and who desires to continue that work, but who ultimately wishes to become a clinician, provided that directorship carries with it certain clinical privileges, so that the incumbent may have an opportunity to gain clinical experience, while at the same time continuing his laboratory work. Many a man would be willing to devote all his time to such hospital work when he would be quite unwilling to engage wholly in pathologic or laboratory investigations. Moreover, in a small hospital, the laboratory work and the hospital work will both be made more efficient if there is some such close relation between the departments. One great difficulty has been in the larger hospitals that the interests of the director of the laboratory, who is generally a man of no clinical attainment or affiliation, and the interests of the men holding clinical positions, are not sufficiently associated. I have heard it said by a distinguished pathologist at an autopsy that "If the clinical man would leave this material undisturbed, we could get much more out of it." This man had many warm friends among the clinicians who were his associates, but his interests were so purely concerned with the laboratory part of the investigations that the interests of the clinicians fell, to a certain extent, into the background.

The leading medical centers have for years recognized the importance of a laboratory training on a man's clinical qualifications, and a plan has been recently brought forward suggesting that every hospital should be provided with a clinical laboratory, and that this clinical laboratory should be under the direction of some member of the staff who also has charge of a ward service, and that this ward service should be continuous throughout the year. The man in charge of these two departments must necessarily have had a thorough laboratory training, so that he can intelligently direct both the laboratory work and the clinical work. The plan further suggests that certain of the assistants be engaged in clinical work, and certain others have their time largely occupied with laboratory work, but to have no assistant who was not at some time in his service engaged in both phases. Such a plan would have a very important bearing upon the education of the young and growing members of the staff of the hospital.

There would be no difficulty in obtaining well qualified young men to serve as assistants in such a department, for even when the laboratory work is more strictly confined to pathology, there are a good many recent medical graduates who are very willing to spend their time and make routine examinations of surgical specimens, bacteriologic cultures, autopsies, etc. A year's training of this sort makes a man especially well prepared for one of the positions as regular interne in the hospital, and a combined service of this sort is becoming more and more desirable.

It does not take a very prolonged laboratory training to enable one to appreciate some of the limitations of the laboratory work, and these limitations are usually not at all appreciated by the practitioner who is without any such training. In consequence some of them place entirely too much dependence upon a laboratory report—so much so that they may even discredit their own observations. Others, because an occasional laboratory report may not coincide with their own findings, forget that it is often only an aid to diagnosis, and become skeptical as to its having any value at all. The laboratory findings should be taken only as one feature of the group of symptoms upon which the final judgment must be based. No one appreciates that so well as the man who has been trained in the laboratory and at the bedside.

Certain features of laboratory work can be satisfactorily accomplished by the regular hospital internes. These are the routine sputum examinations, the blood examinations, the serum tests for typhoid fever, and urinalysis. As a rule, it is much better that this work should be done by the interne on the clinical service, for two reasons, first, because his knowledge of the case makes the work of more interest, and, secondly, because of the training which he thus receives.

Much can be done to increase the efficiency of the laboratory if careful records are made, and made in such a way as to be easily available to the hospital staff. When possible, it is an excellent plan to have the records typewritten, as a record prepared in this way will often be read when otherwise it might be scarcely legible. A plan found very useful is to have at least two copies of the record made—one to be filed as part of the laboratory records, the other to be incorporated into the clinical ward history.

The laboratory records should be bound, indexed, and kept in this way on file, so that at any time they are easily available.

If the hospital is in any way connected with a medical

school, it is, of course, one of its duties to supply pathologic material, and all autopsies and surgical specimens should be numbered, and the material filed away properly preserved, so that it may be obtained for subsequent use if desired. In the ordinary hospital, however, this is of much less importance, although it is always well to preserve tissues from interesting conditions, so that at a subsequent time a series of cases may be studied together. In time such material will accumulate and become unwieldy, and the undesirable material can then be discarded. It is a wise plan to preserve all microscopic slides on which the final diagnosis is based for future reference in connection with individual cases or for use in studying any series of cases.

The question as to whether there should be a small museum or collection of pathologic specimens in connection with the laboratory is a debated one. There is no doubt but that it is very desirable that interesting specimens, either surgical or removed at autopsy, should be preserved, for a time at least; there may be an occasion to exhibit them to illustrate certain pathologic conditions.

One line of work which is still somewhat experimental and in the process of development is the preparation and use of bacterial vaccines. The technic in their preparation, though slightly laborious, is not especially complicated, and it is not difficult to train a man to do this work readily. It does add, however, considerable to the laboratory routine and will make it necessary that there should be a larger laboratory force of workers.

An important thing in any laboratory is that there should be some non-professional individual who can be trained to do considerable of the laboratory technic, for the work of cutting and staining sections and preparation of the culture-media, etc., is too burdensome to be entirely upon professional men. It need not take a great deal of time of the man who has become skilful at it, and usually this work may be done by some man or woman who has certain other hospital duties.

CHAPTER XIX

THE ANNUAL REPORT

By Thomas Howell, M.D.

Hospitals, as a rule, publish annual reports of their work. Institutions under control of the Federal Government, individual states, or civic divisions of the latter are ordinarily required by law to do so. Those under private or ecclesiastic auspices feel it incumbent on them to follow the custom.

In order to secure uniformity the authorities of several of the states designate what shall be presented in the annual reports of the institutions supervised and maintained by them. The city and the county hospitals enjoy more or less latitude in compiling their reports.

Private and ecclesiastic hospitals are free to publish whatever their directors deem proper for the best interests of the institution. As a result, there is a regrettable lack of uniformity in their reports.

Most annual reports are made up largely of statistics —facts numerically stated. The information so compiled is of particular interest to hospital trustees, hospital workers, physicians, and contributors.

As has been frequently pointed out, hospitals are peculiar in that the persons who furnish the funds to establish and maintain them do not thereby acquire any proprietary interest in them. They give for humanitarian purposes without expecting to obtain ownership privileges.

Neither do the trustees, who are responsible to the contributors and incorporators for the proper conduct of

THE ANNUAL REPORT

the hospital, possess any proprietary interest in it. And they are not chosen ordinarily because of expert knowledge of the work, but because of their prominence in business, society, and philanthropy, and because it is believed that they will take an active interest in promoting the welfare of the institution. They are usually busy men and women, and cannot be expected to give the hospital's affairs the same attention which they give to their own business.

They appoint the officers and make occasional inspections of the hospital, but here ordinarily, their contactual knowledge of detail ends. They very properly expect that the administrative and operative details shall be attended to by the officers and employees employed and paid for so doing. But, nevertheless, they recognize that they are held responsible by contributors or taxpayers for the proper conduct of the institution. They also recognize that to intelligently administer the trust imposed on them it is necessary that they shall be kept acquainted with the work of the hospital, including all its departments.

Here is where the value of accurate and coördinated statistics becomes manifest. They present a resumptive view of the work. From this, deductions are drawn which are of material assistance in solving present problems and in forecasting future requirements.

To assist them in intelligently deciding current problems, the trustees must receive information on many matters at their regular monthly or semi-monthly meetings, but in addition they, in common with the contributors, desire to have a comprehensive annual report giving in detail such information as the number of patients cared for, the revenue from different sources, how much was expended for the different classes of supplies, how much for improvements and repairs, and how much for other purposes. They like to know the cost of operating the different departments, the average and total cost of caring for private room, ward, medical, surgical, maternity, dispensary, and accident patients. They are interested to learn how much it costs the hospital to train a nurse and the expense involved in nursing a patient; also what the relative expense is of providing food for nurses, domestics, private and ward patients, and officers. They want to know for what purposes the incomes from the various funds are spent, what it costs to maintain a bed for the year, the average cost per ambulance call, the daily average number of beds occupied, the number of free, part-pay, and private patients.

They expect all this information, and much more, carefully compiled, and so presented that it will be easy to compare the work done by the hospital one year with another. And, if possible, they like to have these statistics so tabulated that they are comparable with those of other institutions of similar organization and doing the same kind of work.

To be of value, it is essential that statistics should be accurately and intelligently compiled. Too often this work is allowed to accumulate until the end of the year and then done under time limit.

Frequently people unacquainted with clerical work and the interpretation of statistical data, internes, for example, are required to tabulate the statistics. They resent being asked to do this class of work, and hurry through it, only anxious to dispose of it as speedily and easily as possible. The result is that the product produced by these amateur statisticians is so full of errors as to render it of little value. I have seen the same glaring inaccuracies repeated in reports for several successive years.

The statistics for the annual report should be compiled by, or under the direction of, a clerk who is capable of collecting, analyzing and tabulating statistical data, and who is likely to remain in the employ of the institution for a number of years. Carefully gotten up in this way, hospital statistics are of real value; inaccurately compiled, they are misleading and useless.

The board of directors of a new institution, or of an institution the annual report of which leaves much to be desired, will do well to study the reports of a number of the leading hospitals before deciding what theirs shall contain, and before adopting a system of statistics. Among many others, those issued by the following institutions are worthy of study: Massachusetts General, Boston City and Homeopathic Hospitals of Boston; Bellevue, Presbyterian, New York, Roosevelt, Mt. Sinai Hospitals of New York; the Hartford Hospital of Hartford, Connecticut; the Rhode Island Hospital of Providence, Rhode Island; the City Hospital of Worcester, Massachusetts; the Pennsylvania Hospital of Philadelphia; the Buffalo General of Buffalo, New York; the Allegheny General Hospital of Allegheny, Pennsylvania; the Evanston Hospital of Evanston, Illinois.

The chapter on Hospital Bookkeeping, and the section on Uniform Hospital Accounting and Statistics, which follows at the end of this chapter, and which gives the headings and rulings of a uniform accounting and reporting scheme adopted by a considerable number of the leading hospitals of New York and other cities, should be carefully studied. The general adoption of the system of accounting and of arranging statistical data therein laid down would result in uniformity of statistics and facility of comparisons.

It is essential to start right, for frequent changes in the arrangement of a hospital's annual report render it of little value for reference. Routinism in the arrangement of a report is of great value, as any one who has searched them or has attempted the reduction of the statistics of different hospitals to a common basis will testify. It expedites and renders comparatively easy what is otherwise tedious and difficult.

What an Annual Report Should Contain.—"What shall be included in our annual report?" is a question often propounded, both by novices and experts in hospital management. It is not an easy one to answer. If all hospitals were supported and supervised in the same manner, and if their organizations and functions were the same, the problem would be easier of solution. As it is, nearly every hospital is surrounded with conditions peculiar to itself, and what would be an ideal report for one, would be wholly unsuitable for another.

Uniformity in hospital reports, of which we hear so much just now, does not mean that all hospitals should publish reports similar in all particulars—far from it. Each hospital has, or should have, an individuality. The reports should reflect this individuality. To make reports identical in all details would not only rob them of their individualities, but would result in a tiresome sameness. This would be undesirable. But they can be uniform in certain particulars, without losing their distinctive characteristics.

There is no reason, however, why a common nomenclature should not be used, and the financial statistics analyzed and compiled in a fairly uniform manner. Unless this be done, it is impossible to make intelligent comparisons of the work done by different institutions.

All hospital reports are published for the same purpose —that is, to furnish information. But authorities differ as to the kind of information which should be published, just as newspaper editors differ as to what constitutes news. Some think that the public wants to know, or has a right to know, all the details; others think not. Some think that the financial aspect of the institution should receive the most attention; others think the non-financial statistics are more entitled to consideration.

Inasmuch as persons of intelligence differ as to just what a report should contain, it would appear best to cover briefly, yet comprehensively, all phases of the hospital's activities, allowing the readers to select what they shall read.

However, it is doubtful whether elaborate amplification is desirable in an annual report. Many hospitals publish their disbursements in great detail. Not content with grouping their expenditures, they use up many pages in stating the amounts paid for nail-files, nipple-shields, crutch-tips, mop-sticks, tin dippers, darning cotton, axle-grease, etc.

The total amount paid in a year for a particular item means nothing unless the inventories are compared.

If instead of publishing the total amounts paid for each of these thousand and one items, the average prices paid for them were published, it would not appear so useless, as this would tend to show whether or not the steward is a close buyer. But it is doubtful if even this is of sufficient interest and importance to justify the time and expense involved.

Hospitals are not founded for the purpose of purchasing goods—this is merely incidental. They are founded for the reception and care of sick persons. The patient should be the unit from which to reckon costs. Accordingly, the annual report should place emphasis, not on the total amount spent for each of the various supplies, but on the cost per day and year of supplying a patient with such items as food, medical supplies, and nursing.

The report is published to be read, to inform the public concerning the work done by the hospital, what it hopes to accomplish, and what its needs are. It should be made interesting. The literary style should be simple. The facts should be clearly and concisely stated. It should be borne in mind that the average person is averse to mental effort, except where his own interests are concerned. His energies are consumed in studying and managing his own affairs. Long, complicated sentences, and big, unusual words should be avoided. Paragraphs should be short and numerous headings introduced.

Where it can be conveniently done, it is well to give the percentage of the increase or decrease, as percentages mean much to the average reader.

Unless the mass of facts contained in the report be well arranged, it will prove uninteresting reading, and soon find its way to the waste-basket. Hospital officials should, therefore, give considerable attention to their reports and should see to it that they are gotten up in the very best manner.

It should be remembered that many people who never

see the hospital or meet its officials have only the annual report to judge it by, and their estimate of the institution will be largely influenced by the general make-up of the report. Cheap paper and poor typographic work will detract from it, no matter how well the reports of the officers are written and the statistics tabulated.

The majority of persons will disregard the statistical tables and content themselves with reading the reports of the president of the board of trustees, the treasurer, and superintendent. The reports of these officers, based largely upon the statistics, should be carefully prepared.

The statistical tables are published for the benefit of those who desire more detailed information, or who, for one reason or another, prefer to draw their own deductions from them.

After the exact form of the tables and their headings have been decided upon by the statistician, the work of tabulating is largely automatic.

The subjoined list of headings, compiled from the reports of half a dozen leading hospitals, shows what the annual report may contain. It is hardly probable that every one of these would be used by any one hospital, but those marked with an asterisk form the basis of all reports.

* Names of officers and members of the board of trustees, standing committees, medical and surgical staffs, internes, executive officers of the institution.
* Report of the president or executive committee.
* Treasurer's report, with statement of funds.
* Report of auditor.
  Report of standing committees.
  Report of medical board.
  Report of ladies' aid association.
* Report of superintendent, including statistical tables and statement of current expenses.
  Report of the principal of the training-school for nurses.
  Report of the district nurse.

- * Training-school information, including curriculum.
- Report of pathologist.
- Report of skiagrapher.
- Report of apothecary.
- Medical and surgical statistics, including list of operations and causes of death.
- * Out-patient department statistics.
- * Contributions.
- * Permanent free beds.
- * Annual free beds.
- * List of articles presented to the hospital.
- * List of donators and members.
- * List of guarantors of deficiency.
- Report of librarian.
- Roll of trustees.
- Roll of nurses.
- Roll of internes.
- * Admission of patients, rules, and rates.
- House rules.
- Act of corporation.
- By-laws, rules, and regulations.

The Trustees' Report.—In nearly all annual reports the first few pages are given up to the names of incorporators, trustees, medical staff, officers, and internes. The report of the board of trustees generally follows this list of names. There are certain hospitals where the trustees make no report except through the superintendent; sometimes the reverse obtains, the trustees making the report for both.

The writer is of the opinion that one well-written comprehensive report, concisely summarizing the year's work, is better than two, both of which must be read in order to obtain an understanding of the hospital's activities and needs. Generally, however, the trustees and superintendent make separate reports, and where this is the case, it will be necessary to have a distinct understanding as to just what each is to discuss, in order to avoid the duplication of subjects.

The report of the trustees should deal broadly, but briefly, with the larger affairs of the hospital, such as the purchase and sale of land, the construction of buildings, bequests, changes in the medical and executive staffs, financial estimates, general administration, and projected improvements. It should discuss the large affairs because these interest the contributors; it should discuss them briefly to insure their being read.

The discussion of matters of detail should be delegated to the executive officers.

Treasurer's Report.—The report of the treasurer should contain detailed information regarding the hospital's finances, the receipts, disbursements, and resources. The condition of the various funds and in what securities they are invested should be fully and clearly stated in order that the public in general, and particularly that part of it which contributes to the support of the hospital, may understand just what its financial condition is. The hospital which does not take the contributing public into its confidence and correctly inform it as to the condition of its finances, should not expect to receive its support.

Either in the treasurer's or in the superintendent's report the total amount of bills receivable should be compared with those on hand at the close of the previous year. This is not ordinarily done, but unless it is done, the statement of the hospital's financial condition is incomplete. No business house would think of compiling a balance sheet which did not show its current assets and liabilities. The publication of this statement will also tend to increase the efficiency of the hospital's collector.

The treasurer's report is largely a matter of bookkeeping, and is thoroughly discussed in a preceding chapter.

The Superintendent's Report.—The superintendent is the chief executive of the hospital. He is the one to whom the heads of all departments report, and he is supposed to be conversant with all administrative affairs. His report will cover most of the important events of the year. The statistical tables are ordinarily a part of it. It will show in tabular form the number of admissions, daily average number of patients, per capita cost, average length of stay in the hospital, number of accidents, out-patient cases treated, nationalities, residences, civil conditions, ages, occupations, and condition at time of discharge of all patients admitted. It will also contain a list of the expenditures for the year, contrasted with those of the preceding year.

The superintendent will be expected to discuss such matters as finances, statistics, improvements and repairs, special needs of the institution, charity and paying patients, ambulance service, etc.

Report of the Principal of Training-school.—The report of the principal of the training-school will be addressed to the trustees or to the superintendent of the hospital, depending upon the manner in which the hospital is organized. In some institutions the superintendent of nurses makes no annual report, the superintendent of the hospital covering in his report the matters ordinarily reported on by the training-school principal.

This report will deal entirely with matters connected with the school, such as the number of graduates employed, the number of pupil nurses, the number of probationers received during the year, the number accepted, the number of nurses assigned to each of the various departments, changes in the curriculum, resignations, promotions, dismissals, etc.

Unless the school issues a prospectus annually, the report of the hospital should contain such information concerning the school, faculty, and curriculum as a woman contemplating entering a training-school would wish to know.

Report of the Medical Board.—The medical board sometimes prepares for publication in the annual report a summary of the professional work accomplished or initiated during the year, together with recommendations for changes and improvements which, in the opinion of the board, will enhance the welfare of the patients and add to the efficiency of the hospital.

It is also customary to have reports from the pathologic and x-ray departments.

Reports of the Standing Committees.—Under this heading are included the reports of the committees on training-school, on investments, on membership, and various other auxiliary committees. In the majority of hospitals committees of this class will make no written reports for publication in the annual report, but in some instances considerable prominence is given to them.

Report of Ladies' Aid Associations.—Ladies' aid associations render valuable services to charitable hospitals conducted on the voluntary system, as are most of the hospitals in the United States. It is customary for this committee to prepare a statement of its work for publication in the annual report.

The Inventory.—In order to ascertain the exact cost of operating the hospital and to determine the average cost per day of caring for patients, it will be necessary to take an inventory of the stock on hand at the close of the year and to compare it with the corresponding inventory of the previous year.

Very few institutions publish their inventories, but it would appear well to do so, as they furnish interesting information. When the heads of the departments who have this work in charge know that it is to be published, they are likely to be more careful in compiling it.

Whether it be published or not, the inventory of stock on hand should be taken each year, as it is impossible to get at the exact costs without doing so.

Private-room Service Statistics.—The demand for hospital privileges on the part of the well-to-do marks a new epoch in hospital development. Until recently hospitals made no attempt to attract private patients, or to furnish them with suitable accommodations. They are now reaching out for this class. Hospital managers think that by so doing they will be enabled to add to their net income, and with the increment thus obtained, care for more charity patients.

However, very few managers of hospitals which maintain private patient services know whether they are conducting them at a profit or at a loss, for the reason that they do not insist on an accurate system of statistics being introduced and maintained.

The manufacturing concern which does not ascertain the cost of manufacturing its goods will ordinarily finally become insolvent; and the hospital which does not know what it costs to care for its private patients will probably be burdened with an increasing deficit.

Hospital officials should have definite, concrete knowledge of the cost of caring for private patients. Having this knowledge, they will then be in a position to establish a suitable schedule of rates, and they will no longer be deceived into believing that their private-room service is producing a profit, when in reality it is increasing the deficit.

Cases Treated, with Results.—The majority of hospitals publish their morbidity statistics in great detail; the minority publish none.

Whether these statistics are valuable enough to justify the labor, time, and money spent on them is a mooted question. At any event, they are only of use to medical men. I have talked with many physicians regarding these statistics; most of them say that while they ordinarily glance over them, they rarely make any use of them. Occasionally a member of the staff, in preparing a paper, will consult them.

The trustees of the Rhode Island Hospital, Providence, about two years ago went into this question very carefully. They addressed letters to the members of their staffs and to the superintendents of other hospitals, in order to obtain, if possible, data that would assist them in deciding whether to continue the publication of their rather elaborate statistical tables. They have summarized the questions and replies as follows:

Staff.—1. Do you think it worth the time and trouble and expense to publish the medical and surgical statistics of the patients treated in the hospital?

2. What advantage are they to the hospital or to the medical staff?

3. What is your own personal feeling in regard to the necessity of publishing these statistics?

	Yes.	Question.	No.
Question 1	8	1	15
Question 2	8	1	16
Question 3	7	4	14

Superintendents of Other Hospitals.—1. Do you publish in detail the medical and surgical statistics of the patients treated in your hospital?

2. If so, do you think it worth the time, trouble, and expense?

3. Who consults these statistics, or what advantage are they to the hospital or to the medical staff?

4. What is your own personal feeling in regard to the necessity of publishing these statistics?

	Yes.	Question.	No.
Question 1	12	2	
Question 2	3	5	7
Question 3	3	3	6
Question 4	2	5	6

It will be seen that fifteen members of the staff and seven superintendents thought that the statistics were of little use and not worth the time, trouble, and expense of compiling and publishing; eight members of the staff and three superintendents thought they were of value; and one member of the staff and five superintendents were in doubt.

These replies do not settle the question. The Rhode Island Hospital trustees, after careful consideration, decided to make no change in their statistics for the present.

Between the two extremes—entire absence of medical and surgical tables on one hand, and elaborate detail on the other—it would seem that a happy mean might be found. If a hospital admitting, say, 5000 patients annually, were to devote from six to ten pages of its report to accurately compiled and carefully tabulated medical and surgical statistics, the probabilities are that this would give general satisfaction.

If, however, the hospital staff comprises several men with wide professional reputations, it probably is best to publish more elaborate morbidity statistics, for in this case they will be frequently referred to by medical men.

Photographs.—There are many who believe that photographs of hospital scenes add much to the attractiveness of a report. They serve to arrest attention, and many people who would not ordinarily read a line of a report will display much interest in the pictures. Having glanced over them, they are much more likely to become interested in the reading matter.

Inasmuch as pictures serve to attract attention to a report, it would seem as though their publication is desirable.

The Average Cost per Day.—Hospitals publish in their annual reports the average cost per day of caring for patients, but under the existing conditions the costs obtained by the different institutions are not comparable, for the reason that identical methods are not employed in obtaining them.

The following methods employed by hospitals in ascertaining the average cost per day per patient, serve to indicate how worthless the per capita costs as arrived at by the different institutions are for the purposes of comparison:

(1) The cost is obtained by dividing the total expenditure for the year by the total number of days' care furnished patients.

(2) The expenditures for improvements and new construction are deducted before dividing.

(3) The out-patient department expenses are deducted, but those of the accident department are included.

(4) The expenditures for extensive improvements, new construction, out-patient, and accident departments are all deducted.

(5) Minor accident cases treated in the accident room are counted as hospital patients.

(6) The income from all sources is deducted.

(7) The inventory is disregarded.

(8) The expenditure for special nursing for private patients is deducted.

(9) The number of patients in the hospital at a certain hour is regarded as the daily average.

(10) The number of patients treated during the entire twenty-four hours, which includes both admissions and discharges, is regarded as the daily average.

These are only a few of the discrepancies, but they will serve to emphasize the necessity of securing uniformity in methods before comparisons will be of value.

Inasmuch as the statement of the per capita cost is the most important one in a report, and attracts the greatest amount of attention, it does seem as though every effort should be made to render it a comparable one.

An excellent method to use in ascertaining the average cost per day of caring for bed patients is to add to the total expense of the hospital for the year the value of the stock on hand at the end of the preceding year, then deduct the expenses of the out-patient and accident departments, and all extraordinary expenses, such as those for land, new construction, etc., and the value of the stock on hand at the close of the year; then divide the result by the total number of days' care furnished patients.

This method is made clear by arranging it in tabular form as follows:

Total expense of hospital for year 1908		$100,000.00
Stock on hand December 31, 1907		10,000.00
		$110,000.00
Deduct:		
Expense of out-patient department	$5,000.00	
Expense of accident room	1,000.00	
Land, new construction, etc	10,000.00	
Stock on hand December 31, 1908	15,000.00	31,000.00
Total expense of caring for bed patients		$ 79,000.00

This sum ($79,000), divided by the total number of days' board furnished, will give the daily per capita cost.

In obtaining the per capita cost of caring for patients it is not ordinarily customary to take into consideration any charge for capital account, interest, or depreciation of plant.

Table of Contents.—If the annual report be of considerable size, an index should be published either on the first or last page, otherwise difficulty will be experienced by persons not familiar with it in promptly obtaining facts they may desire.

Pertinent Facts Relating to Hospital.—It would be convenient if every hospital were to publish on the inside of its cover-page a brief summary of important facts relative to its history, growth, and work. The list might include, among others, the following items:

When founded.

When incorporated.

When important buildings were opened.

Amount of endowment.

Amount of bequests during the year.

Annual expenditures.

When training-school was established.

Total number of bed patients treated since opening of hospital.

Number treated the past year in hospital beds.

Number treated the past year in dispensary.

Amount required to found a free bed.

When ambulance service was established.

Number of beds in hospital.

Per capita cost for the year.

The Publication of By-Laws.—A number of hospitals publish in their annual reports the by-laws of the corporation, and also the rules and regulations governing the officers and employees of the hospital.

It hardly seems necessary to do this. It appears to be almost a waste of labor, paper, and money. Comparatively few people who read the report care anything about the rules and regulations. If they are interested in them, it is an easy matter to procure a copy of them from the hospital.

Books for Statistical Data.—The books used in different institutions for keeping data from which the monthly and annual statistics are compiled, vary greatly. It is difficult to describe any system that will meet with the approval of all superintendents, or even the majority of them. The sources of the financial statistics are described in a previous chapter.

Unless the statistics are kept for each day, it will be impossible to compile them at the close of the year with any degree of accuracy.

Most institutions have a large register in which the names of the patients are entered as they are admitted. This register shows the following facts relative to each patient, when obtainable: Birthplace, age, residence, civil condition, sex, occupation, disease or disability, and physical condition on discharge. The headings and rulings for this book are shown in form No. 1.

Another book, the daily index, gives the number admitted, treated, and discharged. It also gives the service to which the patients are assigned, and whether free, pay, or private. The deaths are entered in this index. At the end of each month the different columns are added, in order to ascertain the number of days' treatment given males and females, medical, surgical, maternity, and private patients, and also the number of each of the same classes admitted and discharged. The daily averages are then obtained by dividing these totals by the number of days in the month. The rulings and headings for the daily index are shown in form No. 2.

In another index a daily record is kept of the number of persons employed as officers, nurses, orderlies, and in other capacities; also the number of officers, nurses, orderlies and other employees boarded. The rulings and headings of this book are shown in form No. 3.

In the out-patient department, in addition to the large register in which the names, ages, occupations, and residences of patients are kept, there will be an index which will show the number of new and returning cases treated each day, and the divisions in which they received treatment. This index is illustrated in form No. 4.

In the postmortem register will be recorded the names of deceased persons, the date and hour of death, together with the causes of death.

The operation book will contain a list of all operations that are done.

The donation book will contain a list of all persons donating flowers, books, magazines, newspapers, etc.

HEADINGS OF UNIFORM ACCOUNTING AND REPORTING SCHEME ADOPTED BY LEADING HOSPITALS OF NEW YORK AND OTHER CITIES

SCHEDULE 1.

DETAILED STATEMENT OF OPERATING, CORPORATION, AND OTHER CURRENT EXPENSES.

Administration Expenses.

Salaries—officers' and clerks'.
Office expenses.
Stationery, printing, and postage.
Telephone and telegraph.
Legal expenses.
Miscellaneous.
 Total administration expenses.

Professional Care of Patients.

Salaries and wages.
Physicians.
Superintendent of nurses, assistant, and instructors.
Nurses.
Special nurses.
Orderlies.
Special orderlies.
Ward employees.
Equipment for nurses.
Uniforms.
Books.
Instruments.
Apparatus and instruments.
Medical supplies.
Surgical supplies.
Alcohol, liquors, wines, etc.

Dispensary:
    Emergency ward: } Salaries and labor.
    Visiting and home (district) nursing: } Supplies.
        Total professional care of patients.

Department Expenses.

Ambulance.
Pathologic laboratory.
Training-school.
Housekeeping.   Salaries and labor.
Kitchen.   Supplies.
Laundry.
Steward's department.
  Labor.
  Provisions:
    Bread.
    Milk and cream.
    Groceries.
    Butter and eggs.
    Fruit and vegetables.
    Meat, poultry, and fish.
      Total: steward's department.
      Total department expenses.

General House and Property Expense.

Electric lighting.
Fuel, oil, and waste.
Gas.
Ice.
Insurance.
Maintenance—real estate and buildings.
Maintenance—machinery and tools.
Plumbing and steam-fitting.
Photography.
Rent.
Miscellaneous.
  Total general house and property expenses.
  Total operating expenses.

Corporation or Other Current Expenses.

Salaries—officers' and clerks'.
Stationery, printing, and postage.
Legal expenses.
Interest on mortgages or loans payable.
Taxes.
Miscellaneous.
  Total corporation expenses.
Current expenses from special funds for stated purposes
  (Show expenditure from each fund separately).
    Grand total current expenses.
Excess of current revenue over current expenses.
  Total.

SCHEDULE 2.

DETAILED STATEMENT OF CURRENT REVENUE.

Hospital Receipts (or Operating Receipts).

Private-room patients.
Board of friends of patients.
Ward pay patients.
Special nursing.
Dispensary.
Emergency ward.
Ambulance fees.
Miscellaneous.
   Total hospital receipts.

Other Revenue or Income.

From the public treasury.
Donations from individuals to meet current expenses.
Donations from churches to meet current expenses.
From hospital Saturday and Sunday Association
Net receipts from entertainments, fairs, fêtes, etc.
Legacies, unrestricted.
Profits in investments sold.
Revenue from investments or funds for current use.
Miscellaneous.
   Total other revenue or income.
Income from special funds for current expenses.
(Show income account of each fund separately).
   Grand total current revenue.
Excess current expenses over current revenue.
   Total.

SCHEDULE 3.

SUMMARY OF FINANCIAL TRANSACTIONS FOR THE YEAR.

Capital Expenditures.

Additions to sites and grounds.
Additions and betterments, buildings.
Furniture and fixtures (if charged to capital account).
New machinery (if charged to capital account)
Apparatus and instruments (if charged to capital account).
Ambulances, live-stock, etc. (if charged to capital account).
Miscellaneous.
   Total capital expenditures.

Surplus Account.

  Grand total current expenses, Schedule 1.
Loss and depreciation.
    (Show items separately if desired).
    Total.
Surplus for the year.
    Total.

Summary of Financial Transactions for Year.

Capital Receipts.

Fully endowed beds.
Partly endowed beds.
General or special funds or gifts for other than current expenses.
(Show receipts account of each fund or gift separately).
 Total capital receipts.

Deficit Account.

Grand total revenue, Schedule 2.
Amount charged off endowed bed fund or other fund reserves account liability of hospital having ceased.
 Total.
 Deficit for the year.
 Total.

SCHEDULE 4.

Comparative Balance Sheet for Years.

Capital Assets.

Hospital properties and equipments:
 Sites and grounds.
 Buildings.
 Furniture and fixtures.
  Machinery and tools.
 Apparatus and instruments.
 Ambulances, live-stock, etc.
 Miscellaneous.
Investments:
 Mortgages receivable.
 Bonds.
 Stocks.
 Other investments.
  Total capital assets.

Current Assets.

Loans and notes receivable.
Accounts receivable.
Accounts receivable from public treasury.
General material on hand.
Cash in hands of treasurer.
Cash in hands of superintendent.
Advances:
 Prepaid insurance.
 Other prepaid expenses.
  Total current assets.
  Grand total assets.
  Deficit.
  Total.

COMPARATIVE BALANCE SHEET FOR YEARS.

Capital Liabilities.

Capital account (hospital properties and equipments).
Endowed bed fund reserves.
Partly endowed bed fund reserves.
Other fund reserves.
  (List each separately).
Bonds outstanding on hospital property.
Mortgages payable.
  Total capital liabilities.

Current Liabilities.

Loans and notes payable.
Audited vouchers unpaid or accounts payable.
  Total current liabilities.
  Grand total liabilities.
    Surplus.
    Total.

SCHEDULE 5.

STATEMENT SHOWING INCREASE OR DECREASE OF PRINCIPAL OF ALL CAPITAL FUNDS DURING YEAR ENDED DECEMBER 31, 1909.

Description of funds.	Amount Dec. 31, 1908.	Received during year.	Expended during year.	Amount Dec. 31, 1909.	Increase.	Decrease.
Total..........						

SCHEDULE 6.

COMPARATIVE STATISTICS FOR YEARS 1910, 1909.

Hospital Wards and Private Rooms.

Patients in hospital first of year:
  In medical wards. ⎫
  In surgical wards. ⎬ Male.
  In private rooms. ⎭
    Total.

Patients admitted during year:
    To medical wards. ⎫
    To surgical wards. ⎬ Female.
    To private rooms. ⎭
      Total.

Total patients treated in hospital wards and private rooms during year:
    Male.
    Female.

Patients discharged during year:
    Cured. ⎫
    Improved. ⎪
    Unimproved. ⎬ Male.
    Transferred to other institutions. ⎪
    Died. ⎭
      Total.

Patients in hospital end of year:
    In medical wards. ⎫
    In surgical wards. ⎬ Female.
    In private rooms. ⎭
      Total.

Total patients days' treatment. ⎫   Free ward.
Percentage.   ⎬   Endowed bed.
Average patients per day.   ⎭   Pay ward.
                                                 Private room.
    Total.

Average time per patient in hospital.
Daily average cost per private-room patient.
Daily average cost per ward patient.

Emergency Ward.

Patients under treatment first of year. ⎫ Male.
Patients admitted during year.   ⎭
Total patients treated during year.   ⎫
Patients discharged during year.   ⎬ Female.
Patients under treatment end of year. ⎭
Visits made to emergency ward during year.
Average visits made per day.
Average visits per patient.
Daily average cost per emergency ward patient.

Dispensary.

Patients under treatment first of year. ⎫ Male.
Patients admitted during year.   ⎭
Total patients treated during year.   ⎫
Patients discharged during year.   ⎬ Female.
Patients under treatment end of year. ⎭
Visits made to dispensary during year.
Average visits per day.
Average visits per patient.
Daily average cost per dispensary patient.

Ambulance.

Ambulance calls during year.
Average calls per day.
Average cost per ambulance call.
Patients treated by ambulance surgeon in emergency ward and transferred.
Patients treated by ambulance surgeon and left at place of call or transferred direct to other institutions.

Visiting of Home (District) Nursing.

Number of patients visited.
Number of visits made.
Average visits per day.
Average cost per visit.

Summary.

Total patients treated during year in all departments.
Average patients per day in all departments.
Daily average number of employees boarded in hospital.
Daily cost per capital for provisions for all persons supported.

422 HOSPITAL MANAGEMENT

Form 77

Number	Name	Ward	When admitted	Age	Civil Cond.	Birthplace	Occupation	Residence	Service

Fig. 155.—Form for daily record.

Form 42 General Hospital

_____ 191_

Day of Month	Treated								Admitted								Discharged							Deaths
	Males	Females	Total	Medical	Surgical	Major	Special	Private	Males	Females	Medical	Surgical	Major	Special	Private		Males	Females	Medical	Surgical	Major	Special	Private	
1																								
2																								
3																								
4																								
5																								
6																								
7																								
8																								
9																								
10																								
11																								
12																								
13																								
14																								
15																								
16																								
17																								
18																								
19																								
20																								
21																								
22																								
23																								
24																								
25																								
26																								
27																								
28																								
29																								
30																								
31																								
Total																								
Daily Average																								

Fig. 156.—Form for monthly report.

HOSPITAL MANAGEMENT

Form #3

General Hospital

_____ 191 ___

Day of Month	Employed						Boarded						
	Males	Females	Officers	Nurses	Orderlies	Other Employees	Males	Females	Officers	Nurses	Orderlies	Other Employees	
1													
2													
3													
4													
5													
6													
7													
8													
9													
10													
11													
12													
13													
14													
15													
16													
17													
18													
19													
20													
21													
22													
23													
24													
25													
26													
27													
28													
29													
30													
31													
Total													
Average													

Fig. 157.—Form for monthly report.

Fig. 158.—Form for monthly report.

General Hospital

....191

Name..

Security	Disease	Duration of Disease	Result	When discharged	Paying		Free		Number	Remarks
					wks	dys	wks	dys		

Fig. 159.—Specimen form.

APPENDIX I

TRAINING-SCHOOL REGULATIONS AND SUGGESTIONS

REPORT OF SPECIAL TRAINING-SCHOOL COMMITTEE

Henry M. Hurd, M.D., Johns Hopkins Hospital, Baltimore, Md.; F. A. Washburn, M.D., Massachusetts General Hospital, Boston, Mass.; Miss Charlotte A. Aikens, 722 Sheridan Ave., Detroit, Mich.; Miss Mary M. Riddle, Newton General Hospital, Newton Lower Falls, Mass.; Miss Mary L. Keith, Rochester City Hospital, Rochester, N. Y.; W. L. Babcock, M.D., The Grace Hospital, Detroit, Mich.

TO THE AMERICAN HOSPITAL ASSOCIATION:

Your Committee, appointed by the President, begs to report on the following resolutions referred to it by the Association at its Tenth Annual Conference:

Resolved, That a committee be appointed, consisting of seven members of this organization and the President Ex-officio, whose duty it shall be—

First: To seek information from leading physicians, surgeons, nurses, and training-school committees, and from every available source, bearing upon the curriculum and length of the course of training of our nurses.

Second: To consider to what extent hospitals should undertake to prepare a class of nurse helpers or assistants.

Third: To prepare a model curriculum, containing only such subjects as they deem necessary for the proper training of a regular nurse or nurse helper, and to report at the next annual meeting of this Association.

The recommendations of this Committee were made after fully considering the needs of both training-schools and hospitals, together with such related factors as required consideration. It is not possible in the present state of hospital work to recommend or bring about certain more or less ideal conditions for a training-school. The Committee recognizes that it might be desirable to have a preparatory course of several months' duration, the teaching of this course to be conducted outside of the hospital by trained paid instructors. Such a preparatory course would enable the pupil to approach her practical hospital work with a substantial foundation of knowledge. Many, at present, unsurmountable conditions, educational, professional, financial, etc., prevent carrying out these and other desirable innovations in all hospitals.

In considering the mutual and related interests of hospitals and training-schools, it was early recognized by the Committee that general hospitals of from twenty-five to fifty or seventy-five beds could not be considered from the same standpoint as large city institutions of two hundred beds or over, whose functions of late years have broadened and diversified along special and sociologic lines. Owing to this fact, the classification of hospitals which follows was found necessary by the Committee in working out a detailed curriculum for the training-school. In this division, the Committee has been careful not to lose sight of the interests of the training-school as a school or, in other words, has tried to consider the interests of the school apart from the hospital, wherever possible. At the same time the Committee recognizes that the training-school is an integral part of and subordinate to the hospital.

CLASSIFICATION OF HOSPITALS

1. Isolated small hospitals.
2. Small hospitals near to, or in affiliation with, large general hospitals.
3. Special hospitals, including eye and ear, skin and cancer, children's and infants', lying-in, tuberculosis, orthopedic hospitals, etc.; sanatoria for nervous and mental diseases, hospitals for contagious diseases; hospitals for the insane, and hospitals for incurables.
4. Large general hospitals.

It is the sense of the Committee that hospitals of less than twenty-five beds, which cannot affiliate or maintain some association with larger institutions, on account of their isolation or financial condition, should not attempt to maintain training-schools for the training of nurses.

The following general recommendations, to cover all classes of hospitals, were adopted by the Committee:

1. That a probationary term of not less than three months be maintained.
2. That probationers be admitted in classes, at regular intervals, preferably twice yearly.
3. That a preliminary course of study, of not less than three months' duration, be given to each class, such course to include practical demonstrations of general nursing methods.
4. That at least two weeks of the preliminary course be given before allowing pupils to assume any nursing responsibility.
5. That pupil nurses should not be called upon to give more than sixty-three hours per week to their work, including class hours and exclusive of time off duty. Emergency work out of hours, or overtime work, should be repaid pupils as soon as possible. All time lost by illness of pupils should be made up at the end of the course.
6. That all hospitals which cannot give one of the courses hereinafter outlined, in its entirety, should seek affiliation with other hospitals in the subjects not covered by the class of patients under treatment.

APPENDIX

7. That paid medical instructors should be employed by all hospitals that can afford to employ them. The Committee has ascertained that a few hundred dollars per year will furnish competent paid instructors for the work. Where paid instructors cannot be maintained, arrangements should be made to have the lectures and strictly medical teaching of the school presented by two or three medical men, rather than by a larger number of physicians.

8. That a vacation of at least two weeks per year for the two years three months' course, and three weeks per year for the three years' course be allowed all pupils during the summer months.

9. That all hospitals maintaining training-schools of any character, including hospitals for the insane, employ a graduate nurse as Superintendent of nurses.

10. That no hospital should attempt to maintain a training-school for nurses if it cannot meet the requirements of the two years three months' minimum course, or arrange affiliations with other hospitals that will provide full equivalents.

11. That training-schools should not be maintained in small hospitals without at least two paid resident instructors being provided for the teaching of nurses, one of whom must necessarily be Superintendent of the hospital and Principal of the training-school. That all hospitals, irrespective of size, have a graduate nurse as night supervisor. This number should be considered the absolute minimum, irrespective of the size of the school.

12. That many large general hospitals can advantageously establish a course of six or nine months in hospital economics administration and institutional nursing. This recommendation is made in response to the great demand for nurses trained in hospital or institutional work to fill positions in training-schools or other hospital departments.

QUALIFICATIONS FOR ADMISSION AS A PROBATIONER TO THE PRELIMINARY COURSE

1. Age, twenty-one to thirty-five years.
2. Height and weight, average.
3. Physical health, sight, and hearing should be normal.
4. Physical examination should be given candidates before final acceptance to the school by a physician appointed by the Training-school Committee or Hospital.
5. Proof of recent vaccination, or vaccination at time of entering the school.
6. Presentation of certificate, giving evidence of one year in a high school or its *equivalent*. *Equivalent* may be defined as:
    (a) Additional educational qualifications.
    (b) Evidence of further mental training, such as courses in business college, stenography, art, music, etc.
    (c) Exceptional personal fitness, combined with desirable home training.

It is not expected that any one or all of the above suggested qualifications be accepted in lieu of a common school education.

It is suggested that occasional candidates may have qualifications or attributes which might be considered equivalent to the first year of high school duty.

An application blank, covering the above necessary qualifications and several other questions that will occur to the Principal, should be devised. It is recommended that a form (specimen of which is given on p. 438) be used for a physician's statement. It may be incorporated as a part of the application blank. Even though the physician's statement be satisfactory, a physical examination should be made by a physician appointed by the Training-school Committee or the Hospital at the time of admission to the preliminary course.

CLASS I

ISOLATED SMALL HOSPITALS

The Committee recognizes that the training-school problem in the isolated small hospital, of from twenty-five to seventy-five beds, is a problem apart from the training-school situation in larger institutions. Numerically, this is the largest division of hospitals in the classification. Hospitals of this size are scattered throughout the entire country. They are most common in the Middle West, South, and Far West, and are less stable in organization than older and larger institutions. They may be municipal, county, private, or semi-private in their management, or, as is frequently the case, organized by village or corporate associations. The professional work and medical departments of these hospitals are usually more or less circumscribed in variety and limited to general medicine, general surgery, and gynecology. A moderate number of these hospitals have small obstetric departments, and a still smaller number have a children's department. Few of the smaller institutions have a contagious department. Many of these hospitals have demonstrated the possibility of maintaining training-schools that compare favorably with schools in larger institutions. Properly managed training-schools in these institutions are recognized as capable of turning out graduates well qualified for general medical and surgical nursing in private families. Many factors entering into the situation of these schools lead the Committee to recommend a two years three months' course, of which three months shall constitute a definite preliminary course of study.

The term of school training should be not less than thirty-eight weeks per year for the two years three months' minimum course hereinafter outlined.

PRELIMINARY COURSES

The preliminary schedule as outlined can be used for the two years three months' course in the smaller hospital, or the complete three years' course in the large general hospital. The teaching of these subjects in the preliminary course must, of necessity, be more or less elementary. It is recommended that the study of the subjects outlined be attempted in a systematic manner. It is not expected that they will be completed during the three months of preliminary training. This course should be amplified and continued throughout the junior year, in association with subjects hereinafter outlined for the first year. This course has been constructed with the hope that it will provide the groundwork of the subsequent practical career of the pupil nurse in the school and in the hospital.

PRELIMINARY COURSE

(a) Practice and theory of nursing (elementary).

(b) Disinfection, sterilization, and protection against bacterial diseases (elementary bacteriology).

(c) Study of common drugs and their administration. (Preferably taught in pharmacy in class sections. See Clinics and Demonstrations, first year, No. 16.)

(d) Dietetics: Classification of foods, care of foods, cooking of foods, serving of foods. (See Clinics and Demonstrations, first year, No. 15.)

(e) Hospital ethics.

(f) Household economy. (See Clinics and Demonstrations, first year, Nos. 1, 2, and 3.)

(g) Hygiene and sanitation.

(h) Bandages and dressings. (See Clinics and Demonstrations, first year, Nos. 9, 10, and 11.)

(i) Elementary study of anatomy and physiology.

JUNIOR YEAR

(a) Continuation of studies of preliminary course.

(b) General medical and surgical nursing.

(c) Ward and bedside clinics and demonstrations.

OUTLINE

CLINICS AND DEMONSTRATIONS (FIRST YEAR)

1. Beds; bedding; bed-making, with and without patient; management of helpless patients; changing beds; bed-making for operative patients; rubber cushions; bed rests; cradles; arrangement of pillows, etc.; substitutes for hospital appliances.

2. Sweeping; dusting; preparing room for patient; disinfection of bedding; furniture, etc.; care of patients' clothing in wards and private rooms; disinfection of infected clothing.

3. Care of linen rooms; refrigerators; bath-rooms and appliances, sinks; hoppers; bath-tubs, etc.

4. Baths—full sponge, to reduce temperatures; foot baths; vapor baths; hot and cold packs.

5. Administration of rectal injections, for laxative, nutritive, stimulating, astringent purposes; care of appliances; disinfection of excreta.

6. Vaginal douches; methods of sterilizing appliances; use and care of catheters; vesical douches; rectal and colonic irrigations.

7. Local hot and cold applications; making of poultices; fomentations, compresses; methods of application; care of hot-water bottles; uses and care of ice-caps and coils.

8. Chart keeping; method of recording bedside observations.

9. Making of bandages—roller, many-tailed, plaster, abdominal, breast; pneumonia jackets.

10. Methods of applying roller bandages.

11. Methods of applying other bandages.

12. Appliances to prepare for ward examinations and dressings; sterilization of ward instruments; nurses' duties during dressings.

13. Preparation of patients for operation; hand disinfection.

14. Preparation and care of surgical dressings, sponges, swabs, etc.

15. Tray setting and food serving; feeding of helpless and delirious patients; management of liquid diet.

16. Administration of medicines; methods of giving pills, tablets, capsules, powders, oils, fluids; application of plasters, ointments, etc.; use and care of medicine droppers and minim glasses, atomizers, inhalers, hypodermic syringes, etc.; management of inhalations, eye drops, suppositories, etc.

17. Care of the dead.

18. Symptomatology—the pulse; correct methods of examining pulse; volume, tension, rhythm, rate, etc.; effect of exercise, emotions, baths, drugs, shock, and hemorrhage.

19. The face in disease—the skin; expression, eyes, mouth, teeth, etc.; variations from normal, care of mouth and teeth; general observations of the body.

20. Respiration—normal and in respiratory affections.

21. Pneumonia—respiration, cough, and sputum; crisis and lysis explained, and charts shown.

22. Typhoid fever—face, rose spots, temperature charts, changes in temperature and pulse explained; danger signals; prophylactic measures; methods of managing delirious patients, proper restraint, etc.

23. Specimens of excreta—urine, sputum, feces, etc.; nurses' duties regarding each; importance and general management.

NOTE.—The numbers signify only headings or divisions, and should not be construed to limit the number of demonstrations or clinics.

SECOND YEAR

LECTURES AND DEMONSTRATIONS

Accidents and emergencies, including poisonings, two hours.

Fractures and head injuries, one hour.

Preparation of patients for anesthesia and their after-care, one hour.

Surgical material, instruments, and operative technic, two hours.

Complication of wounds, two hours.

Infection, inflammation, and immunity, one hour.

Care of orthopedic patients, one hour.

Gynecology, two hours.

Diseases of the digestive organs, two hours.

Diseases of the kidneys, one hour.

APPENDIX

Typhoid fever, two hours.
General fevers, one hour.
Tuberculosis, two hours.
Other diseases of the lungs, two hours.
Diseases of the heart and circulatory system, one hour.
Obstetrics, seven hours.
Contagious, infectious, and genito-urinary diseases, three hours.
Diseases of the skin and morbid growths, one hour.
Care of infants and sick children, four hours.
Diseases of the eye, one hour.
Diseases of the ear, nose, and throat, one hour.
Diseases of the nervous system, insanity, and care of delirious patients, two hours.

OUTLINE

CLINICS AND DEMONSTRATIONS (SECOND AND THIRD YEARS)

1. Surgical technic; preparation for operation; nurses' duties during operations.

2. Preparation of antiseptic gauzes, ligatures, etc.; preparation for hypodermoclysis; for aspirating; preparation of anesthetist's outfit.

3. Management of sutures and ligatures during operation; instruments for common operations.

4. Surgical anatomy and surgical positions.

5. Surgical specimens—appendix, tumors, cysts, bone, etc.; preparation and general care.

6. Methods of preparing patients for examinations; inspection, percussion, auscultation, etc.; abdominal, vaginal, instrumental, and non-instrumental.

7. Methods of arresting hemorrhages, external, internal.

8. Clinic on pulse and affections of the heart and circulatory system.

9. Clinic on respiratory affections—pneumonia, pleurisy, asthma, tuberculosis, etc.

10. Fevers—important symptoms in special cases.

11. Sepsis—charts shown; important symptoms and nursing points.

12. Children's diseases—rickets, teeth, general characteristics; skin affections of children; diseases of the eyes, ears, glandular system; comparison of symptoms in children with adults; marasmus; digestive disorders; adenoids, etc.

13. Orthopedic clinic; bow-legs, Potts' disease; imperfect development; hip-joint disease; spinal curvature; physical exercises; adjustment of braces; extension of apparatus and corrective appliances.

14. Milk modification for infants according to different formulæ; also for fever patients and invalids.

15. Obstetric methods; preparation for normal labor; for instrumental delivery; dressing the cord; care of the baby's mouth and eyes; massage of the mother's breasts; use and care of breast-pump; application of abdominal and breast-binders; bathing and dressing the baby; management of obstetric emergencies, etc.

16. Demonstration of ophthalmic methods; washing out the conjunctival sac; applying eye drops to the eye; eye compresses; preparation for ophthalmic operations, dressings, etc.

17. Nursing methods in aural, mouth, and throat cases; preparation of field of operation in such cases; methods of feeding; uses of syringes, sprays, etc.; nasal douches; taking cultures from the throat; instruments for tracheotomy; intubation, care of tube, etc.

18. The uses of water for remedial purposes; external application; spinal sprays and douches; Schott baths; medicated baths, etc.

19. Internal application of water; lavage; enteroclysis; preparation for intravenous infusions, etc.

20. Massage; demonstration of methods; effleurage; friction; petrissage; tapotement; methods of stroking; management of light and heavy treatments.

21. Massage; kneading, percussion; general massage; contraindications.

22. Local massage—legs and abdomen.

23. Local massage—head and neck.

24. Physical exercises; passive and active movements.

25. Urine and urinalysis; simple tests for albumin, sugar, acidity, specific gravity, etc.

26. First aid methods—bandaging, etc., in case of accident; artificial respiration, etc.

27. Management of delirious and insane patients.

NOTE.—The numbers signify only headings or divisions, not the number of demonstrations or clinics. It is hoped that each school will utilize such patients as the institution provides to give as varied clinical and practical instruction as possible.

It is recommended that, as the facilities and needs of different hospitals vary, several of the above subjects be amplified and others added to suit local requirements. Not less than forty-two hours during the second year should be devoted to the practical teaching of the above subjects. It is recommended that continued and special attention be given, throughout the second year, to dietetics, hygiene, and the management of special diseases. It will occasionally occur that patients suffering from some special disease, epidemic, or infection may be brought into the hospital. If possible, they should be made the occasion of special clinics and demonstrations.

The above outline of the two years three months' course should constitute the minimum teaching course in the isolated small hospital. Hospitals that cannot give this schedule in its entirety should arrange affiliations with larger hospitals.

CLASS II

SMALL HOSPITALS IN PROXIMITY TO LARGE GENERAL HOSPITALS

The Committee recommends that hospitals of from twenty-five to seventy-five beds, in proximity to larger hospitals or large medical centers, arrange for affiliation with these institutions for such training-school work as cannot be given in the local hospital. Hospitals of this class, which cannot give the three years' maximum course, hereinafter outlined, should arrange their affiliation so as to complete the three years' course for the pupil. This gives the services of the pupil to the local hospital for at least two years three months, or two years and six months of the course. It is not expected that affiliation will be sought by many hospitals for more than two or three subjects. If affiliation is sought as outlined, the time devoted by pupils of training-schools of this class should be considered additional to the minimum schedule recommended for the isolated small hospital. The Committee recommends the following periods of affiliation:

Obstetrics, three months.
Diseases of children, three months.
Contagious diseases (optional), two or three months.
General medicine or general surgery, three to six months.
Eye and ear, orthopedic, or out-patient work, three months.

CLASS III

SPECIAL HOSPITALS

This class includes eye and ear, skin and cancer, children's and infants', lying-in, tuberculosis, orthopedic hospitals, etc.; sanatoria for nervous and mental diseases, hospitals for contagious diseases, hospitals for incurables, and for the insane.

On approaching the subject of training-schools for these hospitals, the Committee met with considerable difficulty, incident to the limited character of the work carried on.

The Committee recommends that large hospitals for the insane, giving a two years three months' course, as outlined, seek affiliation or reciprocity with general hospitals in subjects which, from lack of material or other reasons, cannot be given in the parent school.

Other special hospitals in this class should seek pupils from general hospitals desiring to affiliate in their specialty, or employ graduates. The Committee does not consider that special hospitals, whose clientele is limited to one specialty, are in a position to maintain training-schools or to train nurses adequately for general nursing.

CLASS IV

LARGE GENERAL HOSPITALS

The Committee recommends a three years' graded course for training-schools in hospitals of this class, the course to include a probationary period of three months, including the preliminary course, as stated, of from three to six months, for each class of probationers.

The outline for the three years' graded course assumes that a hospital of seventy-five or more beds offers at least, either at home or by affiliation, nursing in the following departments: medicine, surgery, obstetrics, and diseases of children.

PRELIMINARY COURSE OF THREE TO SIX MONTHS

The outline for this course will be found in the two years three months' course on p. 430. It is expected that the work in the preliminary term of the three years' course be amplified and advanced beyond that of the shorter course.

FIRST YEAR THEORETIC WORK

Preliminary course as previously outlined, and in addition:
Principles of Nursing, thirty hours.
(Class recitations from text-books or by topics or by lectures.)
Fever Nursing, including contagion, twelve hours.
Study of Drugs and their Administration, ten hours.
Measuring and Determining Body Fluids, two hours.
Reviews and Examinations, four hours.

FIRST YEAR PRACTICAL WORK

Practical work of the preliminary course (as previously outlined), and in addition:
Medical Nursing, three to five months.
 (Including the nervous and insane, fevers (non-contagious), and all the general medical affections of men and women.)
Surgical Nursing, three to five months.
 (Including gynecology and orthopedics.)
Vacation, three weeks.
It is recommended that two months of night duty be given in this year, one month in medical and one month in surgical wards.

The practical work of this year is also to be supplemented by bedside clinics, and demonstrations as outlined on pp. 431 and 432.

SECOND YEAR THEORETIC WORK

Study of Drugs and their Administration, ten hours.
Massage, one to two hours.
Anatomy and Physiology, twelve to twenty hours.
Foods and Food Values, eight to fourteen hours.
Bedside Clinics or Lectures, eight to fourteen hours.
Obstetric Nursing—
 Class recitations, ten to sixteen hours.
 Lectures, four to six hours.
 Demonstrations included in practical work.
Reviews and Examinations, eight hours.

SECOND YEAR PRACTICAL WORK

Operating-room Experience, two to four months.
Nursing Sick Children, two to four months.
Nursing Services in the special departments of the hospital, such as—
 Department for contagious diseases.
 Department for private patients.

Dispensary or out-patient department, four to five months.
Emergency wards.
Open-air department.
Massage, eight to twelve lessons.
Vacation, three weeks.
Two or three months of night duty are recommended.
The practical work of this year is to be supplemented by bedside clinics and demonstrations as outlined on pp. 433 and 434.

THIRD YEAR THEORETIC WORK

Lectures on Special Subjects, six to twelve hours
    Care of the eye.
    Care of the ear, nose, and throat.
    Care of the nervous and insane.
    Diseases of the skin and venereal diseases.
    Tuberculosis.
    Contagions.
Hospitals not treating any class of cases mentioned above will lack in practical work and should devote more time to theory.
Ethics of Private Nursing, six hours.
Lectures on Subjects Allied to Nursing, seven to fourteen hours.
    Industrial and living conditions of the community.
    Tuberculosis in the community.
    Local milk and food supply.
    Local charitable resources and relief of needy families.
    Social service and charity work.
    Settlements, visiting nurse work, school nursing.
    Preventive work of Board of Health.
    The nurse's obligations to her school and to her alumnæ association.
    Current topics related to nursing.
Lectures on subjects allied to nursing should be given by specialists or experts.

THIRD YEAR PRACTICAL WORK

Obstetric Nursing, two to four months.
Diet Kitchen Practice, including the modification of milk, one to two months.
District Nursing Under Supervision, one to two months.
Executive Work (for pupils who show fitness), five to six months—
    In charge of wards.
    In training-school office.
    As assistant to night supervisor.
Vacation.
One to two months of night duty are recommended.
Each senior pupil should conduct, under supervision, at least one demonstration for the junior class.
The practical work of this year should be supplemented by bedside clinics and demonstrations as outlined on pp. 433 and 434.

STATEMENT OF FAMILY PHYSICIAN

Name of applicant..
Exact date of birth..................Height......Weight......
What serious illnesses has the candidate had?....................
Is she subject to headache?....................................
      To throat disorders?....................................
      To digestive disorders?..................................
      To ovarian or uterine disorders?..........................
What is her heredity, especially in relation to tuberculosis, epilepsy, or mental disease?..
Are her heart and lungs sound?..............................
Is her menstrual function regular and normal?...................
Are her teeth in good order?..................................
Breath odorless, or otherwise?................Complexion?......
Are her sight and hearing good?................................
Has she been successfully vaccinated?..........................
Has she any physical defect which might interfere with the work of nursing?..
Have you carefully examined the applicant, and do you recommend her admission to the school?..................................
        Signature....................................M. D.
        Residence................................
Date......................................
The above is for the Training-school records.

NOTE.—A physical examination will be made by a physician connected with the training-school before the pupil enters the school. (End of Committee's report.)

ADDITIONAL TRAINING-SCHOOL SUGGESTIONS AND SPECIMEN FORMS

GENERAL HOSPITAL TRAINING-SCHOOL FOR NURSES

The General Hospital Training-school for Nurses offers a .... years' course of study and training in the art of nursing. The school is a department of the general hospital, which contains .... beds for patients. Those wishing to receive this course of instruction must apply by letter or personally to the superintendent. Letters of application should contain a brief personal history with the names and addresses of two *responsible* persons, not relatives, to whom the applicant has been known for a number of years, and a statement from a physician certifying to sound health and unimpaired faculties. Pupils are required to have been successfully vaccinated within two years. Applicants are reminded that a thorough English education is essential, and that women of superior education and cultivation will be preferred. The most desirable age for candidates is between twenty-one and thirty-five years. They must be of average height and weight, and a strong physique.

Applications to enter this school (which must be made in writing on blanks which are furnished on request) are placed on file as received. Approved candidates will receive due notice and printed instructions as to necessary preparation for coming. Classes are formed every .... months. A certain number of names are kept on an "emergency list," and these candidates may be sent for on short notice. The period of probation is .... months, during which time candidates are examined as to their education, physical strength, endurance, adaptability to the work, powers of observation, judgment, etc. On the satisfactory completion of .... months' probation they assume the uniform of the school. At the end of .... months they are examined upon the work gone over, and if this examination and their record are both satisfactory they are allowed to continue, and then sign an agreement to conform to all the requirements imposed upon the pupils; if not, they are dropped. The same is true as to the examinations at the end of the first and second years.

The instruction comprises a thorough training in the principles and practice of nursing. Bedside clinical instruction and special lectures are included in the course. Experience in nursing the following classes of patients is provided for: Medical, including contagious diseases; surgical, including general surgery, eye, ear, nose and throat, orthopedic, etc.; obstetric patients and the care of infants and children. A preliminary course extending over .... weeks is devoted mainly to instruction in elementary nursing.

The hours off duty are especially arranged for the preliminary course. During the remainder of the course, two to three hours weekly are allotted for class work, as the schedule may require.

The pupils do the work of nursing in the hospital under supervision, and, in return they receive board, lodging and laundry, and the instruction of the school, and after the completion of the probation term, an allowance of .... per month to provide uniforms and text-books. Should a pupil be ill, she is cared for without charge, but is required to make up time lost. In addition to the daily time, a part of Sunday and one afternoon weekly are allowed for rest and recreation. A vacation of two weeks is allowed the first year, and three weeks the second and third years.

Nurses are subject in all particulars to the rules of the hospital and the discipline of the school. They are under the authority of the superintendent of the hospital and the principal of the school, who have full power to decide as to the propriety of retaining or rejecting a candidate on probation, or to discharge a nurse at any time for any reason that they may judge to be sufficient. Pupils will not be allowed during their course of instruction to nurse sick relatives at home, or to absent themselves for other than personal reasons. Absences are not allowed except for extreme cause.

Candidates when called are expected to report promptly, and to bring with them the means of returning to their homes, should they not successfully pass their probationary term. Any change of plan or of address on the part of a candidate, whose name is on the waiting list, should be immediately reported to the principal of the training-school.

When the full term of three years is ended, and the final examinations have been successfully passed, the nurses thus trained will receive the diploma of the school, and are allowed to wear the badge of the school.

APPLICATION FOR ADMISSION

(To be filled out in the applicant's own handwriting.)

1. Name in full (no initials or pet name)......................
2. Present address..
3. Age............Date and place of birth....................
4. Complexion......Height......Weight......Bust measure....
5. Have you any physical defect, weakness, or blemish?..........
6. Are your sight and hearing perfect?........................
7. Have you always been strong and healthy?..................
8. Are you willing to nurse contagious cases?..................
9. What is your present occupation?..........................
10. Why do you wish to leave it?...............................
11. By whom have you been employed during the last three years?
....
12. Your father's name, address, and occupation................
13. Name and address of nearest relative or friend...............
14. What is your religious belief or denomination?.............
15. Are you single?..Engaged?..Married?..Divorced?..Widowed?
16. Have you children?....How many?....Their ages?........ How provided for?......
17. Have you any responsibility that may call you away during training period?..
18. Where were you educated?................................
19. In what schools and what branches?........................
20. Have you taught school?........How long, and where?......
21. Have you a practical knowledge of housework?............:......
22. Have you had any experience in nursing?....................
23. Have you ever been connected with any hospital or training-school, if so, how long, where, and in what capacity?
....
24. Give names and addresses of two persons, not relatives, as reference.

....

I declare the above answers to be correct and true, and if accepted, I will agree to conform, in all respects, to the rules of the hospital and the requirements of the school.

....
Candidate.

Date...................

Private and confidential.

GENERAL HOSPITAL TRAINING-SCHOOL FOR NURSES

.................191

DEAR........................

    MISS..............................

of.............................is desirous of being received as a pupil-nurse in this school, and has referred us to you for information regarding her fitness.

It is essential that candidates should be women of sound health, thoroughly practical, and of refined and cultivated minds; but it is even more essential that they should be thoroughly conscientious women, of earnest purpose and high aspirations.

They must be obedient and submissive to teaching and discipline, capable of self-sacrifice and of patient, cheerful, kindly devotion to the sick.

It is clearly of great importance both to Miss.................. and to this school that no mistake shall be made regarding her fitness for nursing and for the exacting drill of the training required.

I should be glad, therefore, if you would answer the following questions as fully as possible at your earliest convenience. Your communication will be regarded as strictly confidential, and your candid opinion concerning the candidate in question will greatly assist in making a proper selection of nurses.

Thanking you in advance for your assistance, I remain,
                   Yours very truly,

....

To............................

Respecting Miss...
1. How long have you known her?
2. What is her age?
3. Her history, especially for the last few years?
4. What is your opinion regarding her health?
      Her habits and disposition?
      Her temper?
      Her manner?
      Her intelligence and capabilities?
      Her moral character?
5. Is she of firm and earnest purpose, patient and persevering?
6. What have been your opportunities of forming an opinion of the candidate?

                        Signature......................

Date..........................

GENERAL HOSPITAL

REQUISITION FOR SPECIAL NURSE

(To be filled out and signed by physician in charge or house officer.)

Ward............

Patient's name..
Diagnosis and remarks about case..............................
....
..,...
....
At whose request?..

Signed..

Approved:

....Supt.
Pay or free...
If paid, by whom?...
Day nurse, name.............................Grad. or pupil?
  Supplied, hour........Date..........................
  Omitted, hour........ " ....
Night nurse, name...........................Grad. or pupil?
  Supplied, hour........Date..........................
  Omitted, hour........ " ....

This blank is to be returned to the office when special service is discontinued.

GENERAL HOSPITAL

HEAD NURSE'S REPORT

Excellent............E
Good...............G
Fair................F
Poor...............P

1. General attention and kindness to patients...................
2. Quietness...
3. Thoroughness of work.......................................
4. Interest displayed...
5. Observation...
6. Memory...
7. Method...
8. Teachableness..
9. Punctuality...
10. General behavior...
11. Neatness in person and work...............................
12. Pleasantness, especially when found fault with..............

MONTHLY REPORT OF HEAD NURSE
NURSES' MONTHLY GRADES

Ward.......................... *Date*....................

Nurse	Prac-tical Work	Quiet-ness	Punc-tuality	Neat-ness	Personal Appearance	Deport-ment

Maximum number attainable for each point, 3.

Head Nurse.

WEEKLY RECORD OF RECREATION AND EXTRA DUTY HOURS

Week Ending—

NAMES	SUN.		MON.		TUES.		WED.		THUR.		FRIDAY		SAT.		TOTAL	
	R.	Ex.	R.	Ex.	R.	Ex.	R.	Ex.	R.	Ex.	R.	Ex.	R.	Ex.	R.	Ex.

Head Nurse.

TRAINING-SCHOOL RECORD

Candidate's name....... Date of entrance...... Probation ended....

Address .... Age ....Religion............

Friend's address........ Date of graduation.......................

	1ST YEAR.	2D YEAR.	3D YEAR.	AVERAGES.	REMARKS.
Deportment..............					
Health.................				Practical	
Order and cleanliness...				work ...	
Theory of nursing......					
Hygiene................				1st year...	
Anatomy................					
Physiology.............					
Dietetics..............				2d year ...	
Bacteriology...........					
Cooking................					
Bandaging..............				3d year ...	
Surgical nursing.......					
Gynecology.............				Theory ...	
Obstetrics.............					
Materia medica.........					
Diseases of the nervous system...............					
Diseases of the eye, ear, nose, and throat				1st year ..	
Contagious diseases ...					
Children's diseases....				2d year ...	
Emergencies					
Diseases of the skin...					
General medical nursing................					
Urinalysis.............				Total	
Massage................				average .	
Executive ability......					

Notes.

APPENDIX 445

NURSES MONTHLY RECORD—HOSPITAL OF THE GOOD SHEPHERD, SYRACUSE, N. Y.

Name _____ Year _____

MONTH	MEN		WOMEN		INFANTS and CHILDREN		OBSTET-RICS		PRIVATE PATIENTS		R. R. DISP.	D. K. OPR.	SPECIAL NURSING						Ill-ness	Ab-sence	Vaca-tion
	Med'l & Surg'l		Med'l & Surg'l		Med'l & Surg'l				Med'l & Surg'l				Med.	Surg.	Eye	Ear	Obst.	Nerv's/Conting			
	Day	Night	Day	Night	Day	Night	Day	Night	Day	Night											

Fig. 160.

RECORD OF THEORETICAL INSTRUCTION

SUBJECT	INSTRUCTOR	No. of Lessons	Date of Examination	Rating	SUBJECT	INSTRUCTOR	No. of Lessons	Date of Examination	Rating

REMARKS

Fig. 161.—Form used in Hospital of the Good Shepherd, Syracuse, N. Y. Reverse side of card form shown in Fig. 160.

APPENDIX

RECORD OF INSTRUCTION AND EXAMINATION.

SUBJECT	INSTRUCTOR	No. of Lessons	Date of Examination	Rating

Summary of Work

HOSPITAL RECORD	Rating	SUMMARY	Rating
Reliability		Nursing Ward patients	
Executive ability		" Private patients	
Quality of work		Operating room service	
Observance of Regulations		Night Duty	
Adaptibility		Averages	
Remarks		Theoretical	
		Practical	

Fig. 162.—Form used in Hospital of the Good Shepherd, Syracuse, N. Y.

INSTRUCTIONS AND REGULATIONS FOR SPECIAL AND GRADUATE NURSES

1. Special nurses will report to the principal of the training-school before going on duty and when leaving case.

2. When on duty either wear your regulation school uniform or a white uniform, including cap and rubber heels. A nurse not properly uniformed will not be allowed to come on duty.

3. Stay in patient's room. Do not visit with pupil nurses, house physicians, or others during hours of duty, and never discuss with others the private affairs of your patient.

4. Order special supplies, including linen for the day, from the corridor nurse at 7.30 A. M. Have cot removed from room before 8.00 A. M. Room is to be swept and dusted before 8.30 A. M. Sweeping of dust or dirt from rooms into the corridors is forbidden.

5. All supplies, especially rubber goods, utensils, instruments, etc., must be promptly returned to their proper places after use. Retaining in patient's room or elsewhere articles or supplies in common use is strictly forbidden.

6. The tearing of towels, sheets, etc., is strictly forbidden. Wastefulness in the use of alcohol, cotton, gauze, and various surgical supplies will not be permitted. Nurses known to be habitually wasteful will not be called by the hospital. Use all that is necessary and no more.

7. In case any unusual supplies or articles are needed, such as cannot be furnished by the corridor nurse, you are requested to apply for same to the principal.

8. Garbage must be thrown into receptacles provided for that purpose. Used gauze and bandages must be placed in the gauze pails and all waste removed from the patients rooms' promptly. Special nurses must not leave waste, litter, or dirty utensils scattered about the toilet rooms.

9. Special nurses should provide themselves with *clinical thermometers, hypodermic syringes, fountain pens,* and *scissors.*

10. Report to principal or superintendent at once any complaint on the part of the patients regarding meals or service.

11. The attention of special nurses is especially called to the rules covering diet kitchen issues and extras.

12. Keep your clothing and wraps in your patient's room. Nurses will not be permitted to leave their clothing or apparel in other rooms.

13. Graduate nurses will be expected to give .... hours' service per day. In exceptional or difficult cases, ... hours' relief will be given, when ordered by the physician in charge of the case. Not more than .... hours' relief can be given by corridor nurses. The time for the hours of corridor relief will be entirely at the discretion of the principal.

14. Each special nurse is responsible for the care of her patient and room. No articles of furniture, pillows, etc., should be removed from the room or from any vacant room, without permission of the principal. When your patient is discharged from the hospital the room must be stripped and prepared for the cleaners.

15. Nurses will not be permitted to use the telephone except in the interest of their patients. All messages will be charged to the patient. Nurses will not be called to the phone except for necessary inquiries in reference to their patients. You should instruct your friends not to call you while at the hospital, except while off duty.

16. A charge of .... per week is entered against the patient for the board of the nurse, and use of cot, while in the hospital.

17. Show your loyalty to the hospital and to the physician in charge of your case by avoiding any discussion of the merits of either the hospital or the physician.

18. Nurses are requested not to visit the hospital while caring for contagious diseases outside of the hospital.

19. Special nurses will see that the general rules of the hospital that relate to their work and to their patients are carried out at all times.

20. The principal will immediately call the attention of special nurses to any infringement of the above regulations.

21. Graduates who wilfully violate any of these regulations will not be called to the hospital to care for patients.

APPENDIX II

HOSPITAL DIETARIES

BUFFALO GENERAL HOSPITAL PRIVATE ROOM DIETS

(These diets are not all served to every patient. Patients have their choice of articles.)

SUNDAY.

Breakfast.

Grapefruit. Oranges.
Stewed figs.
Strawberries. Pineapple.
Cream of wheat.
Pettyjohn's food.
Rolled oats.
Boiled shad.
Butter sauce.

Broiled steak.
Coddled eggs.
Potato balls.
Parkerhouse rolls.
Toast.
Bread and butter.
Coffee. Milk.
Cream.

Dinner.

Tomato bisque with whipped cream.
Broiled spring chicken.
Sweet pickle plums.
Boston baked beans.
Mashed potatoes.
Baked potatoes.
Asparagus on toast.
Creamed corn.

Tomatoes with mayonnaise.
Green onions.
Graham bread. White bread.
Toast.
Sponge cake.
Vanilla ice-cream with strawberries.
Sherry-wine jelly.
Coffee. Milk. Tea.

Supper.

Creamed sweetbreads.
Cold roast beef.
Baked potatoes.
Cream toast.
Watercress. Beet salad.
Strawberry shortcake with whipped cream.
Baked apples.

Custard.
Pineapple jelly.
Lemon jelly.
Toast.
Rye bread.
White bread.
Fig tarts.
Tea. Milk. Cocoa.

Monday.

Breakfast.

Grapefruit.
Bananas.
Strawberries.
Stewed prunes.
Shredded wheat.
Rolled oats.
Farina.
Cornmeal mush.

Broiled bacon.
Sauted calf's liver.
Coddled eggs.
Creamed potatoes.
Coffee-cake.
Toast.
Bread and butter.
Coffee. Milk. Cream.

Dinner.

Amber soup.
Creamed crackers.
Soft-shell crabs.
Roast beef. Scraped meat-balls.
Spiced bananas.
Mashed potatoes.
Baked potatoes.
Spinach with hard-boiled eggs.
Creamed oyster-plant.

Celery. Watercress.
Graham and white bread.
Toast.
Chocolate blanc mange with whipped cream.
Ice-cream.
Maple syrup and walnuts.
Orange sherbet.
Tea. Milk. Coffee.

Supper.

Sliced ham.
Creamed chicken.
Baked potatoes.
Fried hominy with maple syrup.
Lettuce salad.
Radishes.
Toast.
Rye and white bread.

Sponge jelly roll.
Strawberries.
Stewed rhubarb.
Baked apples.
Sherry-wine jelly.
Lemon jelly.
Custard.
Tea. Milk. Cocoa.

Tuesday.

Breakfast.

Grapefruit. Oranges.
Baked apples.
Strawberries.
Rolled oats.
Wheatena.
Cream of wheat.
Broiled steak.

Creamed codfish.
Baked potatoes.
Cinnamon rolls.
Toast.
Bread and butter.
Coffee. Milk. Cream.

Dinner.

Rice soup.
Broiled yellow pike.
Butter sauce.
Broiled chicken.
Broiled lamb chops.
Plum jelly.
Mashed potatoes.
Baked potatoes.
Asparagus on toast.

Creamed cabbage.
Tomatoes with mayonnaise.
Green onions.
Toast.
Bread and butter.
Ice-cream with chocolate sauce.
Strawberry sherbet.
Tapioca cream.
Tea. Coffee. Milk.

Tuesday.

Supper.

Cold roast beef.
Broiled squabs.
Creamed potatoes.
Baked potatoes.
Creamed hominy.
Celery.
Watercress.
Toast.

Rye and white bread.
Cocoanut cake.
Strawberries.
Stewed rhubarb.
. Baked apples.
Custard.
Wine jelly.
Tea.　　Milk.

Wednesday.

Breakfast.

Grapefruit.
Bananas.
Strawberries.
Pineapple.
Corn flakes.
Rolled oats.
Cream of wheat.

Broiled ham.
Coddled eggs.
Creamed potatoes.
Boston brown bread.
Toast.
Graham and white bread.
Coffee.　Milk.　Cream.

Dinner.

Purée of peas with
whipped cream.
Broiled perch.
Roast lamb.　Mint sauce.
Scraped meat-balls.
White meat of chicken.
Currant jelly.
Mashed potatoes.
Baked potatoes.
Green peas.

Buttered beets.
Lettuce salad.
Toast.
Graham and white bread.
Ice-cream.
Caramel sauce.
Sponge cake.
Prune soufflé.
Port-wine jelly.
Tea.　Milk.　Coffee.

Supper.

Fricaseed chicken
with toast.
Broiled steak.
Fried potatoes.
Baked potatoes.
Sliced tomatoes with
French dressing.
Boiled rice.

Rye and white bread.
Molasses cup-cake.
Strawberries.
Baked apples.
Rhubarb sauce.
Toast.　Custard.
Sherry wine jelly.
Tea.　Milk.　Cocoa.

APPENDIX 453

Thursday.

Breakfast.

Grapefruit.
Pineapple.
Stewed prunes.
Oranges.
Shredded wheat.
Ralston's food.
Farina.
Rolled oats.

Broiled lamb chops.
Coddled eggs.
Potato-balls.
Parkerhouse rolls.
Toast.
Graham and white bread.
Coffee.   Cream.
Milk.

Dinner.

Tomato bouillon.
Creamed crackers.
Roast chicken with dressing.
Giblet gravy.
Broiled steak.
Spiced figs.
Mashed potatoes.
Baked potatoes.
Asparagus on toast.

Creamed oyster-plant.
Tomatoes with mayonnaise.
Watercress.
Rye and white bread.
Toast.
Ice-cream.
Strawberry sherbet.
Fruit jelly with whipped cream
Tea.   Milk.   Coffee.

Supper.

Cold tongue.
Frogs' legs.
Scraped meat-balls.
Fried potatoes.
Baked potatoes.
Macaroni and cheese.
Watercress.
Egg salad.
Green onions.

Graham and white bread.
Toast.
Strawberries.
Rhubarb sauce.
Baked apples.
Lemon jelly.
Wine jelly.
Custard.
Tea.   Milk.   Cocoa.

Friday.

Breakfast.

Grapefruit.
Baked apples.
Strawberries.
Stewed prunes.
Shredded wheat.
Pettijohn's food.
Cream of wheat.
Rolled oats.

Broiled lamb chops.
Broiled bacon.
Coddled eggs.
Cream potatoes.
Coffee-cake.
Toast.
Bread and butter.
Coffee.   **Milk.**   Tea.

Friday.

Dinner.

Vegetable soup.
Broiled shad with butter sauce.
Broiled steak with Chili sauce.
Curry giblet stew with boiled rice.
Creamed potatoes.
Baked potatoes.

Escalloped tomatoes.
Spinach with hard-boiled eggs.
Lettuce salad. Radishes.
Rye and white bread.
Toast.
Rhubarb pudding.
Ice-cream.
Orange sherbet.
Tea. Milk.

Supper.

Cold sliced chicken.
Stuffed calf's heart.
Fried potatoes.
Baked potatoes.
Sliced tomatoes.
Watercress.
French toast with maple syrup.
Graham and white bread.

Toast.
Strawberries.
Rhubarb sauce.
Baked apple.
Wine jelly.
Lemon jelly.
Custard.
Tea. Milk. Cocoa.

Saturday.

Breakfast.

Grapefruit.
Oranges.
Strawberries.
Stewed figs.
Shredded wheat.
Wheatena.
Rolled oats.
Farina.

Broiled steak.
Cod-fish balls.
Fried potatoes.
Cinnamon rolls.
Toast.
Bread and butter.
Coffee. Milk.
Tea.

Dinner.

Barley soup.
Roast veal with dressing.
White meat of chicken.
Scraped meat-balls.
Spiced plums.
Mashed potatoes.
Baked potatoes.
Buttered lima beans.
Asparagus on toast.

Watercress.
Beet salad.
Green onions.
Graham and white bread.
Toast.
Caramel custard.
Ice-cream. Chocolate sauce.
Lemon sherbet.
Tea. Milk. Coffee.

Supper.

Creamed chicken.
Cornbeef hash.
Baked potatoes.
Corn fritters with maple syrup.
Salmon salad.
Watercress.
Rye and white bread.
Chocolate cake.

Toast.
Baked apples.
Strawberries.
Apple sauce.
Custard.
Wine jelly.
Lemon jelly.
Tea. Milk. Cocoa.

Sunday, May 8th.

NIGHT NURSES.

Supper (11 to 12 P. M.).
Cold ham.
Potato salad.
Strawberries.
Bread and butter.
Coffee.　　Cake.

INTERNES.

Lunch (10.30 P. M. to 12 M.).
Bread and butter folds.
Ham sandwiches.
Coffee.　　Milk.

NIGHT ORDERLIES.

Supper.
Cold meat.
Fried potatoes.
Pickles.　　Cookies.
Bread and butter.
Coffee.

DOCTORS AND NURSES.
Breakfast.
Oranges.
Cereals { Rolled oats.
in　　　 { Shredded wheat.
cream.　{ Toasted cornflakes.
Bacon.　Rolls and coffee.

Dinner.

Barley soup.
Roast chicken and gravy.
Mashed potatoes.
Peas.　　Radishes.
Vanilla ice-cream.
Coffee.

Supper.
Egg salad on lettuce.
Cold boiled ham.
Bread and butter.
Strawberries.　　Sponge cake.
Tea.

EMPLOYEES.

Breakfast.
Oatmeal.
Bacon.
Rolls.　　Coffee.

Dinner,
Roast beef.
Steamed potatoes.
Peas.　Bread and butter.
Ice-cream.
Tea.

Supper.
Cold corned beef.
Bread and butter.
Pickles.　Stewed rhubarb.
Tea.

WARDS.

Breakfast.
Oatmeal.
Toast.　Bread and butter.
Coffee.　Milk.

Dinner.

Roast beef.
Steamed potatoes.
Peas.　Bread and butter.
Cornstarch pudding.
Tea.　　Milk.

Supper.
Steamed rice.
Bread and butter.
Stewed rhubarb.
Toast.　Tea.
Graham wafers.

Monday, May 9th.

NIGHT NURSES.
Supper.
Hamburg steak.
Creamed potatoes.
Shredded cabbage with French dressing.
Baked custard.
Bread. Butter. Coffee.

DOCTORS.
Lunch.
Egg sandwiches.
Fruit sandwiches.
Coffee or milk.

NIGHT ORDERLIES.
Supper.
Hamburg steak.
Bread and butter.
India relish.
Graham crackers.
Stewed rhubarb.
Coffee.

DOCTORS AND NURSES.
Breakfast.
Stewed prunes.
Cereals in cream. { Farina. Shredded wheat. Toasted cornflakes. }
Pork sausage.
Toast and coffee.

Luncheon.
Cold roast beef.
Scalloped potatoes.
India relish.
Bread and butter.
Stewed rhubarb.
Tea.

Dinner.
Vegetable soup.
Beef-steak.
Bread and butter.
Baked corn.
Mashed potatoes.
Cocoanut custard pie.
Coffee.

EMPLOYEES.
Breakfast.
Farina.
Pork sausage.
Toast. Coffee.

Dinner.
Irish stew.
Steamed potatoes.
Tapioca pudding.
Tea.

Supper.
Bologna sausage.
Fried potatoes.
Stewed prunes.
Bread and butter.
Tea.

WARDS.
Breakfast.
Farina.
Toast. Coffee.
Milk.

Dinner.
Irish stew.
Bread and butter.
Steamed potatoes.
Tapioca pudding.
Tea. Milk.

Supper.
Creamed fish on toast.
Tea. Milk.
Bread and butter.

Tuesday, May 10th.

NIGHT NURSES.

Supper.

Scalloped chicken.
Mashed potatoes.
Peas.
Prune souffle.
Baking powder biscuits.
Coffee.

DOCTORS.

Lunch.

Chicken sandwiches.
Rye bread sandwiches.
Coffee.   Milk.

NIGHT ORDERLIES.

Supper.

Bologna.
Fried potatoes.
Cake.
Stewed rhubarb.
Bread and butter.
Coffee.

DOCTORS AND NURSES.

Breakfast.

Bananas.
Cereals in cream. { Hominy. Shredded wheat. Toasted cornflakes. }
Boiled eggs.
Muffins and butter.
Coffee.   Milk.

Luncheon.

Creamed codfish.
Baked potatoes.
Maple cream cake.
Tea.   Bread and butter.

Dinner.

Tomato soup.
Roast lamb with mint sauce.
Mashed potatoes.
Buttered parsnips.
Cabbage salad. Bread and butter.
Bread pudding with hard sauce.
Coffee.

EMPLOYEES.

Breakfast.

Hominy.
Boiled eggs.
Toast.   Coffee.

Dinner.

Roast lamb (shoulder).
Mashed potatoes.
Green onions.
Rice pudding.
Bread and butter.
Tea.

Supper.

Meat pie.
Bread and butter.
Stewed rhubarb.
Tea.

WARDS.

Breakfast.

Hominy.
Toast.
Coffee or milk.

Dinner.

Roast lamb (shoulder).
Steamed potatoes.
Corn.   Bread and butter.
Rice pudding.
Tea or milk.

Supper.

Cereal.
Toast.
Prunes.   Tea and milk.
Bread and butter.

Wednesday, May 11th.

NIGHT NURSES.

Supper.

Lamb chops.
Baked potatoes.
Stewed tomatoes.
Lemon jelly.
Cake.   Bread and butter.
Coffee.

DOCTORS.

Lunch.

Cheese sandwiches (made with rye bread).
Bread and butter folds.
Coffee.   Milk.

NIGHT ORDERLIES.

Supper.

Eggs.
Potatoes.
Stewed tomatoes.
Bread and butter.
Coffee.

DOCTORS AND NURSES.

Breakfast.

Baked apples.
Cereals ⎧ Cornmeal mush.
in   ⎨ Shredded wheat.
cream. ⎩ Cornflakes.
Bacon.
Rolls and butter.
Coffee.

Luncheon.

Omelet.
Creamed potatoes.
Radishes.
Bread and butter.
Rhubarb pie.
Cookies.   Milk and tea.

Dinner.

Vermicelli soup.
Roast veal with dressing.
Browned potatoes.
Lima beans.
Bread and butter.
Cornstarch blanc mange.
Coffee with whipped cream

EMPLOYEES.

Breakfast.

Cereal.
Bacon.
Rolls and Coffee.

Dinner.

Roast beef.
Steamed potatoes.
Lima beans.   Bread and butter.
Ginger bread and vanilla sauce.
Tea.

Supper.

Macaroni with tomato sauce.
Hashed brown potatoes.
Bread and butter.
Tea.   Stewed prunes.

WARDS—HOUSE DIETS.

Breakfast.

Cereal.
Toast.
Coffee.   Milk.
Bread and butter.

Dinner.

Hamburg steak.
Creamed potatoes.
Stewed tomatoes.
Gingerbread and vanilla sauce.
Tea and milk.

Supper.

Macaroni and cream sauce.
Stewed rhubarb.
Toast.   Bread and butter.
Tea.   Milk.

Thursday, May 12th.

NIGHT NURSES.

Supper.
Baked eggs.
Potatoes au gratin.
Lettuce with cream dressing.
Bread and butter.
Coffee.
Fruit.
Chocolate cake.

DOCTORS.

Lunch.
Chicken sandwiches.
Brown bread sandwiches.
Coffee.   Milk.

NIGHT ORDERLIES.

Supper.
Bacon.
Potatoes.
Coffee.
Bread and butter.
Fruit.

DOCTORS AND NURSES.

Breakfast.
Bananas.
Cereals { Rolled oats.
in { Shredded wheat.
cream. { Toasted cornflakes.
Liver and bacon.
Toast (buttered).
Coffee.

Luncheon.
Minced lamb on toast.
Rice croquettes.
Lettuce with French dressing.
Bread and butter.
Chocolate cake.
Milk and tea.

Dinner.
Beef soup with rice.
Roast beef.
Browned potatoes.
Spinach.   Bread and butter.
Strawberry ice.
Coffee.

EMPLOYEES.

Breakfast.
Rolled oats.
Fried liver.
Toast and coffee.

Dinner.
Roast shoulder of veal.
Browned potatoes.
Parsnips.   Bread and butter.
Bread pudding.
Tea.

Supper.
Wieners.   Saurkraut.
Rye bread and butter.
Mustard.
Fruit and tea.

WARDS.

Breakfast.
Rolled oats.
Fruit.
Bread and butter.
Coffee and milk.

Dinner.
Beef stew.
Steamed potatoes.
Peas.   Bread and butter.
Bread pudding.
Tea and milk.

Supper.
Hominy.
Toast.   Stewed prunes.
Tea and milk.
Bread and butter.

Friday, May 13th.

NIGHT NURSES.
Supper.
Creamed fish.
Oak Hill potatoes.
Buttered toast.
Stewed fruit.
Coffee.

DOCTORS.
Lunch.
Sardine sandwiches.
Egg sandwiches.
Milk and coffee.

NIGHT ORDERLIES.
Supper.
Cold meat.
Bread and butter.
Stewed tomatoes.
Rhubarb pie and cheese.

DOCTORS AND NURSES.
Breakfast.
Strawberries.
Cereals { Farina.
in   { Shredded wheat.
cream. { Toasted cornflakes.
Boiled eggs.
Popovers.   Coffee.

Luncheon.
Scalloped chicken.
Baked potatoes.
Bologna.
Baking powder biscuits.
Plum jam.   Tea.

Dinner.
Vegetable soup.
Fried blue pike.
Beef steak.
Potato puff.
Scalloped tomatoes.
Bread and butter.
Rhubarb pie.   Cheese.
Coffee.

EMPLOYEES.
Breakfast.
Farina.
Fried eggs.
Toast.   Bread and butter.
Coffee.

Dinner.
Fried fish.
Steamed potatoes.
Stewed tomatoes.
Cornstarch pudding.
Tea.   Bread and butter.

Supper.
Baked beans.
Fried potatoes.
Bread and butter.
Tomato catsup.
Fruit.   Tea.

WARDS.
Breakfast.
Farina.
Toast.
Bread and butter.
Coffee and milk.

Dinner.
Baked fish.
Steamed potatoes.
Stewed tomatoes.
Cornstarch pudding.
Milk.   Tea.   Bread and butter.

Supper.
Baked potatoes and cream gravy.
Stewed apricots.
Toast.   Bread and butter.
Tea.   Milk.

Saturday, May 14th.

NIGHT NURSES.

Supper.
Broiled ham.
Creamed potatoes.
Bread and butter.
Radishes.
Snow pudding.
Soft custard.
Coffee.

DOCTORS.

Lunch.
Tongue sandwiches.
Brown bread sandwiches.
Coffee or milk.

NIGHT ORDERLIES.

Supper.
Hamburg steak.
Potatoes.
Bread and butter.
Fruit. Pickles.
Coffee.

DOCTORS AND NURSES.

Breakfast.
Stewed rhubarb.
Cereals { Hominy.
in { Shredded wheat.
cream. { Toasted cornflakes.
Bacon.
Buttered toast.
Coffee.

Luncheon.
Macaroni with tomato sauce.
Hashed brown potatoes.
Chops. Bread and butter.
Stewed apricots.
Ginger snaps.
Tea. Milk.

Dinner.
Split pea soup.
Corned beef.
Steamed potatoes.
Hot slaw.
Bread and butter.
Rice pudding.
Coffee.

EMPLOYEES.

Breakfast.
Hominy.
Hash.
Toast. Coffee.
Bread and butter.

Dinner.
Corned beef.
Steamed potatoes.
Cabbage. Bread and butter.
Chocolate bread pudding.
Tea.

Supper.
Cold meat.
Baked potatoes.
India relish.
Bread and butter.
Fruit. Tea.

WARDS.

Breakfast.
Hominy.
Toast.
Bread and butter.
Coffee. Milk.

Dinner.
Pot roast.
Browned potatoes.
Lima beans.
Chocolate bread pudding.
Bread and butter.
Milk and tea.

Supper.
Pea soup.
Toast. Bread and butter.
Cereal.
Tea and milk.

THE WORCESTER CITY HOSPITAL, PATIENTS' DIET

HOUSE DIET

Breakfast.—Coffee (milk and sugar), bread and butter, rolls, or toast. Cereals—Oatmeal, cream-of-wheat, grapenuts, or force. Meats—Hash, eggs, salt fish, minced meat, or warmed-over cold meat.

Dinner.—Bread and butter. Meats—Beef (roast or boiled), or mutton (roast or boiled), or corned beef, or fresh fish or Irish stew. Vegetables—Potatoes and tomatoes, baked beans, turnips, beets, lettuce, rice, or macaroni. Pudding—Rice, bread, tapioca, farina, cornstarch, or custard.

Supper.—Tea (sugar and milk). Bread and butter. Fruit—Apples (stewed or baked), prunes, or pears.

NITROGENOUS DIET

Breakfast.—Tea or coffee (milk). Bread and butter or graham bread. Meats—Eggs, fresh fish, stew *without* vegetables, meat hash *without* potatoes.

Dinner.—Soup—Stock or chowder, graham bread. Meats—Beef (roast or boiled), mutton (roast or boiled), fresh fish, or Irish stew. Vegetables—Spinach, lettuce, celery, or string beans. Pudding—Custard.

Supper.—Tea (milk), graham bread and butter, bread and milk, eggs, or cold meat.

FARINACEOUS DIET

Breakfast.—Tea or coffee (milk and sugar). Bread and butter, corn bread, rolls, toast and hominy, farina, or Indian meal.

Dinner.—Soup (vegetable). Bread. Baked potatoes and tomatoes, French beans, rice, or macaroni. Pudding—Rice, bread, tapioca, or cornstarch.

Supper.—Tea (milk and sugar). Bread and milk, milk toast, hominy, boiled rice, or farina. Fruit—Apples (stewed or baked), prunes, or pears.

OBSTETRIC DIET

First Day After Confinement

Milk, gruel, cocoa, or broth, 4 oz. every two hours.

Second Day

Breakfast.—Cereal and cocoa, 6 oz.
10 A. M.—Milk or gruel, 6 oz.
Dinner.—Soup or broth, with toast, rice, or cornstarch.
3 P. M.—Milk or gruel, 6 oz.
Supper.—Milk-toast, tea, or cocoa.
8 P. M.—Milk or gruel, 6 oz.
Milk, cocoa through night p. r. n.

Third Day

Breakfast.—Cereal, cocoa, toast.
10 A. M.—Milk or gruel, 6 oz.
Dinner.—Steak and baked potatoes, cornstarch, rice, or some milk pudding. Bread and butter. Milk and cocoa.
3 P. M.—Milk, broth, or gruel, 6 oz.
Supper.—Milk-toast, custard, or baked apple.
8 P. M.—Milk or gruel.
Liquid nourishment through night.

Fourth Day

Breakfast—Dropped egg, cereal, cocoa, tea, or milk.
10 A. M.—Milk, 6 oz.
Dinner.—Steak, chop, chicken, potato, milk pudding, bread and butter, tea, cocoa, or milk.
3 P. M.—Milk or gruel, 6 oz.
Supper.—Bread and butter, sauce, baked apple, or custard.
8 P. M.—Milk or gruel, 6 oz.
Liquid nourishment through night.

Fifth Day.

Breakfast.—Oyster stew, dropped egg, cocoa, tea, or milk, cereal, bread, or toast.
10 A. M.—Milk, 6 oz.
Dinner.—Roast or boiled meat, potato, bread and butter, dessert.
3 P. M.—Liquid nourishment, 6 oz.
Supper.—Bread or toast, sauce or custard.
8 P. M.—Liquid nourishment, 6 oz.
The succeeding days' diet remain about the same in character unless there is a special written order to the contrary.

LIQUID DIET

Milk (2 pints), broth, gruel, beef-tea (kind and quantity as ordered by the attending physician or surgeon), beef juice, koumyss, oyster broth, mutton broth, chicken broth, bouillon, barley-water, oatmeal gruel, malted milk.

Usually 4 pints of liquid nourishment is allowed for each patient, so that 6 oz. every two hours may be given.

MILK DIET

Breakfast.—1 pint of milk.
Dinner.—1 pint of milk.
Supper.—1 pint of milk.

SEMISOLID DIET

Breakfast.—Cocoa, coffee, or tea, cereal with milk-toast.
Dinner.—Soup with toast, any milk pudding.
Supper.—Tea or coffee, cream-toast, custard, or junket.
Amounts for twenty-four hours: Milk, 2 pints; sugar, 2 oz.; soup, 1 pint; cocoa, 1 pint.
Patients on this diet should have milk or some liquid nourishment at 10, 3, and 8 o'clock and during night.

SPECIAL DIETS

(Ordered by Attending Physician or Surgeon)

Breakfast.—Oysters (raw), oysters (stew), cream of wheat, shredded wheat, eggs (raw), eggs (dropped), eggs (scrambled), eggs (boiled), toast (dry), toast (milk), cocoa, milk (pints extra).

Dinner.—Beef-steak, mutton chops, chicken, mashed potato, baked potato, soup (milk) with croutons, oysters (raw), oysters (stew), dropped eggs, scrambled eggs, toast (dry), toast (milk), boiled rice, cornstarch, blanc mange, custard, tapioca pudding, cocoa.

SOME SPECIAL DIETS, MASSACHUSETTS GENERAL HOSPITAL

HOUSE DIET WITH CARE

No coarse vegetables. No brown bread or beans. No salt fish or hash.

Give strained soups. Oatmeal, strained.

EXTRA DIET WITH CARE

Chicken, egg, toast, stale bread, blanc mange, scraped-beef sandwiches, all soft custards (without raisins), raw oysters, crackers, ice-cream, jelly, milk, broths, gruels, soups, whey, slip, oranges, weak tea and coffee, cocoa.

SPECIAL DRY, SALT-FREE DIET

Morning.—Salt-free bread, two slices (toasted, if desired). Plenty of salt-free butter. Maple syrup, if desired. Two soft-boiled eggs without salt.

10 A. M.—Rice, with a little cream and sugar or syrup.

Noon.—Mashed potato, with butter. No salt. Salt-free bread, two slices. Salt-free butter (plenty).

4 P. M.—Rice, tapioca, or custard (hard).

Night.—Salt-free bread, two slices. Salt-free butter (plenty). Soft-boiled eggs, two.

One orange a day. Limit liquids to 1 pint a day, including milk and water.

HYPERCHLORHYDRIA (HEWES)

Olive oil, $\frac{1}{2}$ to 1 oz. at 7.30 A. M.

Breakfast.—Toast. Milk. Low proteid cereal—rice, wheat.

Lunch, 10 A. M.—Crackers, with or without milk.

Dinner.—Meat, potato, rice, macaroni, squash, etc. Custard, tapioca, sago, ice-cream.

Lunch, 3 P. M.—Crackers.

Supper.—Same as breakfast. Oil again in evening.

DIET FOR ACUTE COLITIS (DYSENTERY)

Purge and starve for one day; then lean meat, 10 oz., three times a day. Albumin-water (2 eggs), six to eight times a day. Continue for four days, then add skimmed milk, 1 pint a day. Toast (no butter), 3 slices a day, with maple syrup. Rice, 1 saucer daily. After ten days increase toast, give butter, macaroni, tapioca, cream-cheese, Indian-meal mush.

DIET FOR GASTRIC AND DUODENAL ULCER (HEWES)

Milk, 2 oz.; 1 soda-cracker (powdered), and sugar, 1 oz., every two hours. Give for two or three days, then increase to milk, 6 to 8 oz., with 4 crackers and sugar, 1 to 2 oz., every two hours. Eight feedings in twenty-four hours. Continue for two to three weeks, then adopt following:

1. Milk and crackers.
2. Indian-meal mush, with cream or salt.
3. Potato purée, jelly.
4. Milk and white of 2 eggs.
5. Soft custard.
6. Chocolate.
7. Pea purée.
8. Milk and crackers.

Continue for two months.

SCHMIDT DIET (HEWES)

Morning.—50 gm. zwieback; 1 pint of oatmeal gruel, 40 gm. oatmeal; 10 gm. butter; 200 gm. milk; 300 gm. water; 1 egg.

11 A. M.—1 pint milk.

Noon.—125 gm. chopped beef, broiled, and made palatable with 20 gm. butter; 250 gm. mashed potato, using 10 gm. butter. Serve meat on 50 gm. toast.

4 P. M.—1 pint of milk.

Night.—Same as morning.

SPECIAL DIET LIST

YES	NO
Bread twenty-four hours old.	Tea, coffee.
Crackers.	Cake, candy.
Milk.	Doughnuts, pie.
Eggs (not fried).	New bread.
Broiled or roast-beef, mutton, chicken.	Kidneys, liver.
	Beer, wines, and liquors.
Broiled or boiled fish.	Tomatoes, rhubarb.
Potato, very little.	Asparagus.
Peas, spinach, beans.	Sour fruits.
Baked apple, squash.	Pork or salt meat.
Soups, macaroni.	Fried meat.
Oatmeal or cracked wheat.	Cabbage.
Cocoa.	Pickles.

Do not eat meat or soup more than once daily. Drink plenty of water. Eat slowly and chew carefully.

DIET LIST

YES	NO
Bread twenty-four hours' old.	Tea, coffee.
Crackers.	Cake, candy.
Milk.	Doughnuts, pie.
Eggs (not fried).	Beans, new bread.
Broiled or roast-beef, mutton, chicken.	Pork or salt meat. Fried meat.
Broiled or boiled fish.	Salt fish.
Potato, very little.	Cabbage.
Peas, spinach.	Pickles.
Baked apple.	
Soups.	
Oatmeal or cracked wheat.	
Cocoa.	

TYPHOID FEVER DIETS

Dr. Shattuck's Enteric Diet:

Milk.
Mellin's Food.
Ice cream.
Milk whey.
Slip.
Finely minced chicken.
Eggs, soft boiled or raw.
Milk-toast without crust.
Macaroni.
Blanc mange.
Broths.

Special Enteric Diet:

Steak; chop; white meat of chicken in small amounts.
Toast; bread; cereals.
Eggs in any form.
Mashed potato.
Tomatoes, strained.
Oysters.
Stewed fruits.
Crackers.
Patients must be told to chew all food well.

LIQUIDS AND SOFT-SOLID DIET (HEWES). WEAK STOMACH. WEAK HEART. TYPHOID

First Day

Breakfast.—Indian meal mush with cream and sugar, or with salt only (hot); milk, three ounces.

10 to 11 A. M.—Crackers and milk, or egg-nog.

Dinner.—Pea purée or potato; soft or cream toast, and soft-boiled egg.

3 to 4 P. M.—Custard or tapioca.

Night.—Rice; milk.

Second Day

Breakfast.—Wheat germs; milk.
10 to 11 A. M.—Crackers and milk.
Noon.—Finely cut chicken; wine jelly.
3 to 4 P. M.—Chocolate or crackers and milk.
Night.—Cream-toast; apple sauce.

Third Day

Breakfast.—Wheat flakes; milk.
10 to 11 A. M.—Crackers and milk.
Dinner.—Two soft-boiled eggs; rice (custard or cornstarch at 3 to 4 P. M.).
Night.—Potato purée; toast.
Alternate diets.

DIET FOR ACUTE NEPHRITIS. No. 1

Uric Acid Gravel

Four days.—Milk, 800 c.c.; cream, 300 c.c.; bread, 200 gm.; butter. Feed six times a day with mixture milk, 150 gm.; cream, 1 oz.; bread, ½ slice.

Fifth day.—Adopt following: Milk, 800 c.c.; cream, 300 c.c.; rice, 50 gm.; tapioca, 50 gm.; bread, 100 gm. Occasionally ice cream, custard. Vary diet from day to day in above limits.

If edema present and fails to go, change above diet to **Dry Salt-free Diet**.

At start give no more liquids than above; after edema has gone may give water as desired.

SPECIAL NEPHRITIC DIET. No. 2

(Not for very acute stages)

(See Diet No 1)

Breakfast.—Toast, with salt and butter; milk, 4 oz.; 1 soft-boiled egg, with salt
Noon.—Toast and butter; 1 soft-boiled egg; 50 gm. rice, with milk and sugar, or custard.
Night.—Tapioca or rice; toast; apple sauce; milk. Limit liquids to 1000 c.c.

DIET FOR OXALURIA

Avoid spinach, rhubarb, figs, cocoa and chocolate, tea and coffee, potatoes, green beans, plums, tomatoes, berries
Cut carbohydrates low.
This diet:
1. Eggs; toast; milk.
2. Meat or fish; green vegetables, except those forbidden; peas; onions; custard; fruit; ice cream.
3. Cereals; cold meat; cooked fruit (except forbidden form).

Diabetic Diet. (Strict—Sugar Free.)

Contains about 20 gm. of carbohydrate; calories, 2800; proteid, 110 gm.

Breakfast.—Bacon, 100 gm.; eggs, 2; orange, 1; coffee, with saccharin and cream.

11 A. M.—Cheese, cream or Swiss, 50 gm.

Noon.—Beef, veal, lamb, or chicken, 100 gm.; lettuce or tomato salad, with oil; spinach, onions, or cabbage, cauliflower, olives; custard made of eggs and cream, with saccharin or ice cream made the same way.

4 P. M.—Soft-boiled eggs, with butter.

Night.—Fish, 100 gm.; cucumber salad, asparagus, or beet tops; mushrooms; almonds. Give all cream and butter possible. Vary diet daily within above limits.

At start give above diet, with addition of 200 gm. bread. After two to four days cut bread gradually 100 gm.; 50 gm. to strict diet. If acidosis increases with strict diet give large doses of soda. Control in this way and change of diet as long as possible.

If patient has increasing acidosis on strict diet and soda, 8 oz. a day, try method of starvation one day, vegetable diet (no carbohydrate) one day, oatmeal, 250 gm., one day, alternating.

Same plan may be tried if failure to get sugar free on strict diet, but first try plan of cutting down proteid on strict diet, replacing with more cream and butter, as sugar is made from proteid.

Keep on strict diet one month after using sugar free, then add bread, 25 gm., etc.

Diet for Diabetics

1. *Foods Allowed*

Eggs, fish, fowl, and meat of all kinds, except liver; butter, olive oil, and fats of all kinds: cheese; nuts of all kinds, except chestnuts; olives, cucumbers, mushrooms, young onions, string beans, watercress, asparagus tips, tomatoes, pickles, sauer kraut, sea-kale, dandelions, turnip tops, spinach, lettuce, cabbage, cauliflower, Brussels sprouts. (The green-colored parts of vegetables are the most harmless.) Bread made from genuine gluten flour, or almond or soja-bean meal; custard, blanc mange; milk in moderate quantities; buttermilk, cream, koumiss, tea, coffee, cocoa-shells, plain soda-water, Vichy, Apollinaris. To sweeten tea, coffee, custard, etc., glycerin or saccharin may be used instead of sugar.

2. *Foods Forbidden*

White-colored vegetables and those which grow below ground; turnips, beets, parsnips, carrots, radishes, celery, potatoes, wheat, oatmeal, rye, corn, rice, sago, tapioca, squash, peas, beans; fruit of all kinds, except lemons, sour oranges, sour cherries, cranberries, and red currants; bread, "crackers," pastry, macaroni, and vermicelli; sugar and sweetened foods, jam, syrup, molasses; sweet pickles; cocoa, chocolate. Soups must not be "thickened."

Remarks

Many samples of gluten flour are harmful, as they contain a large amount of starch.

APPENDIX III

MISCELLANEOUS

SPECIMEN FORMS AND STATEMENTS

METHODIST EPISCOPAL HOSPITAL, BROOKLYN, N. Y.

THE hospital is open for the treatment of general medical or surgical diseases, excepting those of a contagious or incurable character.

The charge for ward patients shall be, for adults $10 per week, or $1.50 per day, and for children $6 per week, or $1 per day, payable in advance, or in such proportions of these sums as they or their friends may be able to pay, provided, however, that no one ever be refused admission on account of inability to pay unless the resources of the hospital shall have become exhausted.

The charge for board in private rooms shall be at rates fixed by the Executive Commitee, and payable in advance, and shall include adequate nursing, which, as a rule, means one nurse for every four patients. If patients require or their friends desire that they shall have the exclusive services of a nurse, such nurse or nurses will be provided at the patient's expence. Rare or expensive medicines, special articles of diet, instruments or appliances not ordinarily supplied, must be provided at the patient's expense. In both wards and private rooms the day of entering and the day of leaving are both counted as full days.

The regular charges made by the hospital for the care of patients shall cover only the ordinary diet and nursing, together with the services of the House Staff.

The customary charges shall be made for the use of the operating room and for the private use of the ambulance.

The attending physicians and surgeons shall receive no compensation from patients treated in the wards of the hospital, which are intended only for those whose circumstances will not permit the use of private rooms.

The attending and consulting physicians and surgeons are expected to make definite private arrangement as to their professional fees with those patients whom they recommend to the hospital authorities for treatment in private rooms *before* such patients are sent to the hospital.

Whenever a patient applies directly to the hospital for treatment in a private bed, and it shall appear that an ability exists to pay for

COMPARATIVE WAGES PAID BY HOSPITALS, U. S. AND CANADA.

NAME	Chicago	Mg. w'tee	New York City	To- ronto	Boston	Wash- ington	Buf- falo	De- troit	Cleve- land	Philadelphia	Pat- terson, N.J.	Balti- more	Hade- ton, Pa.	Lon- don, Ont.	Minne- apolis	St Paul Minn	Win- nipeg	Mon- treal	Salt Lake City	St Louis, Mo.	Macon, Ga.	AVERAGE WAGES PAID
Matron	$55.00	$40.00	$60.00	$30.00	$83.33	$40.00	$75.00	$50.00	$33.00	$35.00	$35.00	$75.00	$50.00	$30.00	$41.50	$66.00	$65.00		$50.00	$40.00	$30.00	$52.54
Assistant Matron	44.00	34.00	50.00		100.00	50.00		50.00			30.00	40.00			40.00			26.67			15.00	32.82
Clerk	80.00	40.00	50.00	40.00	160.00	20.00		75.00	$50.00		35.00	160.00		40.00	40.00	40.00	75.00	193.33	45.00	20.00		52.82
Cashier and Bookkeeper			*51.66		75.00		40.00	78.00	*75.00		35.00	150.00				50.00	52.50					59.42
Stenographer	50.00	50.00	60	55.00	100.00	125.00	35.00	*20.00	40.00		25.00	135.00		40.00	60.00	25.00	35.00	45.00	40.00			43.25
Clerk and Bookkeeper	168.00	65.00	90.00	165.00	148.33	164.00	40.00	140.00	*75.00		25.00	*65.00	160.00		60.00	50.00	145.00	180.00		20.00		87.84
Pharmacist	134.67	60.00	60.00	130.00	75.00		50.00	75.00	75.00	40.00	25.00	155.00	160.00	50.00		33.00	140.00	100.00		40.00		57.84
Steward	50.00	45.00	125.00	60.00	183.33			35.00	50.00		25.00	75.00		40.00	60.00	45.00	60.00					63.05
Telephone Operator	170.00	*23.00	*45.00			25.00	60.00	30.00	35.00		12.00	*25.00					27.50	60.00			40.00	26.04
Door Keeper		30.00	30.00	25.00	117.00		60.00	30.00		15.00		*25.00		25.00		30.00	30.00	15.00	25.00		10.00	30.15
Bell Boy	127.50		35.00	60.00	135.00	*25.00	15.00					35.00		16.00				15.00		25.00	18.00	16.00
Orderlies	†52.50	*25.00	*30.00	18.00	60.00		25.00	14.00	*30.00	18.00	*30.00	*25.00	18.00	18.00	20.00	20.00	15.00	10.00			20.00	25.60
Night Watchman	115.00		*15.00	6.00		15.00	27.00	27.00	35.00	18.00		*65.00				30.00	23.00	25.00		25.00	30.00	39.30
Store Keeper	42.00	20.00	*24.00	10.00		25.00	22.00	25.00	35.00	18.00		*35.00				40.00						37.00
Chef	40.00		*40.00	22.00				75.00	30.00	35.00	35.00	30.00			25.00		40.00	30.00	25.00		40.00	48.53
Assistant	15.00	28.00	*100.00	22.00	23.00		40.00		80.00		35.00	*55.00		50.00	35.00	40.00		20.00	20.00	20.00	25.00	28.82
Cook	†50.00	30.00	50.00	25.00	70.00		35.00	25.00	25.00		20.00	25.00	25.00	30.00	30.00			30.00	35.00			37.00
Kitchen Boy	42.50		*25.00		60.00		20.00	20.00	30.00	25.00	15.00	15.00	15.00		18.00			10.00		25.00	12.50	21.05
Assistant	35.00	43.00	*25.00	18.00	33.00		20.00	15.00	15.00	15.00		18.00	14.00		18.00	18.00	16.00	30.00	16.00	20.00	15.00	16.56
Kitchen Maids	18.00	28.00	*18.00	14.00	30.00	18.00	18.00	15.00	15.00	14.00		14.00	15.00		16.00	18.00	18.00	13.00	20.00	15.00	9.00	16.38
Dining Room Maids	22.00	17.24	18.00	14.00	20.00		14.00	15.00	15.00	14.00		14.00	15.00		16.00		16.00	13.00	15.00	16.00	9.00	16.16
Floor Maids	18.00	83.00	15.00		14.00	*30.00	13.00	15.00	*30.00				15.00					14.00		20.00		17.75
Operating Room Maids	22.00	17.84	15.00	14.00		13.00	28.00	*28.00	*25.00	20.00	15.00	*30.00	15.00		20.00	20.00	190.00	13.00			9.00	13.52
Scrub Girls	18.00	132.50	*30.00		75.00	14.00	14.00	18.00	*40.00	25.00	15.00	*25.00	14.00		18.00	22.00	25.00	25.00	30.00			44.15
Head Laundryman	163.00	*65.00	*60.00				20.00	15.00	*45.00	14.00		*35.00			18.00	18.00	24.00	16.00	25.00			17.37
Assistant	†30.00			14.00			15.00	15.00	15.00	15.00	15.00	130.00	13.00	40.00	16.00	18.00	24.00	12.00	†25.00			18.04
Mangle Girls	18.00	128.67	15.00		16.00	*14.00	14.00	15.00	*30.00	15.00	15.00	130.00		15.00			40.00	18.00			10.00	21.50
Ironing Girls	22.00	127.50	15.00		16.00	14.00	18.00	14.00	14.00		20.00	120.00					24.00	18.00			12.50	20.33
Washer Man			15.00		16.00		18.00	20.00	*30.00	20.00	18.00			40.00			28.00				12.50	20.54
Porter	25.00		*18.00		15.00	25.00		15.00	15.00	16.00	17.00	17.00			15.00		24.00	14.00		50.00		19.04
Linen Room Sorter	27.00	20.00	15.00		25.00		15.00	14.00		15.00	14.00	17.00			30.00	20.00				14.00		20.23
Sewing Girls	32.00	*25.00	*24.00		15.00		20.00	20.00	*32.00	15.00	20.00	125.00	20.00	20.00	25.00	25.00	50.00	14.00	25.00	18.00		25.61
Elevator Men	25.00		*24.00		30.00	*22.00	25.00	20.00	*40.00	15.00	*14.20	*33.00			23.00	30.00	*40.00	17.50		14.00		24.82
Yard Men			*24.00		30.00		25.00		25.00		15.00	*83.00				30.00	50.00					81.55
Ambulance Man		20.00	40.00		33.00	45.00	35.00				20.00	133.33	170.00			100.00	116.66	11		60.00	35.00	42.60
Chief Engineer	163.00	*100.00	120.00	80.00	125.00	160.00	130.00	*40.00	*40.00	25.00	70.00	*44.00	150.00	50.00	70.00		116.66	35.00	75.00	60.00		54.37
Carpenter	32.00	17.24	*55.00	40.00		125.00	*30.00	*40.00	25.00	25.00		150.00				40.00	160.00	40.00	25.00			46.71
Painter	35.00	*40.00	*40.00	23.00	1100.00	180.00	*60.00	*45.00	*45.00	40.00	40.00	*65.00				25.00		45.00		20.00		23.00
Window Washer	30.00	*27.00	*24.00	14.00			20.00					*40.00		40.00				15.00			10.00	51.45
Painters	50.00	*100.00	60.00	80.00	1100.00	*23.00	*35.00	30.00	38.00			*65.00			30.00	30.00	57.50	50.00				

† With board, without lodging
‡ Without board and lodging

Each column represents a leading hospital and the figures given are the highest wages paid.
Figures given include room and board unless marked.

Fig. 163.—This table was prepared by Mr. Asa Bacon, Superintendent of Presbyterian Hospital, Chicago, and presented to the American Hospital Association in 1907. There has been no *general* or decided change in the rates given. Where change has been made the tendency is for the rate of wages to increase.

professional services, in whole or in part, over and above the hospital charges, for board and nursing, which must in every case be met first, the superintendent shall arrange in regard to the fee, and collect the same; and no bill will be presented by the attending physician or surgeon.

(Section from rules regarding admission of patients.)

BUFFALO GENERAL HOSPITAL

The rates for wards include board, nursing, medical and surgical care, surgical dressing, and drugs of the United States Pharmacopœia. Ward patients must wear the clothing of the hospital.

The rates for semi-private ward and private rooms include the services of the house staff, corridor nursing (one nurse to four patients), surgical dressings, and medicines of the United States Pharmacopœia. Oxygen gas when used as a tonic, proprietary medicines, wines, mineral waters, and foods when out of season, when ordered by the physician, or to supply the demands of the patients, will be charged for as extras.

If a special nurse is wanted, the same charge will be made to the patient that the hospital has to pay the nurse, plus $5.00 per week for the board of the nurse.

Friends of patients are permitted to occupy private rooms at the regular rate of the rooms, when the rooms are not wanted for patients. When the rooms are needed they *must vacate at once.* Extra meals are served at the rate of 75 cents for breakfast and supper, and $1 for dinner. For a friend occupying a cot in a private room with a patient a charge of $5 per week is made. Ambulance service for private patients $3 per trip within the city limits, when patients are coming or going from the hospital. The hospital does not launder private patients' personal clothing.

The rates charged for semi-private ward or private rooms do not include the services of the attending physicians and surgeons. These should be arranged for on their first visit.

Patients are received at any hour during the day or night.

Contagious or infectious patients are not received at the hospital.

The hospital reserves the right to dismiss a patient when his condition becomes such as to be detrimental or disturbing to other patients in the hospital.

(Section from rules.)

NEW YORK HOSPITAL

INFORMATION CIRCULAR FOR ORDERLIES

Wages

The pay is $30 per month, with board and laundry, 18 pieces per week (no lodging). Wages increase 5 per cent. for each six months of continuous and satisfactory service until a maximum service of five years is reached, when the pay becomes $50 per month and remains stationary.

Hours of Duty and Leave of Absence

Day orderlies are on duty from 7 A. M. to 7 P. M. Night orderlies from 7 P. M. to 7 A. M. No orderly may leave his post until his relief actually reports in the ward.

No leave of absence is promised. It is the aim of the hospital authorities, however, to arrange business so that day orderlies may be excused from duty one afternoon each week after 3 P. M., and the whole of each alternate Sunday after 9 A. M. This is a concession, not a right, and it should be thoroughly understood in order that undue disappointment may not follow when leaves of absence are withheld. Night orderlies are excused from duty one night in each month, under the same conditions.

Uniforms.

Uniforms are furnished by the hospital and remain the property of the hospital.

In order that orderlies may present a neat appearance the following requirements must be strictly observed:

(1) Uniforms must be changed as often as directed by Head Ward Nurse, and underclothes at least twice weekly.

(2) Those who shave must do so daily.

(3) Tub baths (provision for which has been made) must be taken three times a week.

A report of the observance of all rules will be made monthly by the Head Ward Nurse.

Advancement will depend on the number of points thus received.

Assignment to Duty

Orderlies are not employed for any special duty. They are assigned to duty and changed from time to time in the discretion of the superintendent of the training-school. They are the assistants to the nurses in charge of the wards and subordinate to them. They are not engaged for any stipulated period. Their employment may be terminated by the hospital at any hour, without previous notice. They also may leave the hospital service at any hour, without previous notice, except in the case of those who are on night duty. These having served through the night, may leave on the following morning.

Tardiness, drinking liquor, being asleep on duty, harshness to patients, accepting bribes or fees from patients or their friends, appropriating food or drink intended for patients, are offenses justifying immediate dismissal.

Letters of Recommendation

The hospital will not give letters of recommendation to those who are discharged for cause, nor will it give reasons for dismissals. The orderly, likewise, need simply announce his intention when he leaves the hospital employ, and will not be called upon for reasons.

The Presbyterian Hospital in the City of New York, N. Y.

*Position Wanted*_____ *Date*_____

*Age*_____ *Birthplace*_____ *Married, Single, Widowed*

*Religious Belief*_____

*Name and Address of last Employer*_____

_____

*In what capacity were you employed?*_____

*How long were you in that position?*_____

*Why did you leave?*_____

*Name and Address of other employers during past three years,*_____

_____

*Do you drink?*_____ *Smoke?*_____ *Chew?*_____

CONTRACT.—I, the undersigned, if employed, agree to do faithfully the work assigned to me, and to conform to all the rules of the hospital while in its employment, and it is distinctly understood and agreed, that whether I am paid by the day, week, or month, my engagement is to terminate upon notice by the Superintendent that my services are no longer required; and upon payment being made to me for the actual time of service rendered, I agree to accept and receipt for the same in full for all demands against the hospital. The hospital reserves the right to deduct for absence from whatever cause and for any damage done to property while in its service.

*Name*_____

*Address*_____

*Name and Address of nearest relative or friend*_____

ST. LUKE'S HOSPITAL, NEW YORK

CONTRACT: I, the undersigned, accept the terms herein mentioned, agree to do faithfully the work assigned to me, and to conform to all the rules of the hospital while in its employment; and it is distinctly understood and agreed, that, whether I am paid by the day, week, month, or year, my engagement is to terminate upon notice by the superintendent that my services are no longer required; and upon payment being made to me for the actual time of service rendered, I agree to accept and receipt for the same in full consideration for all demands against said institution. The hospital reserves the right to deduct for absence from whatever cause.

NOTE.—The above contract is printed in good large type at head of each page of the employees' book, which is signed by each employee on engagement.

TORONTO GENERAL HOSPITAL

RULES FOR EMPLOYEES IN THE MATRON'S DEPARTMENT

Hours for Rising and Meals

The rising bell will ring at 5.30 A. M., and all employees who sleep at the hospital must rise promptly, put their rooms in order, and be ready for duty at 6 A. M.

Breakfast at 6 A. M., dinner at 12 M., supper at 6 P. M.

Punctuality at all meals is enjoined, and tardiness or impropriety of conduct in the dining room must be promptly reported to the matron.

Employees in passing through the corridor to and from meals must avoid loud talking or laughing, or any other action calculated to produce disturbance.

Promptness at work will be required, and the right is reserved to make a deduction from the daily wages of such as are tardy without a good reason.

Working Hours

From 7.30 A. M. to 6.00 P. M.

Retiring Hour

Employees are expected to retire at 9.30 P. M., unless special permission is given otherwise.

Gas in bedrooms must be used at all times carefully, and promptly extinguished at the hour for retiring to bed.

Washing.

The clothing of employees who sleep in the hospital will be washed at the laundry. Such clothing will be collected each Tuesday at 7 A. M., and cannot be washed if sent at any other hour, without special permission from the matron. Every article of clothing must be marked with the full name of the owner. Twelve pieces are allowed each week. No white dresses or skirts will be washed.

Sunday

All employees are expected to attend some religious service on Sunday, and their hour of work on that day will be arranged accordingly.

Sickness

In case of illness report must be made to the matron at once. No drug shall be supplied without an order from the house physician. If employees require attention from physicians or nurses, by reason of illness, they will be cared for in one of the medical or surgical wards.

Visits from Friends

Employees are not expected to receive calls from their friends during working hours.

Ex-employees

Ex-employees shall not be allowed to visit the hospital.

Relation to Patients

Employees shall not hold any communication with patients.

Vacation

A vacation of two weeks will be allowed during each year to all employees who have been in the employ of the hospital for one year.

Violation of Rules

Any employee violating any of the above rules shall be liable to instant dismissal.

APPENDIX 475

DEPARTMENT	Daily Average Number of Patients		TEA (OUNCES)		COFFEE (OUNCES)		COCOA (OUNCES)		SUGAR (OUNCES)		LEMONS	
	Public	Private	Total Quantity used during Month ..... Days	Used per Capita per Diem	Total Quantity used during Month ..... Days	Used per Capita per Diem	Total Quantity used during Month ..... Days	Used per Capita per Diem	Total Quantity used during Month ..... Days	Used per Capita per Diem	Total Quantity used during Month ..... Days	Used per Capita per Diem
Annex												
Eye and Ear												
Wards 1, 2, 3, 4												
Wards 5, 6, 7												
Wards 8, 9, 10, 11												
Wards 12, 25, R. S.												
Fourth Floor												
Bermuda												
Pavilion												
West Wing												
Private Wards												

Fig. 164.—Table showing the quantities of various items used, per capita per diem for public and private patients with average per patient, Toronto General Hospital.

476 HOSPITAL MANAGEMENT

DEPARTMENT	Total Number of Patients during Month		MILK (Pints)		CREAM (Pints)		EGGS		BUTTER (Ounces)		BREAD (Loaves)	
	Public	Private	Total Quantity used during Month ....Days	Used per Capita per Diem	Total Quantity used during Month ....Days	Used per Capita per Diem	Total Quantity used during Month ....Days	Used per Capita per Diem	Total Quantity used during Month ....Days	Used per Capita per Diem	Total Quantity used during Month ....Days	Used per Capita per Diem
Annex												
Eye and Ear												
Wards 1, 2, 3, 4												
Wards 5, 6, 7												
Wards 8, 9, 10, 11												
Wards 12, 13, 14, 15												
Fourth Floor												
Burnside												
Pavilion												
West Wing												
Private Wards												

Fig. 165.—Table showing the quantities of various items used per capita per diem for public and private patients with average per patient, Toronto General Hospital.

T. G. H.

Daily Orders ....19......

Ward....................

Private ....
Semi-Private ....
Total ....

Rec'd	Ord'd		Rec'd	Ord'd	
.....	.....	qts. Milk	.....	.....	Cereals ....
.....	.....	pts. Cream	.....	.....	....
.....	.....	doz. Eggs	.....	.....	Fruits ....
.....	.....	lbs. Butter	.....	.....	....
.....	.....	Bread White	.....	.....	Canned Goods....................
.....	.....	Brown	.....	.....	....
.....	.....	lbs. Tea	.....	.....	Other Items.... ....
.....	.....	" Coffee	.....	.....	....
.....	.....	tins Cocoa	.....	.....	....
.....	.....	lbs. Sugar	.....	.....	....
.....	.....	Lemons	.....	.....	....
.....	.....	Oranges	.....	.....	....
.....	.....	Bananas	.....	.....	....
.....	.....	Grapefruit	.....	.....	....
.....	.....	qts. Buttermilk	.....	.....	Salt
.....	.....	pts. Oysters	.....	.....	Pepper
.....	.....	lbs. Beef	.....	.....	Mustard
.....	.....	....	.....	.....	Vinegar
.....	.....	Canned Chicken	.....	.....	**WEEKLY ORDER**
.....	.....	" Tomatoes	.....	.....	Soap.................... ....
.....	.....	" Corn	.....	.....	" ....
.....	.....	" Peas	.....	.....	" Brown
.....	.....	Biscuits Soda	.....	.....	" Carbolic
.....	.....	"	.....	.....	Sapolio
.....	.....	Corn Starch	.....	.....	" Hand
.....	.....	Chickens	.....	.....	Matches
.....	.....	Olives	.....	.....	Candles
.....	.....	Jam	.....	.....	Brass Polish
.....	.....	Marmalade	.....	.....	Toilet Paper
.....	.....	Jelly Powder	.....	.....	....
.....	.....	Essence	.....	.....	....

Ward Diet........................Soft............................Liquid...........................

Requested by............................ Approved.......................................
  Head Nurse

Received...

RULES FOR RESIDENT PHYSICIANS, COLUMBIA HOSPITAL, PITTSBURG

1. Resident physicians shall be selected by competitive examination by the Committee on Residents, subject to the approval of the Staff and election by the Board of Managers. Applicants shall sign an agreement binding themselves, if elected, to accept the appointment, to serve the full term prescribed by the hospital and to observe the rules and regulations governing their conduct while in the institution. All residents shall, on entering upon their services, be graduates of regular medical schools in good standing.

2. Residents shall reside in the hospital and shall receive board, lodging, and laundry. They shall otherwise serve without compensation, they shall do no outside medical or surgical work, and shall not charge or receive fees for attending patients during their terms of service in the hospital.

3. Each resident shall be responsible for all patients under his care in the absence of the chief and assistant (if any).

4. He shall follow strictly the instructions of his chief and equally so those of the assistant.

5. In case of emergency or in case of doubt as to the course to be pursued, he shall communicate at once by telephone with the chief or assistant, but shall not, except for good and sufficient reasons, interfere with the orders of the chief or assistant.

6. No resident shall absent himself from the hospital without first arranging with a fellow-resident for the proper care of his patients, acquainting him thoroughly with the condition and needs of those which may require attention. He shall also notify the office of his intended absence and of its probable duration, and shall register in the book provided for the purpose the dates and hours of his departure and return.

Leave of absence for a longer period than twelve hours may be granted only by the superintendent, with the approval of the Committee on Residents, and after satisfactory provision has been made for the proper performance of the duties of the absentee.

7. One resident shall always be in the hospital, except at the time of an emergency ambulance call, when the other resident is out.

8. Each resident shall visit all patients under his care twice daily (morning and evening). He shall record all his prescriptions and directions for their administration, and all his orders for the treatment of patients, in books provided for the purpose in each ward.

9. He shall keep a list of all cases under his care and shall furnish a daily list to each of his chiefs and assistants when so requested.

10. He shall keep accurate histories of all patients treated in his service to the satisfaction of his chief and the management.

11. He shall not prescribe potent drugs in the absence of the chief or assistant except by direction or in emergency.

12. He shall attend his chiefs on their rounds, giving preference in case of conflict according to the rules mutually agreed upon by his chiefs.

13. He shall have prompt access to such dressings and instruments as may be necessary in the course of his prescribed work and

in emergency, but he shall not perform any surgical operation except as shall be designated by the attending surgeon, and neither shall he employ any obstetric instruments with a view to delivery except upon the specific instructions of the attending obstetrician.

14. He shall avoid visits to the women's private rooms, except when attended by a nurse.

15. He shall not make vaginal examinations without the knowledge and upon the advice of the chief of the department concerned, except in an emergency case, when it will be necessary to report the same to the superintendent and afterward to his chief. All such examinations shall be made in the presence of at least one nurse.

16. Patients shall not be moved from one ward to another or from one bed to another in the same ward without a written order from the superintendent or her clerk. Neither shall private room patients be moved from one room to another without the consent of the physician or surgeon in charge of the case, and then only upon written order of the superintendent or clerk.

17. Residents shall not dismiss patients without the specific directions of their chiefs.

18. The medical resident shall admit all patients to the hospital by filling out the blanks provided for the purpose and shall at once turn the same into the office for the approval of the superintendent or clerk. He shall examine each patient sufficiently to determine whether or not it is a proper case for admission, and if so, to further determine to what department the case shall be assigned.

19. Each resident shall be responsible for the making of such analyses as may be ordered by the attending physician or required in routine hospital work. The urine of each patient shall be examined within twenty-four hours following admission. When necessary the patient shall be catheterized for this purpose.

20. Immediately following the discharge, death, or transfer of a patient, the resident in charge shall collect all the case history sheets, fill in the necessary data, and deliver them, either in person or by messenger, to the office of the superintendent.

21. Permission to perform an autopsy shall be obtained, when possible, from the patient's relatives, and if such permission is obtained, the pathologist and attending physician or surgeon shall be promptly notified.

22. All patients dying under suspicious circumstances or as the result of an accident shall be immediately reported to the coroner by telephone and the coroner's blank filled out and left at the office. Upon the death of any patient (except in coroner's cases) a death certificate shall be promptly filled out and left at the office.

23. Residents shall not publish reports of cases or exhibit pathologic specimens at the meetings of societies without the consent of the physician or surgeon having charge of the case, and neither shall they give information to newspaper reporters or others concerning anything which occurs in the hospital, or to patients without consultation with the management.

24. Residents are expected to have morning rounds and daily dressings completed by 11 A. M. Evening rounds shall be made before 8 P. M., except when unavoidable.

25. Residents shall give such instructions to orderlies and male nurses as may be necessary for the proper performance of their duties with patients.

26. Residents shall give such instructions to nurses as may be necessary to carry out orders and secure efficient service, but shall not reprove or discipline them for dereliction of duty. Any complaints concerning nurses shall be promptly reported to the superintendent of nurses.

27. Relations between resident physicians and pupil nurses of the training-school shall be of a professional character only.

28. Residents shall not prescribe for nurses or visit them when ill except when requested to do so by the superintendent. In all such cases the resident shall be accompanied by a nurse.

29. Each resident, on the completion of his term of service, shall be given a certificate, stating the time spent in the hospital, and signed by the president of the Board of Managers and the members of the hospital staff. The management and the staff reserve the right, however, to withhold the certificate from any resident for good and sufficient reasons.

30. Residents shall comply with the requests of the superintendent. Misunderstandings and grievances between the residents on the one side and the staff and management on the other shall be referred for adjustment to the Committee on Residents. This committee is responsible to both the staff and management for the conduct of residents, and when necessary will refer to them such serious troubles as call for discipline or dismissal. The Board of Managers, on recommendation of the medical staff, may at any time dismiss a resident for inefficiency, neglect of duty, violation of rules, or improper conduct.

31. Smoking in the hospital, except in the resident's private rooms, will not be permitted. Any resident found in any degree of intoxication shall be suspended by the superintendent, pending the investigation of the Committee on Residents.

INDEX

ABUSE, dispensary, 200, 382
Accommodation, 201, 391
Accountant, 206
Accounting, 76, 415
Accuracy, 48, 53
Adhesive plaster 297
Administration building, 52, 131
Admission of patients, 92
Admitting physician, 100
Advisory committee, 74
Aid societies, 193
Alcohol, 314
Alcoholic cases, 32
Allowance, ward, 142
Ambulance, 90, 229, 473
America, 17, 19, 52, 110
American Hospital Association, 67, 76, 118, 371
    field, 21, 24
  hospitals, 52
  Medical Directory, 23, 32
Anesthetics, 308
Anesthetist, 114
Anesthetizing room, 135, 173
Architects, 52
Architecture, 43, 51, 358
Asylums, 20, 34, 38
Atlantic, 125
Atomizers, 303
Auditor, 74
Austria, 18
Auxiliaries, Woman's, 159

BABIES, 37, 159, **160**
  bath-room for, 159
  cot for, 160
  room, 132
Bacon, 245
Bags, hot-water, **301**
  ice-, 301
  soiled clothes, 164
Balconies, 56, 61
Bandages, 296, **299**
Banking institutions, **194**
Barrel, 245
Basket, 323
Bath thermometers, 305
Bath-rooms, 119, 159, 360
Baths, 230
Bed lifters, 157
  rests, 152
  springs, 149
  trucks, 153
Beds, 24, 111, 147, 148, 150
Bedside tables, 156
Beef, 245
Bequests, 201
Bills, 223, 225, **243**
Bins, 176
Blackboard, 182
Blank, 219
Blankets, 291
Blood counter, 18*2*, 305
Blueing, 293
Board, 204

Board book, 209, 211
  medical, 88, 407
  of directors, 72
  of managers, 72, 106
  of public charities, 197
  of trustees, 81
Body ironer, 286
Boiler-house, 140
Boilers, 113
Bookcase, 156
Bookkeeping, 207
Books, 84, 156, 208
  general, 209
  receiving, 244
  sheet, 244
Bowl immersion, 171
  set, 277
Bread, 255
  cutter, 177
Brooms, 236
Buildings, 110
  administration, 131
  operating, 134
  outpatient, 380
Bunker, coal, 276
Business, 225
Butter, 240, 241
  cutter, 178

CABBAGE, 245
Calcium chlorid, 314
Canned goods, 225
Card system, 228
Cases, acute, 28
  chronic, 44
  medical, 32
  surgical, 32
  tuberculous, 34
Cash balance, 209
  blotter, 209
  book, 209
  rebates, 209

Cashier, 243, 244
Castor oil, 313
Castors, 150, 161, 168, 184
Catgut, 305
Catheters, 302
Cauliflower, 285
Charities, 23, 44, 101, 197
Chart, 156, 341
Checks, 216
Cheese, 225
Chief of clinic, 96
  of service, 68
  of staff, 99
Children's hospitals, 37, 42
  wards, 194
Chloroform, 104
Church, 19, 194
  institutions, 19, 47
Circulator, 112
City hospitals, 40
Clergyman, 67
Clinic, 48, 61, 95, 96
  chief of, 96
Clinical examinations, 104
  laboratory, 123
  registrar, 92
Clinics, 39
  and demonstrations, 431
Closets, 54, 123, 173
Clothes, 280, 290
  soiled, bag for, 164
Coal, 276, 277
Cocain, 309
Coffee, 225
Cold storage, 250
Collections, 195
Committee, 74, 340
  advisory, 74
  executive, 74, 75
  finance, 74
  medical, 74
  publicity, 74

Committee, standing, 404, 408
    training-school, 74, 80, 337, 339
        special, 407
Condenser, 113
Conduits, 131
Construction of hospital, 28, 52, 55, 60, 110, 126
Contagious diseases, hospital for, 43
Contract, employees, 473
Convalescent homes, 33, 38, 43, 130
  patients, 38
Convalescents, 139
  homes for, 43
Cost per day, 411
Course, preliminary, 436

DEACONESS homes, 41
Delivery bed, 160
Departments, 103, 387
Dependencies, 119, 127, 136
Dictionary, 23
Dietaries, 259, 450
Dietitian, 253, 259, 260, 269
Diet kitchens, 57, 119, 132, 167
  orders, 263
Diets, 266, 462, 464
Dining-room, 127, 350
Directors, board of, 72
Directory, 23
Discipline, 82, 85, 264
Diseases, acute, 39
  chronic, 49
  contagious, 43, 55
  infectious, 54
Dishwasher, 179
Dishwashing, 252
Dispensary, 200, 323
Doctor, 40, 41, 43
Donations, 192
Drainage-tubes, 301

Dressing materials, 295
Druggist, 325
Drugs, 295, 310, 325, 328, 364
Dynamo, 276

EGGS, 225, 240
Electric light, 187, 258
  plant, 140
  work, 145
Electricity, 145, 181
Elevators, 61, 70, 87, 120, 123, 137, 247
Employees, 75, 124, 132, 145, 191, 192, 251, 277, 288
  rules, 473
Endowment, 19, 205
Engine, 28, 87, 282
Engineer, 87, 274, 275, 279
English hospitals, 56
Equipment, 110, 182, 251, 285
Etherizing room, 173
Ethyl chlorid, 309
Executive committee, 74, 75
Exhaust fans, 117
Expenditures, 207, 208
Extractor, 180, 286, 288

FANS, exhaust, 117
Fees, 94, 386
Field hospital, 17, 18
Finance committee, 74
Flannels, 291
Floors, 116
Flowers, 166
Food, 131, 168
  carrier, 252
  complaints, 167, 261
Form, monthly report, 227
    specimen, 469
Formaldehyd, 311
Fuel, 275, 277
  economy of, 277

Funds, public, 196
  trust, 201
Furniture for hospital, 69, 147

GARBAGE, 129, 248, 255, 262
Gauze bandages, 296
  iodoform, 297
  purchase of, 295
  washing of, 295
German hospitals, 55
Germany, 51
Glassware, 305
Glycerin, 312
Green soap, 313

HEAD nurse, 337
Heating, 112, 275
Homes for convalescents, 43
  for nurses, 141, 349
Hopper room, 163
  sterilizing, 136
Hospital architecture, 43, 51, 358
  association, 72, 201
  beds, 24, 111, 147, 150
  bookkeeping, 207
  construction, 28, 52, 55, 60, 110, 126
  cost of, 125
  field, 17, 18
  furniture, 69, 147
  income, 190
  laboratory, 390
  organization, 191
  plans, 129
  schools, 332
  site, 109
Hospitals, 18
  children's, 37, 42
  city, 40

Hospitals, classification of, 428
  English, 56
    for chronic diseases, 49
    for contagious diseases, 43
  general, 64
  German, 55
  isolated small, 430
  maternity, 37, 46
  multi-storied, 111
  municipal, 40
  Pasteur, 55
  small, 434
  special, 435
  tent, 183
Hot-water bags, 301
Hours of duty, 90, 345
Housekeeper, 86, 265
House staff, 101
Hydrogen peroxid, 312
Hydrotherapeutic room, 181

ICE-bag, 301
Ice crusher, 179
Immersion bowl, 171
Incinerator, 187
Income of hospital, 190
Incubator, 391
Infectious building, 139
Institutions, 22, 25, 36
Instruments, 122, 161, 165
  surgical, 306
Internes, 67, 78
Inventory, 218, 408
  of material, 224
  of stock, 236, 237, 241
Iodoform gauze, 297
Isolation room, 138

JARS, specimen, 182
Journal, 209

INDEX

KETTLES, 175, 180
Kitchen, 124, 127, 145, 175, 246, 248, 259
  equipment, 175
  help, 253
  plans, 247, 249
  serving, 251
  table, 176

LABORATORY, 182, 382
  clinical, 123
  equipment, 182, 391
  hospital, 390
  pathologic, 390
  records, 396
  training, 393
Labor-saving devices, 177
Laundry, 129, 180, 359
  apparatus, 284
  construction, 283
  employees, 288
  equipment, 286
  plans, 124, 285
  rules, 287
  work, 284
Lavatory, 59, 182, 360
Ledger, 214
  card, 233
  purchase, 225
  training-school, 228
Lessons, cookery, 266
Library, 131, 356
Light, 109, 119
  electric, 187, 258
  plant, 140
Lighting, 121, 185
Linen, 289
  closet, 159
  discarded, 298
  infected, 292
  room, 138
Linen, table, 289
Liquors, 315

MAID, 265
Managers, board of, 72, 106
Mangle, 287
Maternity department, 159
  hospital, 37, 46
  ward, 37, 159
Mattresses, 150
Medical board, 88, 407
  cases, acute, 24
  charity, 101
  college, 108
  committee, 74
  institutions, 28
  patients, 39
  students, 40
Medicine cupboards, 187
Medicines, 88, 317
Menus, 254, 269
Microscope, 182, 391, 392
Microscopy, 60
Microtome, 182, 391
Monthly report form, 227, 469
Municipal hospitals, 40

NEEDLE holder, 308
  hypodermic, 307
Nitrous oxid, 309
Nurses, 64, 65
  allowances, 345
  head, 337
  home, 141, 349
  pupil, 62, 342
  room, 354
  school, 64
  special, 201, 448
Nursing course, 331

OPERATING, 93
  building, 134

Operating equipment, 171
  pavilions, 51
  rooms, 120, 170, 235
Orange sticks, 315
Orderlies, 90, 471
Organization of hospital, 191
Out-patient department, 95, 378
  fees, 386
  records, 385
  staff, 384
Out-patients, 128
Oxygen, 309

PASTEUR hospitals, 55
Pathologic building, 139
  department, 91
  laboratory, 390
  specimens, 397
  work, 393
Pathologist, 91
Patients, 19, 33, 42, 128, 183, 198
  cost of, 411
  out-, 95
  pay, 200
  pneumonia, 58
  private, 94, 135
  register, 211
  ward, 92
Pavilion, 60, 65, 112, 132
  main, 137
  plan, 60
  ward, 135
Pay-rolls, 217
Pharmacy, 318, 329
Photographs, 411
Physician, 94
  admitting, 100
  resident, 105
  visiting, 101, 106
Physicians, 96, 97
Plaster, adhesive, 297
  bandages, 299

Plenum system, 111, 114, **381**
Posters, 194
Pot washer, 263
Preliminary course, **436**
Prescription, 321, 323
Probation period, 342, 369
Probationer, qualifications of, **429**
Public, 192
  funds, **196**
Publicity committee, **74**
Pupils, 62, 342

RADIATORS, 114
Razor, 309
Rebates, 234
Reck system, 112
Refrigeration, artificial, **250**
Refrigerator, 145, 179
Register, patients', 211
Registrar, clinical, 92
Report, annual, **195**, **398**
  engineer's, **280**
  head nurse's, **442, 443**
  monthly, 207
  nurses' monthly, **445**
  statistical, 207
  superintendent's, **406**
  training-school, **407**
  treasurer's, **405**
  trustees', **405**
Requisitions, 236, 253
  for special nurse, **442**
Resident physician, 105
Röntgen-ray burns, 105
  department, 181
  expert, **104**
  room, 181
  treatments, **201**
Roof gardens, 61, 109, 142
Room, anesthetizing, 135, **173**
  baby, 132

Room, dining-, 127, 350
  etherizing, 135, 173
  hopper, 163
  hydrotherapeutic, 181
  isolation, 138
  linen, 138
  nurses', 354
  operating, 120, 170
  private, 162
  scrubbing-up, 135, 174
  serving, 137, 167
  sterilizing, 121, 132, 135 173
  utility, 159
  waiting, 131, 382
  x-ray, 181
Rubber goods, 299
Rules, 84, 287, 362
  for orderlies, 471
  for resident physicians, 478

SALARY, apothecary's, 317
  dietitian's, 260
Sanatoria, 32, 45
Scissors, 306
Screen, 154
Scrubbing-up room, 135, 174
Scullery, 145
Service building, 144
Shacks, tuberculosis, 143
Sink, 139, 175
Site for hospital, 109
Soap, 180, 287, 292, 293
  green, 313
Social service, 150, 388
Solarium, 174
Soup kettle, 175
Splints, 316
Starch, 293
Steam tables, 251
Sterilization, steam, 307
Sterilizer, 173
Sterilizing hopper, 136

Sterilizing room, 121, 132, 135, 173
  washer, 292
Stock, 218, 224, 236, 306
Stomach-tube, 302
Storage, cold, 258
Store, 236
Storekeeper, 218, 220, 236
Storeroom, 222, 236, 242, 250
Sugar, 243
Sun-parlor, 59
Superintendent, 67, 73, 79, 84, 207, 335
  assistant, 384
  medical, 336
  nurse, 335
  training-school, 85, 335
Supervising nurse, 335
Supplies, apothecary's, 319
  engineer's, 277
  food, 254
  surgical, 294
Surgical instruments, 306
Suture material, 303
Syringe, bulb, 303
  hypodermic, 307
System, card, 208
  of training, 330

TELEPHONE, 188, 192
Tents, 183
Test-tubes, 182
Training of nurses, 62
Training-school, 64, 82, 330
  committee, 74, 80, 337, 339, 407
  equipment, 339
  forms, 448
  for nurses, 61
  instructors, 361, 368
  ledger, 228
  principal, 336

Training-school records, 373, 444
   regulations, 427
   rules, 362
   superintendent, 336
   supervisors, 337
Trust funds, 201
Trustees, 75, 80, 81
Tuberculosis shacks, 143
Tubes, drainage-, 301
   stomach-, 302
   test-, 182

URINALS, 59, 163, 165
Urine tray, 182
Urinometer, 182
Utensils, 55, 58, 178
   stand for, 164, 171
Utility room, 159

VACUUM, 115
   cleaning system, 186, 360
Ventilation, 113, 115, 127
Visiting physician, 101, 106
Visitors, 95
Vouchers and checks, 216
   record, 190
   register, 190

WAGES, 470
Waiting room, 131, 382
Ward, 53, 55
   alcoholic, 142
   children's, 132
   dependencies, 119, 136
   direction of, 118
   maternity, 37, 132
   open-air, 61
   partitions, 53
   patients, 92, 124
   pavilion, 135
   rules, 92
   semiprivate, 127, 199
   size of, 117
   women's, 136
Washing machines, 284
Waste, 60, 255
Windows, 117
Women's aid societies, 159
   auxiliary, 159

X-RAY burns, 105
   department, 181
   expert, 104
   room, 181
   treatments, 201

SAUNDERS' BOOKS FOR NURSES

	PAGE
Aikens' Clinical Studies for Nurses	3
Aikens' Hospital Management	3
Aikens' Primary Studies for Nurses	3
Aikens' Training School Methods and the Head Nurse	3
Beck's Reference Handbook for Nurses	4
Boyd's State Registration for Nurses	4
Davis' Obstetric and Gynecologic Nursing	5
DeLee's Obstetrics for Nurses	5
Dorland's Medical Dictionaries	7, 8
Fiske's Anatomy and Physiology for Nurses	4
Fowler's Operating Room and the Patient	4
Friedenwald and Ruhrah on Diet	6
Galbraith's Four Epoch's of Woman's Life	6
Galbraith's Hygiene and Physical Training for Women	6
Grafstrom's Mechanotherapy (Massage)	8
Griffith's Care of the Baby	8
Hoxie's Medicine for Nurses	8
Lewis' Anatomy and Physiology for Nurses	7
Macfarlane's Gynecology for Nurses	5
Manhattan Hospital Eye, Ear, Nose and Throat Nursing	6
McCombs' Diseases of Children for Nurses	7
McKenzie's Exercise in Education and Medicine	5
Morris' Essentials of Materia Medica	8
Morrow's Immediate Care of Injured	8
Nancrede's Essentials of Anatomy	8
Paul's Materia Medica for Nurses	8
Paul's Nursing in the Acute Infectious Fevers	8
Pyle's Personal Hygiene	8
Register's Fever Nursing	8
Stoney's Bacteriology and Surgical Technic	2
Stoney's Materia Medica for Nurses	2
Stoney's Nursing	2
Wilson's Reference Handbook of Obstetric Nursing	7

W. B. SAUNDERS COMPANY

925 Walnut Street   Philadelphia

London: 9, Henrietta Street, Covent Garden

Stoney's Nursing NEW (4th) EDITION

In this excellent volume the author explains the entire range of *private* nursing as distinguished from *hospital* nursing; and the nurse is given definite directions how best to meet the various emergencies. *The American Journal of Nursing* says it "is the fullest and most complete" and "may well be recommended as being of great general usefulness. The best chapter is the one on observation of symptoms which is very thorough." There are directions how to *improvise* everything ordinarily needed in the sick room.

> Practical Points in Nursing. By EMILY M. A. STONEY, Superintendent of the Training School for Nurses in the Carney Hospital, South Boston, Mass. 12mo, 495 pages, illustrated. Cloth, $1.75 net.

Stoney's Materia Medica NEW (3d) EDITION

Stoney's Materia Medica was written by a head nurse who knows just what the nurse needs. *American Medicine* says it contains "all the information in regards to drugs that a nurse should possess. * * * The treatment of poisoning is stated in a manner that will permit of its being carried out thoroughly and intelligently."

> Materia Medica for Nurses. By EMILY M. A. STONEY, Superintendent of the Training School for Nurses in the Carney Hospital, South Boston, Mass. 12mo volume of 300 pages. Cloth, $1.50 net.

Stoney's Surgical Technic NEW (3d) EDITION

The first part of the book is devoted to Bacteriology and Antiseptics; the second part to Surgical Technic, Signs of Death, Autopsies, Bandaging and Dressings, Obstetric Nursing, Care of Infants, etc., Hygiene and Personal Conduct of the Nurse, etc. The New York *Medical Record* says it "is a very practical book which presents the subjects stated in its title in a concise manner."

> Bacteriology and Surgical Technic for Nurses. By EMILY M. A. STONEY. Revised by FREDERIC R. GRIFFITH, M. D., New York. 12mo volume of 300 pages, fully illustrated. Cloth, $1.50 net.

Aikens' Hospital Management   JUST READY

This is just the work for hospital superintendents, training-school principals, physicians, and all who are actively interested in hospital administration. Each chapter has been written by one specially fitted to write upon that particular phase of the subject; and Miss Aikens has brought the various chapters into a harmonious whole.

> Hospital Management. Arranged and edited by CHARLOTTE A. AIKENS, formerly Director of Sibley Memorial Hospital, Washington, D. C. 12mo of 488 pages, illustrated.

Aikens' Primary Studies for Nurses

Trained Nurse and Hospital Review says: "It is safe to say that any pupil who has mastered even the major portion of this work would be one of the best prepared first year pupils who ever stood for examination."

> Primary Studies for Nurses. By CHARLOTTE A. AIKENS, formerly Director of Sibley Memorial Hospital, Washington, D. C. 12mo of 435 pages, illustrated. Cloth, $1.75 net.

Aikens' Training-School Methods and the Head Nurse

This work not only tells how to teach, but also what should be taught the nurse and *how much*. The *Medical Record* says: "This book is original, breezy and healthy."

> Hospital Training-School Methods and the Head Nurse. By CHARLOTTE A. AIKENS, formerly Director of Sibley Memorial Hospital, Washington, D. C. 12mo of 267 pages. Cloth, $1.50 net.

Aikens' Clinical Studies for Nurses

ILLUSTRATED

This new work is written on the same lines as the author's successful work for primary students, taking up the studies the nurse must pursue during the second and third years.

> Clinical Studies for Nurses. By CHARLOTTE A. AIKENS, formerly Director of Sibley Memorial Hospital, Washington, D. C. 12mo of 512 pages, illustrated. Cloth, $2.00 net.

Fowler's Operating Room NEW (2d) EDITION

Dr. Fowler's work contains all information of a surgical nature that a nurse must know in order to attain the highest efficiency. *Canadian Journal of Medicine and Surgery* says: "We find compactly and clearly stated just those thousand and one things which when required are so hard to locate."

> The Operating Room and the Patient. By RUSSELL S. FOWLER, M. D., Professor of Surgery, Brooklyn Postgraduate Medical School. Octavo of 284 pages, with original illust tions. Cloth, $2.00 net.

Fiske's Anatomy and Physiology JUST READY

Miss Fiske weaves the physiology in with the anatomy, and in such a way that both anatomy and function are readily understood and retained by the reader.

> Anatomy and Physiology for Nurses. By ANNETTE FISKE, A.M., Graduate of the Waltham Training School for Nurses, Massachusetts. 12mo of 250 pages, Illustrated.

Beck's Reference Handbook NEW (2d) EDITION

This book contains all the information that a nurse requires to carry out any directions given by the physician. The *Montreal Medical Journal* says it is "cleverly systematized and shows close observation of the sickroom and hospital regime."

> A Reference Handbook for Nurses. By AMANDA K. BECK, Graduate of the Illinois Training School for Nurses, Chicago, Ill. 32mo volume of 200 pages. Bound in flexible leather, $1.25 net.

Boyd's State Registration for Nurses

This book tells the nurse just what she must know in order to obtain a certificate in any State. It presents comparative summaries of the laws, requirements, fees, exceptions and restrictions, violations and their penalties. The work will also form a serviceable basis for the drafting of laws.

> State Registration for Nurses. By LOUIE CROFT BOYD, R.N., Graduate Colorado Training School for Nurses. Price, 50 cents net.

DeLee's Obstetrics for Nurses THIRD EDITION

Dr. DeLee's book really considers two subjects—obstetrics for nurses and actual obstetric nursing. *Trained Nurse and Hospital Review* says the "book abounds with practical suggestions, and they are given with such clearness that they cannot fail to leave their impress."

> Obstetrics for Nurses. By JOSEPH B. DELEE, M. D., Professor of Obstetrics at the Northwestern University Medical School, Chicago. 12mo volume of 512 pages, fully illustrated.   Cloth, $2.50 net.

Davis' Obstetric & Gynecologic Nursing

THE NEW (3d) EDITION

The Trained Nurse and Hospital Review says: "This is one of the most practical and useful books ever presented to the nursing profession." The text is illustrated.

> Obstetric and Gynecologic Nursing. By EDWARD P. DAVIS, M. D., Professor of Obstetrics in the Jefferson Medical College, Philadelphia. 12mo volume of 436 pages, illustrated.   Buckram, $1.75 net.

Macfarlane's Gynecology for Nurses
ILLUSTRATED

Dr. A. M. Seabrook, Woman's Hospital of Philadelphia, says: "It is a most admirable little book, covering in a concise but attractive way the subject from the nurse's standpoint. You certainly keep up to date in all these matters, and are to be complimented upon your progress and enterprise."

> A Reference Handbook of Gynecology for Nurses. By CATHARINE MACFARLANE, M. D., Gynecologist to the Woman's Hospital of Philadelphia. 32mo of 150 pages, with 70 illustrations.   Flexible leather, $1.25 net.

McKenzie's Exercise in Education and Medicine

> Exercise in Education and Medicine. By R. TAIT MCKENZIE, B.A., M.D., Professor of Physical Education, and Director of the Department, University of Pennsylvania. Octavo of 406 pages, with 346 illustrations.   Cloth, $3.50 net.

Manhattan Hospital Eye, Ear, Nose, and Throat Nursing ILLUSTRATED

This is a practical book, prepared by surgeons who, from their experience in the operating amphitheatre and at the bedside, have realized the shortcomings of present nursing books in regard to eye, ear, nose, and throat nursing.

> Nursing in Diseases of the Eye, Ear, Nose and Throat. By the Committee on Nurses of the Manhattan Eye, Ear, and Throat Hospital: J. EDWARD GILES, M. D., Surgeon in Eye Department; ARTHUR B. DUEL, M. D., (chairman), Surgeon in Ear Department; HARMON SMITH, M. D., Surgeon in Throat Department. Assisted by JOHN R. SHANNON, M. D., Assistant Surgeon in Eye Department; and JOHN R. PAGE, M. D., Assistant Surgeon in Ear Department. With chapters by HERBERT B. WILCOX, M. D., Attending Physician to the Hospital; and Miss EUGENIA D. AYERS, Superintendent of Nurses. 12mo of 260 pages, illustrated. Cloth, $1.50 net.

Friedenwald and Ruhrah's Dietetics for Nurses NEW (2d) EDITION

This work has been prepared to meet the needs of the nurse, both in training school and after graduation. *American Journal of Nursing* says it "is exactly the book for which nurses and others have long and vainly sought."

> Dietetics for Nurses. By JULIUS FRIEDENWALD, M. D., Professor of Diseases of the Stomach, and JOHN RUHRAH, M. D., Professor of Diseases of Children, College of Physicians and Surgeons, Baltimore. 12mo volume of 395 pages. Cloth, $1.50 net

Friedenwald & Ruhrah on Diet THIRD EDITION

> Diet in Health and Disease. By JULIUS FRIEDENWALD, M.D., and JOHN RUHRAH, M.D. Octavo volume of 764 pages. Cloth, $4.00 net.

Galbraith's Personal Hygiene and Physical Training for Women JUST ISSUED

> Personal Hygiene and Physical Training for Women. By ANNA M. GALBRAITH, M. D., Fellow New York Academy of Medicine. 12mo of 371 pages, illustrated. Cloth, $2.00 net.

Galbraith's Four Epochs of Woman's Life

THE NEW (2d) EDITION

> The Four Epochs of Woman's Life. By ANNA M. GALBRAITH, M.D. With an Introductory Note by JOHN H. MUSSER, M. D., University of Pennsylvania. 12mo of 247 pages. Cloth, $1.50 net.

McCombs' Diseases of Children for Nurses
JUST ISSUED—NEW (2d) EDITION

Dr. McCombs' experience in lecturing to nurses has enabled him to emphasize *just those points that nurses most need to know*. *National Hospital Record* says: "We have needed a good book on children's diseases and this volume admirably fills the want." The nurse's side has been written by head nurses, very valuable being the work of Miss Jennie Manly.

> Diseases of Children for Nurses. By ROBERT S. MCCOMBS, M. D., Instructor of Nurses at the Children's Hospital of Philadelphia. 12mo of 470 pages, illustrated. Cloth, $2.00 net

Wilson's Obstetric Nursing

In Dr. Wilson's work the entire subject is covered from the beginning of pregnancy, its course, signs, labor, its actual accomplishment, the puerperium and care of the infant. *American Journal of Obstetrics* says: "Every page empasizes the nurse's relation to the case."

> A Reference Handbook of Obstetric Nursing. By W. REYNOLDS WILSON, M.D., Visiting Physician to the Philadelphia Lying-in Charity. 32mo of 355 pages, illustrated. Flexible leather, $1.25 net.

American Pocket Dictionary NEW (6th) EDITION

The *Trained Nurse and Hospital Review* says: "We have had many occasions to refer to this dictionary, and in every instance we have found the desired information."

> American Pocket Medical Dictionary. Edited by W. A. NEWMAN DORLAND, A. M., M. D., Loyola University, Chicago. Flexible leather, gold edges, $1.00 net; with patent thumb index, $1.25 net.

Lewis' Anatomy and Physiology SECOND EDITION

Nurses Journal of Pacific Coast says "it is not in any sense rudimentary, but comprehensive in its treatment of the subjects." The low price makes this book particularly attractive.

> Anatomy and Physiology for Nurses. By LEROY LEWIS, M.D., Lecturer on Anatomy and Physiology for Nurses, Lewis Hospital, Bay City, Mich. 12mo of 375 pages, 150 illustrations. Cloth, $1.75 net.

Dorland's Illustrated Dictionary — NEW (5th) EDITION

The American Illustrated Medical Dictionary. Edited by W. A. N. DORLAND, M.D. Large octavo of 876 pages, 293 illustrations, 119 in colors. Flexible leather, $4.50 net; thumb indexed, $5.00 net.

Paul's Materia Medica

A Text-Book of Materia Medica for Nurses. By GEORGE P. PAUL, M.D., Samaritan Hospital, Troy, N. Y. 12mo of 240 pages. Cloth, $1.50 net.

Paul's Fever Nursing

Nursing in the Acute Infectious Fevers. By GEORGE P. PAUL, M.D. Cloth, $1.00 net.

Hoxie's Medicine for Nurses

Practice of Medicine for Nurses. By GEORGE HOWARD HOXIE, M.D., University of Kansas. With a chapter on Technic of Nursing by PEARL L. LAPTAD. 12mo of 284 pages, illustrated. Cloth, $1.50 net.

Grafstrom's Mechano-therapy — SECOND EDITION

Mechano-therapy (Massage and Medical Gymnastics). By AXEL V. GRAFSTROM, B.Sc. M.D., 12mo, 200 page.. Cloth, $1.25 net.

Nancrede's Anatomy — NEW (7th) EDITION

Essentials of Anatomy. CHARLES B. G. DENANCREDE, M.D., University of Michigan. 12mo, 400 pages, 180 illustrations. Cloth, $1.00 net.

Morrow's Immediate Care of Injured

Immediate Care of the Injured. By ALBERT S. MORROW, M.D., New York City Home for Aged and Infirm. Octavo of 340 pages, with 238 illustrations. Cloth, $2.50 net.

Register's Fever Nursing

A Text Book on Practical Fever Nursing. By EDWARD C. REGISTER, M.D., North Carolina Medical College. Octavo of 350 pages, illustrated. Cloth, $2.50 net.

Pyle's Personal Hygiene — NEW (4th) EDITION

A Manual of Personal Hygiene. Edited by WALTER L. PYLE, M.D. Wills Eye Hospital, Philadelphia. 12mo, 472 pages, illus. $1.50 net.

Morris' Materia Medica — NEW (7th) EDITION

Essentials of Materia Medica, Therapeutics, and Prescription Writing. By HENRY MORRIS, M.D. Revised by W. A. BASTEDO, M.D., Columbia University, N. Y. 12mo of 300 pages, illustrated. Cloth, $1.00 net.

Griffith's Care of the Baby — NEW (4th) EDITION

The Care of the Baby. By J. P. CROZER GRIFFITH, M.D., University of Pennsylvania. 12mo of 455 pages, illustrated. Cloth, $1.50 net.

Titles in This Series

1   Charlotte Aikens, editor. *Hospital Management*. Philadelphia, 1911.

2   American Society of Superintendents of Training Schools for Nurses. *Annual Conventions*, 1893–1919.

3   John Shaw Billings and Henry M. Hurd, editors. *Hospitals, Dispensaries and Nursing: Papers and Discussion in the International Congress of Charities, Correction and Philanthropy*. Baltimore, 1894.

4   Annie M. Brainard. *The Evolution of Public Health Nursing*. Philadelphia, 1922.

5   Marie Campbell. *Folks Do Get Born*. New York, 1946.

6   *Civil War Nursing:* Louisa May Alcott. *Hospital Sketches*. Boston, 1863. BOUND WITH *Memoir of Emily Elizabeth Parsons*. Boston, 1880.

7   Committee for the Study of Nursing Education. *Nursing and Nursing Education in the United States*. New York, 1923.

8   Committee on the Grading of Nursing Schools. *Nurses, Patients and Pocketbooks*. New York, 1928.

9   Mrs. Darce Craven. *A Guide to District Nurses*. London, 1889.

10 Dorothy Deming. *The Practical Nurse.* New York, 1947.

11 Katharine J. Densford & Millard S. Everett. *Ethics for Modern Nurses.* Philadelphia, 1946.

12 Katharine D. DeWitt. *Private Duty Nursing.* Philadelphia, 1917.

13 Janet James, editor. *A Lavinia Dock Reader.*

14 Annette Fiske. *First Fifty Years of the Waltham Training School for Nurses.* New York, 1984. BOUND WITH Alfred Worcester. "The Shortage of Nurses—Reminiscences of Alfred Worcester '83." *Harvard Medical Alumni Bulletin 23*, 1949.

15 Virginia Henderson et al. *Nursing Studies Index, 1900–1959.* Philadelphia, 1963, 1966, 1970, 1972.

16 Darlene Clark Hine, editor. *Black Women in Nursing: An Anthology of Historical Sources.*

17 Ellen N. LaMotte. *The Tuberculosis Nurse.* New York, 1915.

18 Barbara Melosh, editor. *American Nurses in Fiction: An Anthology of Short Stories.*

19 Mary Adelaide Nutting. *A Sound Economic Basis for Schools of Nursing.* New York, 1926.

20 Sara E. Parsons. *Nursing Problems and Obligations.* Boston, 1916.

21 Juanita Redmond. *I Served on Bataan.* Philadelphia, 1943.

22 Susan Reverby, editor. *The East Harlem Health Center Demonstration: An Anthology of Pamphlets.*

23 Isabel Hampton Robb. *Educational Standards for Nurses*. Cleveland, 1907.

24 Sister M. Theophane Shoemaker. *History of Nurse-Midwifery in the United States*. Washington, D.C., 1947.

25 Isabel M. Stewart. *Education of Nurses*. New York, 1943.

26 Virginia S. Thatcher. *History of Anesthesia with Emphasis on the Nurse Specialist*. Philadelphia, 1953.

27 Adah H. Thoms. *Pathfinders—A History of the Progress of Colored Graduate Nurses*. New York, 1929.

28 Clara S. Weeks-Shaw. *A Text-Book of Nursing for the Use of Training Schools, Families, and Private Students*. New York, 1885.

29 Writers Program of the WPA in Kansas, compilers. *Lamps on the Prairie: A History of Nursing in Kansas*. Topeka, 1942.